University of Iowa
The Family Practice Handbook

University of Iowa
The Family Practice Handbook

JOHN E. LITTLER, M.D.
Co-Chief Resident
Department of Family Practice
University of Iowa College of Medicine
Iowa City, Iowa

TIMOTHY MOMANY, M.D.
Co-Chief Resident
Department of Family Practice
University of Iowa College of Medicine
Iowa City, Iowa

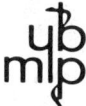

YEAR BOOK MEDICAL PUBLISHERS, INC.
Chicago • London • Boca Raton • Littleton, Mass.

Copyright © 1990 by Year Book Medical Publishers, Inc. All rights reserved. No part of this publication may be reproduced, stored in a retrieval system, or transmitted, in any form or by any means—electronic, mechanical, photocopying, recording, or otherwise—without prior written permission from the publisher. Printed in the United States of America.

Permission to photocopy or reproduce solely for internal or personal use is permitted for libraries or other users registered with the Copyright Clearance Center, provided that the base fee of $4.00 per chapter plus $.10 per page is paid directly to the Copyright Clearance Center, 21 Congress Street, Salem, MA 01970. This consent does not extend to other kinds of copying, such as copying for general distribution, for advertising or promotional purposes, for creating new collected works, or for resale.

1 2 3 4 5 6 7 8 9 0 R P 94 93 92 91 90

Library of Congress Cataloging-in-Publication Data
Littler, John E.
　The family practice handbook / John E. Littler,
　　Timothy Momany.
　　　p.　cm.
　At head of title: University of Iowa.
　Includes bibliographical references.
　ISBN 0-8151-8944-3
　1. Family medicine—Handbooks, manuals,
　　etc.　I. Momany, Timothy.
　II. University of Iowa.　III. Title.
　[DNLM: 1. Family Practice—
　　handbooks.　WB 39 L777f]
　RC55.L57　　1990
　616—dc20　　　　　　　　　　89-70697
　DNLM/DLC　　　　　　　　　CIP
　for Library of Congress

Sponsoring Editor: Kevin M. Kelly
Associate Managing Editor, Manuscript Services: Deborah Thorp
Production Project Coordinator: Karen Halm
Proofroom Supervisor: Barbara M. Kelly

Contributors

All contributors are residents at the Department of Family Practice, University of Iowa College of Medicine, Iowa City, Iowa.

Charles A. Bolick, M.D.
Shelley A. Breyen, M.D.
Katherine M. Broman, M.D.
Pamela L. Brown, M.D.
John J. D'Amore, M.D.
Eric Evans, M.D.
Tom Francis, M.D.
J. Matthew Johnson, M.D.

Becky Leidal, M.D.
John E. Littler, M.D.
Mark J. Mabee, M.D.
Timothy Momany, M.D.
Candace F. Shanks, M.D.
Ann Stein, M.D.
Blaise P. Vitale, M.D.
Garry R. Weischedel, M.D.

Foreword

Family medicine is a difficult topic for a pocket-sized handbook. As evidenced by this volume, even when done well it takes a pretty deep pocket to carry it in! The residents of the University of Iowa Department of Family Practice were challenged by the publisher to create a guide for a resident or student who needs quick information on the variety of medical problems encountered in primary care. Family practice is the logical specialty to write such a book because of the breadth of medical care provided to all ages of either sex. Drs. Littler, Momany, and colleagues have put together their ideas in a way that certainly meets the goals of the challenge.

What should be included? What has to be left out? Those were the most difficult questions that had to be answered at the outset. Utilizing the network of seven family practice residency programs in Iowa, the editors wisely solicited advice about the most common problems seen by other family practice residents during training and discovered which ones required a "look-it-up" approach. The result was this handbook, which does a superb job of bringing together the needed data that previously had to be sought from a number of different sources.

With the rapid changing of medical knowledge, a guide for primary care will have to be fluid in its content. After this excellent first effort, the residents of the University of Iowa Family Practice Program must prepare for future editions. If you discover that an important aspect of care has been omitted, write to the residency program so that your idea may be considered for future editions. My 14 years as a family practice educator have shown me the potential of this specialty to attract increasingly talented and motivated people. This book is evidence of that talent and is a successful beginning that will allow those who follow the opportunity to contribute their scholarship to their chosen specialty of family practice.

Charles E. Driscoll, M.D.
Professor and Head
Department of Family Practice
University of Iowa College of Medicine

Preface

We, as chief residents at the University of Iowa Department of Family Practice, were approached by Year Book Medical Publishers to consider preparing a handbook of family practice analogous in intent and structure to *The Harriet Lane Handbook* in pediatrics and *The Mont Reid Handbook* in surgery. In undertaking this project, our goal has been to provide concise, practical information appropriate for the wide variety of clinical situations experienced by family practice residents. To the extent that we have succeeded, this handbook should prove useful also to residents in other primary care specialties and to medical students during their clinical years, as well as to physicians who require a quick reference in the office. We recognize that the practice of clinical medicine is not a science and that many acceptable alternatives in diagnostic and therapeutic strategies exist. Our contributing authors are all resident colleagues and have discussed issues from the perspective of family practice residents who have the benefit of training in both a community hospital (Mercy Hospital, Iowa City) and a tertiary care center (The University of Iowa Hospitals and Clinics). We do not intend to claim that "our way" is the "only" or "right" way.

The specialty of family practice encompasses such a large area of medical practice that exhaustive coverage in a handbook would be unrealistic. We have attempted to include those conditions that are either commonly encountered or, if uncommon, require prompt recognition. Undoubtedly we have overlooked topics that could legitimately be included. Suggestions or comments are welcome and may be sent to the Chief Residents, Department of Family Practice, University of Iowa, Iowa City, IA 52242.

x   Preface

We would like to thank our contributing authors for their efforts. Our department has provided the support necessary for a project such as this and has our gratitude. In particular, thanks to Dr. Charles Driscoll, M.D., our department head, mentor, and friend, for his support and advice. Dr. Driscoll and James Karboski, Pharm.D, reviewed the entire manuscript and made many valuable suggestions. In addition, the efforts of Pam Hoogerwerf in organizing and processing the sometimes nearly illegible material were essential in actually bringing this project to fruition. Our illustrator, David Pepper, M.D., provided many useful comments and suggestions in addition to considerable time and effort preparing illustrations and algorithms.

Finally, we would like to express special thanks to our wives, Karen and Betsy, and our children for their support and for tolerating the many hours of work involved in preparing this handbook.

John E. Littler, M.D.
Timothy Momany, M.D.
Co-Chief Residents
Department of Family Practice
University of Iowa College of Medicine

Contents

Foreword vii

Preface ix

PART I: The Practice of Family Medicine

1 / EMERGENCY MEDICINE   1

   John E. Littler

   Advanced Cardiac Life Support   1
   Pediatric Advanced Life Support   10
   Trauma   15
   Airway Management   26
   Orotracheal Intubation   28
   Nasotracheal Intubation   29
   Tactile Orotracheal Intubation   30
   Percutaneous Transtracheal Ventilation   32
   Cricothyrotomy   33
   Respiratory Distress   35
   Shock   38
   Coma   41
   Poisoning and Overdose   46
   Environmental Illnesses   53

2 / CARDIOLOGY 60

John J. D'Amore, John E. Littler, and Timothy Momany

Ischemic Heart Disease 60
Ischemic Heart Disease—Inpatient 64
Complications of Acute Myocardial Infarction 68
Congestive Heart Failure 71
Hypertension 74
Syncope 78
Evaluation of Heart Sounds and Murmurs 81
Dyslipidemias 85

3 / PULMONARY MEDICINE 90

Shelley A. Breyen

Pulmonary Function Tests 90
Ventilators and Oxygen Therapy 96
Viral Upper Respiratory Tract Infections 102
Pneumonia 104
Asthma 112
Chronic Obstructive Pulmonary Disease (COPD) 117
Pulmonary Embolism 122
Pleural Effusion (Hydrothorax) 126
Hemoptysis 129

4 / GASTROENTEROLOGY 133

Blaise P. Vitale and John E. Littler

Gastrointestinal Bleeding 133
Dyspepsia/Peptic Ulcer Disease 136
Esophageal Diseases 138
Acute Pancreatitis 141

Chronic Pancreatitis 143
Liver Disease 144
Acute Diarrhea 147
Chronic Diarrhea 150
Constipation 152
Colorectal Tumors 154
Anorectal Diseases 156

5 / HEMATOLOGIC, ELECTROLYTE, AND METABOLIC DISORDERS 159

J. Matthew Johnson, Becky Leidal, and John E. Littler

Bleeding Disorders 159
Anemia 165
Potassium 172
Sodium 177
Hypoglycemia 180
Diabetes Mellitus 184
Diabetic Ketoacidosis 192
Hyperglycemic-Hyperosmolar Nonketotic Syndrome 195
Thyroid 197
Thyroid Enlargement 204

6 / RHEUMATOLOGY/ORTHOPEDICS 207

Charles A. Bolick

Rheumatoid Arthritis 207
Osteoarthritis 212
Chondrocalcinosis 215
Gout 217
Ankylosing Spondylitis 221
Metabolic Bone Disease 223
Systemic Lupus Erythematosus 226
Low Back Pain 231
Overuse Syndromes 237

xiv Contents

    Orthopedic Injuries   *242*
    Fractures   *249*
    Septic Arthritis   *251*

7 / GYNECOLOGY   *258*

Timothy Momany and Candace F. Shanks

    Contraception   *258*
    Pelvic Pain   *262*
    Adnexal Masses   *265*
    Dyspareunia   *268*
    Pediatric Gynecology   *272*
    Abnormal Vaginal Bleeding   *276*
    Dysmenorrhea   *279*
    Infertility   *283*
    Endometriosis   *288*
    Pelvic Inflammatory Disease   *291*
    Spontaneous Abortions   *294*
    Ectopic Pregnancy   *298*
    Premenstrual Tension Syndrome   *301*
    Menopause   *304*

8 / OBSTETRICS   *307*

Pamela L. Brown

    Prenatal Care   *307*
    Prenatal Patient Education   *310*
    Rh Screening and Rho-GAM   *314*
    Hepatitis Screening in Pregnancy   *316*
    Alpha-Fetoprotein   *317*
    Antenatal Fetal Surveillance   *319*
    Hyperemesis Gravidarum   *324*
    Diabetes in Pregnancy   *326*
    Hypertension in Pregnancy   *330*
    Early Antepartum Hemorrhage   *335*
    Late Antepartum Hemorrhage   *338*
    Intrauterine Growth Retardation
    (IUGR)   *341*

Vaginal Birth After Cesarean
(VBAC)   *342*
Preterm Labor   *345*
Premature Rupture of Membranes
(PROM)   *350*
Postdate Pregnancy   *352*
Evaluation of Labor   *354*
Intrapartum Monitoring and
Management   *358*
Pelvimetry   *362*
Induction of Labor   *364*
Vaginal Delivery   *367*
Episiotomy   *375*
Malpresentations   *377*
Shoulder Dystocia   *379*
Cesarean Section   *381*
Postpartum Care   *383*
Postpartum Hemorrhage   *386*
Puerperal Fever   *389*

9 / GENERAL SURGERY   *392*

Ann Stein

Wound Management   *392*
Preoperative Care and Evaluation   *401*
Postoperative Care   *405*
Abdominal Pain   *408*
Appendicitis   *414*
Gallbladder Disease   *416*
Evaluation of Breast Mass   *419*
Burn Injury   *421*

10 / PEDIATRICS   *427*

Katherine M. Broman and Eric Evans

Neonatal Respiratory Problems   *427*
Neonatal Infections   *430*

Metabolic/Hematologic Disorders of the Newborn   *434*
Fever   *439*
Vomiting/Diarrhea   *442*
Febrile Seizures   *445*
Pediatric Meningitis   *447*
Stridor and Dyspnea in the Young Child   *450*
Childhood Exanthems   *453*
Breast Feeding   *457*
Failure to Thrive   *459*
Constipation   *461*
Anemia   *463*
Bites   *466*
Parasites   *470*

11 / GENITOURINARY   472

John E. Littler and Garry R. Weischedel

Lower UTI—Female   *472*
Lower UTI—Male   *474*
Acute Pyelonephritis   *479*
Sexually Transmitted Diseases   *481*
Benign Prostatic Hypertrophy (BPH)   *487*
Hematuria   *489*
Urolithiasis   *491*
Acute Scrotal Pain and Scrotal Masses   *493*
Renal Failure   *497*

12 / EYES, EARS, NOSE, AND THROAT   501

J. Matthew Johnson and John E. Littler

Red Eye   *501*
Conjunctivitis   *505*

Glaucoma *507*
Vertigo *509*
Otitis Media *512*
Pharyngitis *516*
Sinusitis *518*
Rhinitis *520*

13 / DERMATOLOGY *523*

John E. Littler

Acne *523*
Urticaria *525*
Eczema *527*
Contact Dermatitis *528*
Decubitus Ulcers *530*
Skin Cancers and Precancers *532*

14 / NEUROLOGY *535*

Mark J. Mabee

Headache *535*
Dementia *537*
Meningitis *539*
Seizures *541*
Cerebrovascular Disease *545*

15 / PSYCHIATRY *548*

John E. Littler

Principles of Counseling *548*
Affective Disorders *551*
Anxiety Disorders *555*
Substance Abuse *559*
Acute Psychosis *563*
Schizophrenic and Schizophrenic-like Disorders *565*
Eating Disorders *567*

PART II: Procedures

16 / EMERGENCY PROCEDURES 569

Tom Francis

Defibrillation/Cardioversion 569
Tube Thoracostomy 571
Venous Cutdown 573
Intraosseous Infusion 576
Culdocentesis 579
Paracentesis and Peritoneal Lavage 582

17 / HOSPITAL PROCEDURES 585

Tom Francis

Fetal Scalp Electrode 585
Fetal Scalp pH Sampling 587
Circumcision 589
Local and Regional Blocks 592
Arterial Line 597
Central Lines 599
Intrauterine Pressure Catheter 602
Thoracentesis 604
Lumbar Puncture—Adults 606
Urine Collection 608

18 / OFFICE PROCEDURES 610

Tom Francis

Foreign Body Removal—Ear 610
Foreign Body Removal—Eye 611
Excision of Skin Lesions 613
Cryotherapy 615
Electrodesiccation 618
Tympanometry 620
Flexible Nasopharyngoscopy 622
Fine Needle Breast Biopsy 624

Endometrial Biopsy *626*
Arthrocentesis *628*
Ingrown Toenails *632*
Vasectomy *634*
Flexible Sigmoidoscopy *636*

Reference Data *639*

Index *665*

1/ EMERGENCY MEDICINE

John E. Littler, M.D.

ADVANCED CARDIAC LIFE SUPPORT

I. **Overview**

Sudden death occurs in the prehospital setting nearly 1,000 times per day in the United States. The majority of these victims have no warning symptoms prior to collapse. The three main factors that are most important for successful resuscitation of the patient with no pulse are:

- rapid defibrillation of ventricular fibrillation (VF) or pulseless ventricular tachycardia (VT).
- effective CPR, with secure and effective airway and administration of 100% oxygen.
- epinephrine given every 5 minutes to maintain coronary and cerebral perfusion.

Throughout resuscitative measures, the patient must be constantly evaluated. This should include frequent assessment of the adequacy of ventilation and chest compressions. After each intervention, such as defibrillation, the patient must be evaluated by checking for a pulse. This is a more accurate assessment of the patient than is the cardiac monitor.

II. **Pulseless Rhythms**

A. Ventricular fibrillation (VF) pulseless ventricular tachycardia (VT).

1. Survival depends upon rapid defibrillation. As soon as the monitor-defibrillator is available and the rhythm is determined to be VF or pulseless VT, the patient should receive immediate defibrillation with 200 J. If the patient remains pulseless, defibrillation should be repeated at 200-300 J, followed rapidly by 360 J if the patient has not responded. If the equipment is immediately available, this should be done before CPR is initiated.

2. If initial attempts at defibrillation are not successful, or if monitor-defibrillation equipment is not immediately available, CPR should be instituted, with

attention directed to providing an adequate airway with 100% O$_2$ and effective chest compressions. IV access and endotracheal intubation may then be pursued. As soon as an appropriate route of administration has been secured (ET tube or IV), epinephrine 0.5 mg-1.0 mg should be given. This should be repeated every 5 minutes as long as CPR is in progress. Defibrillation should again be attempted at 360 J. If this is not successful in restoring a perfusing rhythm then pharmacologic therapy is instituted as outlined in Figure 1-1.

B. Electromechanical dissociation (EMD).

1. Diagnosed by the absence of a pulse in spite of organized electrical activity on the monitor. Prognosis is poor unless a cause can be found and corrected. The most common correctable causes are hypovolemia, cardiac tamponade, tension pneumothorax, hypoxemia and acidosis. Other causes include massive infarction, pulmonary embolism, and severe shock.

2. Treatment should begin with CPR, including 100% O$_2$, IV access and endotracheal intubation. As soon as an appropriate route for administration has been secured (ET or IV), epinephrine 0.5-1.0 mg should be administered and repeated every 5 minutes. If bradycardia is present, atropine 0.5-1.0 mg may be administered and repeated every 5 minutes up to 2.0 mg total. Fluid bolus should be considered to treat for possible hypovolemia. Patient should be evaluated for other potential causes of EMD (Fig 1-2).

C. Asystole.

1. Prognosis is poor regardless of etiology. Diagnosis should be confirmed in at least two leads as fine ventricular fibrillation may appear to be asystole. If there is any doubt as to the diagnosis, the rhythm should be treated as VF.

2. Treatment should begin with CPR, including 100% O$_2$, IV access and intubation when possible. Epinephrine 0.5-1.0 mg and atropine 1.0 mg should be administered as soon as a route for administration

ACLS

has been established (ET or IV). Epinephrine should be repeated every 5 minutes, and atropine should be repeated in 5 minutes to a total dose of 2 mg. Pacing with temporary external pacer may be considered

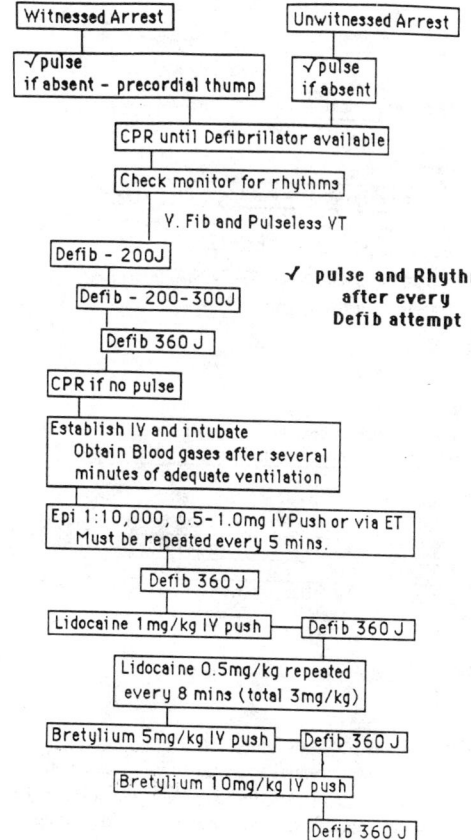

Fig 1-1. Ventricular fibrillation

although recent studies have not shown increased survival with the use of this device in patients that are pulseless (Fig 1-3).

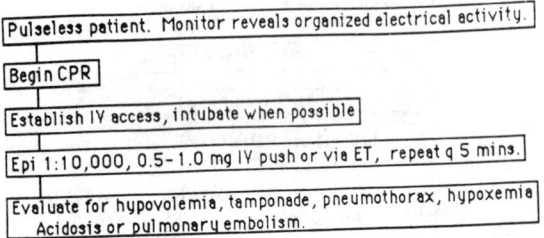

Fig 1-2. EMD

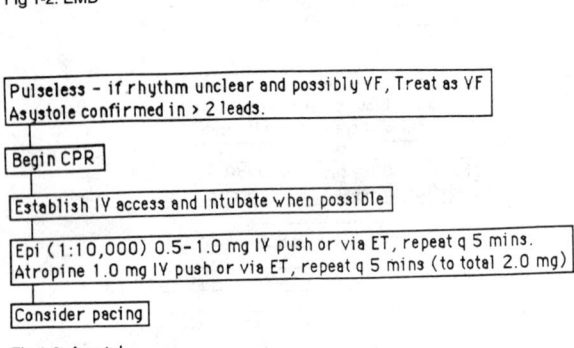

Fig 1-3. Asystole

III. Life-Threatening Dysrhythmias

A. Sustained Ventricular Tachycardia (VT) (with a pulse).
   1. Ventricular tachycardia may be well-tolerated if there is not associated myocardial dysfunction. However, it should be treated without delay because of the risk of developing hemodynamic compromise

or degeneration into ventricular fibrillation. Diagnosis can be difficult because of possible confusion with aberrantly conducted supraventricular tachycardia. Fusion beats are nearly diagnostic of VT, but are not commonly seen. If the patient is stable, vagal maneuvers may help diagnosis of SVT. A trial of lidocaine should be considered next. Verapamil should not be used if the diagnosis is uncertain.

2. In all patients with wide-complex tachycardia initial measures should include O_2 and IV access. If there is dyspnea, hypotension, congestive heart failure, or angina, the patient should be considered to be unstable and treated with synchronized cardioversion. If the patient is *in extremis*, unsynchronized cardioversion should be used. As ventricular tachycardia is generally quite responsive to electrical therapy, initial cardioversion may be done at 50 J. If the patient is stable, pharmacologic therapy is warranted. Lidocaine is the drug of choice.

3. Torsade de pointes is a variant of ventricular tachycardia that requires a different approach to therapy. It is generally nonsustained and without significant hemodynamic effect. However, on occasion it will be sustained and require emergent treatment. Treatment must include identification and correction of predisposing abnormalities. Torsades is generally caused by prolongation of the QT interval with antiarrhythmics such as quinidine, procainamide, and disopyramide, other drugs such as tricyclics and phenothiazines, and pathophysiologic processes such as hypokalemia, hypomagnesemia, hypocalcemia, intracerebral hemorrhage, and myocardial disease. Treatment for hemodynamically significant or sustained torsades is with cardioversion, lidocaine or phenytoin, or overdrive pacing (Fig 1-4).

B. Supraventricular tachycardias require emergency treatment with synchronized cardioversion in the event of cardiovascular compromise, such as angina, dyspnea, hypotension, or congestive heart failure. O_2 should be provided and IV access obtained. If time permits, a short-acting sedative should be used. Recommended initial energy levels for cardioversion are:

- atrial flutter: 25 J.
- PSVT: 75-100 J.
- atrial fibrillation: 100 J.

Underlying causes for the tachycardia should be sought and corrected. The most common causes are congestive failure, hypoxemia, electrolyte and acid/base imbalance. Digitalis, verapamil, or beta blockers may be used to slow the ventricular response.

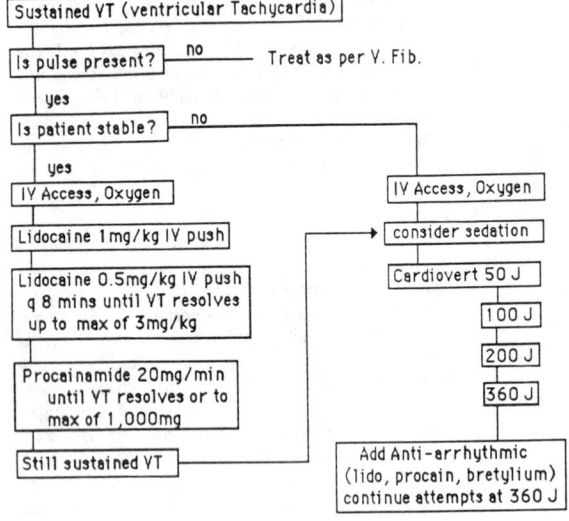

Fig 1-4. Sustained VT

1. Paroxysmal supraventricular tachycardia (PSVT).
    a. Occurs in distinct paroxysms with abrupt onset and usually abrupt cessation. Rate generally is from 160 to 240 beats/minute and the rhythm is regular. P waves may not be discernible. If there is associated bundle-branch block or aberrant conduction, this dysrhythmia can be very dif-

ACLS

ficult to distinguish from ventricular tachycardia. If there is any question, it should be treated as VT.

b. In an unstable patient, treatment of choice is synchronized cardioversion. All patients who are symptomatic should receive O_2. Vagal maneuvers be may tried while oxygen therapy is started and IV access obtained. If the patient is hemodynamically stable, IV verapamil is the drug of choice unless the patient has recently received IV beta blockers. Initial dose is 5 mg. If the initial dose is not successful a second dose of 10 mg may be given about 15 minutes after the first. If this is unsuccessful, digitalis or cardioversion can be used (Fig 1-5).

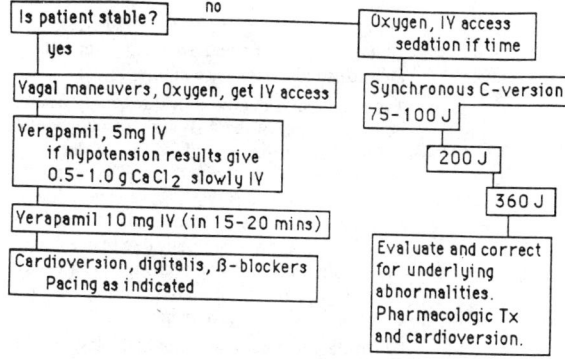

Fig 1-5. PSVT (Paroxysmal supraventricular tachycardia)

IV. Bradydysrhythmias

A. Bradycardia requires urgent treatment only when the patient is symptomatic with angina, dyspnea, hypotension, congestive failure, or if there is significant ventricular ectopy associated. Treatment should include

O_2 and IV access. Atropine is the drug of choice and is given IV in 0.5 mg increments as needed up to 2.0 mg. (In the case of inferior wall MI higher doses may be needed.) An external pacemaker may be used if atropine fails to relieve symptoms (or may be used instead of atropine if immediately available).

1. Sinus bradycardia is due to slowing of the sinus node and may be secondary to sinus node disease, increased parasympathetic tone, or drug effect.
2. A-V node dysfunction may result in bradycardia.
    a. First-degree block is a delay of the sinus impulse generally occurring at the level of the A-V node. By itself, first-degree block will not result in bradycardia as the sinus node maintains control of the rate.
    b. Type I second-degree block occurs at the level of the A-V node and is commonly due to increased parasympathetic tone or drug effect. Progressive prolongation of the PR interval until an atrial impulse is completely blocked is the characteristic feature. This dysrhythmia is generally transient and requires temporizing measures only in the case of symptoms.
    c. Type II second-degree block generally occurs below the level of the A-V node (usually at the bundle branch level) and is usually due to a lesion in the conduction pathway. Characteristic of this dysrhythmia is that P waves are followed by a consistent PR interval until the blocked beat. Because this is generally due to a lesion in the conduction pathway and may progress to third-degree block, therapy generally will require insertion of a pacemaker.
    d. Third-degree block may occur at the level of the A-V node, bundle of His, or at the bundle branch level. If the block is at the A-V node, it is generally temporary and due to increased parasympathetic tone (as may occur in inferior wall MI) or drug effect. In this case it will usually have a narrow QRS complex because the ventricles will be paced by a junctional escape

mechanism. Block below the level of the A-V node indicates the presence of conduction system disease and will usually require a pacemaker (Fig 1-6).

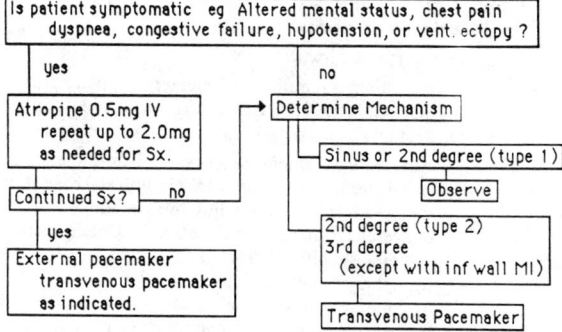

Fig 1-6. Bradycardia (heart rate <60)

Reference

Albarron-Sotelo R, *et al*, eds. Textbook of Advanced Cardiac Life Support. Dallas: American Heart Association, 1987.

PEDIATRIC ADVANCED LIFE SUPPORT

I. **Neonatal Resuscitation**

Evaluation and treatment of newborns requiring resuscitation proceeds in a fashion very similar to that of adults. However, one must keep in mind that most pediatric cardiopulmonary arrests are primary respiratory arrest and attention to airway and adequate ventilation is extremely important. Also, it is especially important with newborns to provide an appropriately warmed environment for maintenance of body temperature. All newborns require maintenance of body temperature and airway suctioning. This will be adequate resuscitation in the vast majority of cases. A few newborns will also require supplemental O_2 and perhaps bag-mask ventilation. Very few infants will require chest compressions or medications for resuscitation.

A. Environment/Airway.

1. All neonates require an adequately warmed environment and should be quickly dried to prevent further heat loss by evaporation.

2. Airway management ideally starts before the infant is delivered by suctioning of the mouth and nose after the head is delivered but before the thorax is delivered. If meconium is present a DeLee suction catheter should be used to thoroughly suction the hypopharynx before delivery of the thorax. If the meconium is thick and particulate, the trachea should be suctioned through an endotracheal tube.

B. Assessment.

1. Respiratory effort should respond to the stimulation produced by vigorous drying and suctioning of the airway. If respirations are not adequate (too slow, shallow or absent) after brief attempts at stimulation, the infant should be ventilated via bag and mask at a rate of 40 breaths per minute.

2. Heart rate should be assessed after adequate respiratory effort has been established. If the heart rate is < 100 beats/minute, assisted ventilations should be started immediately. If the initial heart rate is 60-80 beats/minute, assisted ventilations will usual-

ly produce a rapid increase in heart rate. If this fails to occur after 15-30 seconds of ventilation, chest compressions should be started at a rate of 120 per minute. If the initial heart rate is < 60, chest compressions should be started immediately. If the heart rate does not respond to ventilations and chest compressions after 1 or 2 minutes, medications should be administered.

3. Central cyanosis in a child with adequate respiratory effort and heart rate should be treated with blow-by oxygen.

C. Pharmacologic interventions are required if the neonate fails to respond to adequate ventilations and chest compressions, or if the child has adequate heart rate but fails to develop spontaneous respirations.

1. Epinephrine is indicated in the case of asystole or heart rate of < 80 beats/minute in spite of adequate ventilation and chest compressions. Dose is 0.1cc/kg of 1:10,000 solution (0.01 mg/kg) via ET tube or IV. This should be repeated every 5 minutes as long as the clinical indication persists.

2. Volume expanders are indicated for hypovolemia as evidenced by 1) pallor that persists after oxygenation, 2) weak pulse with a good heart rate, 3) poor response to resuscitation. 10ml/kg of normal saline, lactated ringer's, or plasmanate should be administered intravenously via the umbilical vein over 5-10 minutes.

3. Naloxone is indicated for respiratory depression in the neonate if the mother has been given narcotics during the latter part of labor. The recommended dose is 0.01 mg/kg (of the 0.02 mg/ml neonatal solution) which can be given via ET tube or IV and repeated every 2-3 minutes as needed.

4. Sodium bicarbonate is indicated for acidosis that does not respond to hyperventilation. Dose is 2 mEq/kg (4 ml/kg) of the 0.5 mEq/cc solution, given by slow intravenous push.

Emergency Medicine

II. **Infant and Child Resuscitation**
   A. Assessment:
      1. Respiratory--increased or decreased rate of respirations, increased respiratory effort, depressed level of consciousness, and cyanosis are signs of respiratory distress and possible impending respiratory failure.
      2. Cardiovascular--tachycardia is a common response to stress. Bradycardia is evidence of impending cardiac arrest. Blood pressure remains normal until cardiopulmonary collapse is imminent. Capillary refill, skin color and temperature, urine output and level of consciousness are indicators of end-organ perfusion.
   B. Airway management.
      1. Any child with evidence of respiratory distress or cardiovascular failure should receive humidified oxygen. Airway should be protected by proper positioning and suctioning. An oropharyngeal airway may be used in an unconscious child (appropriate size can be estimated by measuring from the mouth to the angle of the jaw). Nasopharyngeal airway can be used in either conscious or unconscious children. Size is estimated by measuring from the tip of the nose to the tragus.
      2. If ventilations must be supported, a bag-valve-mask device should be used first. Generally this will provide adequate ventilations. If prolonged ventilation is required the child should be intubated after adequate ventilations have been established with the bag-mask device. Size of the ET tube can be estimated by the formula ET size = (16 + patient's age)/4. The laryngoscope blade should be straight for children less than 3 years of age because of the configuration of the upper airway.
   C. Circulation.
      1. Vascular access is important for administration of certain medications that cannot be given via ET tube and for fluid resuscitation. Infusion pumps are recommended because of the ease with which inadvertently large volumes of fluid can be given. The femoral vein is perhaps the most suitable site during resuscitation because cannulation of this vein does

not require interruption of CPR and it provides access to the central circulation. Intraosseous cannulation is a rapid, safe and effective route for infusion of fluids, blood products, and all medications commonly used during resuscitation. It can generally be performed with ease in children under 3 years of age (See Procedure Section). Volume expansion should be based upon frequent reassessment of the patient following each bolus of fluid. Initial bolus should be 20 ml/kg of L.R. or saline. If perfusion is still diminished this may be repeated. If reassessment shows the need for additional fluid, consideration should be given to the use of colloids as they are more efficient at volume expansion.

2. Pharmacologic support.

   a. O_2 is essential in all situations requiring resuscitation.

   b. Epinephrine is indicated in any patient undergoing CPR to improve its effectiveness, and specifically for any pulseless rhythm and bradycardia. Dose is 0.1 ml/kg of 1:10,000 solution given IV, ET, or intraosseous route. This is repeated every 5 minutes as long as the clinical indication persists.

   c. Sodium bicarbonate is indicated only for that part of acidosis that does not respond to hyperventilation. Dose is 1 mEq/kg via IV or intraosseous route.

   d. Atropine is indicated for symptomatic bradycardia and to diminish the vagal response to intubation attempts. Dose is 0.01-0.02 mg/kg via ET, IV, or intraosseous route. Minimum dose is 0-0.1 mg. This may be repeated to maximum dose of 1.0 mg in a child, 2.0 mg in an adolescent.

3. Dysrhythmias.

   a. SVT is a relatively common arrhythmia in children and can cause cardiovascular collapse in infants. Rate is generally above 230 beats/minute. Treatment of choice for patients with cardiovascular instability is synchronized cardioversion (0.5-1.0 J/kg). Verapamil (0.1-

0.15 mg/kg/dose, maximum dose 5 mg) can be used in children older than 1 year of age and who are stable.

b. VT is best treated with synchronized cardioversion in the presence of instability. Initial dose is 0.5-1.0 J/kg. This may be doubled if necessary. Lidocaine bolus of 1 mg/kg prior to cardioversion will increase effectiveness.

c. V-fib is uncommon in children. It is treated with defibrillation at 2 J/kg, with doubling of the dose if unsuccessful.

d. Bradyarrhythmias are treated if symptomatic with oxygen, chest compressions if necessary. Atropine and epinephrine are the drugs of choice.

e. EMD is treated as asystole with ventilation, chest compressions, and epinephrine. Underlying cause should be sought.

f. Asystole is treated with ventilation with 100% oxygen, chest compressions, and epinephrine.

Reference

Albarron-Sotelo R, *et al*, eds. Textbook of Advanced Cardiac Life Support, Dallas: American Heart Association, 1987.

TRAUMA

I. **Overview**

A. Incidence--Minor trauma is extremely common. Only 1 to 5% of all trauma is life- or limb-threatening. However, this percentage still represents a leading cause of death overall, and the major cause of death for persons age 1 to 40 years.

B. Mortality--deaths caused by trauma occur in a trimodal distribution.

1. Death within seconds or minutes from the time of injury is usually due to severe central nervous system injury, cardiac rupture, or injury to major vascular structures. These deaths occur at the scene before emergency medical services arrive.

2. The second group occurs within minutes to a few hours after the injury. Common causes of death include intracranial hemorrhage, chest injuries such as pneumo- or hemothorax, intra-abdominal injury, or combined multisystem injury. Victims in this group represent the population that the emergency medical system can significantly influence in terms of decreasing mortality.

3. The third peak of trauma-related deaths occurs days to weeks after the injury, usually due to sepsis and/or multisystem failure.

C. Assessment: trauma victims must be continuously reassessed for any changes in mental status, vital signs, and physical exam findings.

II. **Primary Survey**

During the primary survey injuries that are immediately life threatening are detected and treated as they are identified.

A. Airway (with cervical spine control):

1. Check for obstruction, which may be anatomical in the unconscious patient requiring only jaw lift, oral or nasopharyngeal airway. Check for blood, secretions, or other foreign matter present in the oropharynx.

2. Respiratory arrest requires a secure airway.

B. Breathing:
   1. Evaluate pattern and rate of respirations in spontaneously breathing patients.
   2. Inspect and palpate the chest wall for evidence of flail segments, penetrating wounds, position of trachea.
   3. Auscultate for evidence of hemo- or pneumothorax
C. Circulation:
   1. Assess adequacy of cardiac output by color of skin, capillary refill, presence of pulses (systolic BP roughly $\geq$ 60 if carotid pulse present, $\geq$ 70 if femoral pulse present, $\geq$ 80 if radial pulse present)
   2. Control hemorrhage. With the exception of scalp wounds blind clamping of arterial bleeding is not appropriate. Direct pressure is the method of choice for controlling hemorrhage.
D. Disability:
   1. Brief neurological exam to evaluate pupil size, position and responsiveness, mental status in terms of responsiveness (ranging from alert, responsive to verbal stimuli, responsive to painful stimuli, unresponsive), gross motor assessment, gross sensory exam.
   2. Formal scales have been developed for evaluating mental status and should be used as they can reduce the variability between observers. See page 41 on evaluation of coma.
E. Expose patient for full evaluation.

III. **Resuscitation**
A. O_2 should be provided to all trauma victims.
B. Fluid - IV access essential. Should have as a minimum two large-bore IVs and begin replacement with Lactated Ringer's or normal saline. Initial fluid therapy can be based upon patient weight, with the average adult requiring 30 ml/kg, or approximately 2 liters. Children should receive initially 10-20 ml/kg. Vital signs and response to initial fluid bolus can be used to classify severity of hemorrhage using the following table (Table 1-1).

Boluses should be repeated up to 40 ml/kg after which blood should be used.

Table 1-1. Classification of Hemorrhage

Parameter	Class I	Class II	Class III	Class IV
blood loss (ml)	up to 750	750 to 1500	1500 to 2000	2,000
% blood volume loss	up to 15%	15-30%	30-40%	40%
pulse	<100	100	120	140
BP	normal	normal	decreased	decreased
capillary refill	normal	prolonged	prolonged	prolonged
respiratory rate	14-20	20-30	30-40	35
urine out-put	30 ml/hr	20-30 ml/hr	5-15 ml/hr	negligible

Adapted from: Asensio J, et al. American Family Physician. Sept. 1988, pg. 105.

Patients that respond promptly and then stabilize after initial fluid bolus usually have less than 20% blood volume loss (Class I or Class II less than 20%). These patients will probably not require transfusion. Patients that initially respond but then have destabilization of vital signs usually have blood loss between 20 and 40% (Class II to Class III), and will require blood. Patients that do not respond to the initial fluid bolus have greater than 40% blood volume loss (Class IV) and require rapid fluid and blood replacement and immediate surgical intervention.

C. Cardiac monitor.

D. Decompression.

1. Foley catheter to monitor response to resuscitative measures. Should not be placed until the urethral meatus has been examined for the presence of blood and the rectal exam has been done to evaluate for high-riding prostate. Either of these suggests the possibility of urethral disruption and a catheter should not be placed until a retrograde urethrogram has been performed.

2. Nasogastric tube to decompress the stomach and reduce the risk of regurgitation and aspiration. Should not be placed nasally if there is evidence of

possible basilar skull fracture such as epistaxis, CSF rhinorrhea or otorrhea, significant facial trauma.

IV. Secondary Survey

A. History: (if circumstances permit this is obtained during resuscitation.)
   1. Allergies.
   2. Medications.
   3. Past medical history.
   4. Last meal.
   5. Events of the injury -EMS personnel at the scene will have valuable information regarding the events of the injury.

B. Physical examination, complete.

V. Head Trauma

A. Significant head or face trauma indicates possible C-spine injury and cervical spine immobilization and evaluation are required.
   1. Most important parameter for evaluating head injury is mental status. In the unconscious patient factors other than the injury may account for the change in mental status (and may have accounted for injury in the first place) such as hypoglycemia, seizure, intoxication or overdose. See page 41, evaluation of coma.
   2. Examine scalp for lacerations, control hemorrhage as needed.
   3. Palpate for depressed fractures.
   4. Re-examine pupils for position, size, reactivity.
   5. Level of alertness should be reassessed frequently, as should motor and sensory exams.
   6. Facial trauma that does not compromise airway does not require immediate treatment.
   7. Focal neurological signs, altered mental status, and depressed skull fractures are indications for CT scan when the patient has been stabilized.

VI. Neck

A. In a conscious, alert patient, the absence of neck pain and tenderness with a normal neurological exam is considered by many to be adequate for ruling out cervical spine injury.

1. Blunt trauma--greatest concern is injury to the airway. Vascular injury is not as likely with blunt trauma as with penetrating injury. Cervical spine injury must be considered. Laryngeal fracture or other airway injury should be suspected if patient demonstrates any of the following:

   a. stridor.
   b. hoarseness.
   c. dyspnea.
   d. tenderness.
   e. subcutaneous emphysema.
   f. flattening of the anterior neck contour, inability to palpate the thyroid prominence. Laryngotracheal injuries are best managed by emergent consultation with an otolaryngologist. Endotracheal intubation can result in further damage and cricothyrotomy may be nearly impossible because of distorted anatomy.

2. Penetrating trauma--may damage airway, vessels, cervical spine or spinal cord. In an obtunded or unconscious patient, or a patient with obvious neurological deficit, cervical spine injury should be assumed. Vascular injuries are of great concern and evalaution will require consultation with a vascular or head and neck surgeon.

VII. Chest

A. During primary survey flail chest, tension pneumothorax and hemothorax were identified and treated as part of initial stabilization. Chest X-ray should be performed early when significatn trauma is present.

1. The patient with significant blunt or penetrating chest trauma that arrests immediately prior to arrival at the emergency department should be treated with definitive airway control, CPR, and rapid infusion of 2L of

crystalloid. Lack of rapid response is indication for immediate thoracotomy for treatment of tamponade, cardiac or great vessel laceration, and for open cardiac compression.

2. The patient with pulse present but with hypotension requires resuscitative measures (oxygen and rapid fluid infusion), and evaluation for source of hypotension. In the case of chest trauma evaluation for cardiac tamponade and myocardial injury is essential.

   a. Tamponade is indicated by Beck's triad of hypotension, jugular venous distension, and muffled heart sounds, along with pulsus paradoxus and Kussmaul's sign (increase in jugular venous distension with inspiration). Jugular venous distension will not occur in a patient that is significantly hypovolemic. Penetrating trauma and physical signs suggestive of tamponade require thoracotomy, although pericardiocentesis may be a temporizing measure.

   b. Myocardial contusion may result from blunt trauma with consequences identical to myocardial infarction. Myocardial laceration is not likely with blunt trauma but may occur and will generally result in tamponade.

   c. Additional evaluation should include a chest x-ray, EKG, and angiography or echocardiogram as indicated.

VIII. Abdomen

A. In multisystem trauma, injury to abdominal organs can be very difficult to detect. In the stable, alert, conscious patient without spinal cord injury, serial abdominal exams and laboratory studies will help detect serious injury. The use of diagnostic procedures will be determined by the clinical situation. Any patient with signs of abdominal trauma and shock that persists or worsens in spite of resuscitative measures requires rapid exploration in the OR. Serious intrathoracic injury must be ruled out by examination and CXR before surgery.

   1. Penetrating trauma.

- a. High-velocity missile injury (gunshot wound) requires laparotomy if the patient is unstable. Some feel that all patients with this type of injury should undergo laparotomy. Others feel that stable patients in whom there are not obvious signs of peritoneal violation may not require laparotomy. If the wound is obviously superficial, treatment is local debridement and disposition is determined by the nature of associated injuries. If penetration of the peritoneum is suspected, peritoneal lavage may be useful in determining if laparotomy is needed. A negative lavage indicates the need for further observation.

- b. Abdominal stab wounds require laparotomy if the patient is unstable and does not respond to initial resuscitation, or if there is obvious peritoneal penetration with evisceration, signs of peritonitis, or free intraperitoneal air. Stab wounds to the lower chest are an indication for peritoneal lavage. Flank, back or anterior abdominal wounds should be explored. If findings suggest peritoneal penetration or are equivocal, lavage should be performed. If the offending instrument is still present, it should be removed in the OR.

2. Blunt trauma - hemodynamically unstable patients with blunt trauma require laparotomy. In the stable patient, serial exams, serial hematocrit, and other laboratory studies as indicated are appropriate. Peritoneal lavage should be considered if the patient is intoxicated, unconscious, has spinal cord injury, demonstrates equivocal exam, or will be undergoing general anesthesia for any reason. If the lavage is positive or if repeated exams demonstrate the development of shock or peritonitis, laparotomy should be performed.

IX. **Pelvis/Genitourinary**

  A. Pelvic fracture - in the immediate evaluation and treatment of trauma, pelvic fractures are of importance because of the possibility of associated hemorrhage, abdominal, vascular or genitourinary injury. Injury to other major organ systems is much more likely to be life threatening, but because of the risk of significant hemorrhage from pelvic fracture, x-ray evaluation of the pelvis should be performed early.

B. Genitourinary trauma--should be considered if any of the following are present:
   1. obvious injury to external genitalia.
   2. hematuria.
   3. pelvic fracture.
   4. oligouria or anuria.
   5. trauma to abdomen, flank, back.
   6. pedestrian struck by motor vehicle.

C. Evaluation.
   1. X-ray of pelvis in all patients with significant trauma or findings listed above. Urine analysis is also essential.
   2. Finding of blood at urethral meatus or dislocated prostate should be evaluated with retrograde urethrogram when patient is stable. Foley catheter should not be placed in light of these physical findings until properly evaluated.
   3. If bladder injury is suspected by lower abdominal blunt or penetrating trauma or pelvic fracture, retrograde cystogram should be performed.
   4. IVP should be obtained in all patients with significant hematuria or penetrating trauma in flank or lower abdomen.
      a. if IVP shows no dye excretion renal fragmentation or pedicle injury is suggested. Further evaluation should include CT scan or angiography if the patient's condition allows.
      b. if contrast is extravasated there is a tear of the collecting system and surgical repair will probably be required.
      c. delayed excretion suggests renal contusion which generally will require only close observation.

Trauma

X. **Extremities**

A. Goal is accurate diagnosis and correction of limb-threatening disorders. Definitive treatment of orthopedic injuries is not an appropriate goal during the initial management of a trauma victim. Neurovascular status distal to the site of the injury must be carefully assessed.

B. Fractures/dislocations.

1. Grossly angulated fractures should be aligned with firm, gentle axial traction and splinted. This should not be done if the deformity is close to or involves a joint.

2. Dislocations should be reduced as soon as possible after examination and x-rays have confirmed the diagnosis.

C. Amputation.

1. Replantation should be considered possible until the appropriate consultant has determined otherwise.

2. Hemorrhage from the amputation stump should be controlled with elevation and direct pressure. A sterile compression dressing should be applied. A tourniquet should only be used if other methods for controlling hemorrhage are unsuccessful.

3. The amputated part should be preserved by wrapping in a sterile dressing moistened with sterile saline. It should be sealed in a clean dry container such as a plastic bag. The plastic bag may be placed in ice water. The amputated part should not be placed directly in water or ice and should not be frozen.

D. Open fracture.

1. Any break in the skin near a fracture site should be considered evidence for an open fracture.

2. Open fractures should be covered with a sterile dressing and splinted in position unless there is evidence of neurovascular compromise distally. In this case, gross realignment should be established by gentle axial traction. If bony fragments are thereby retracted

back into the wound, the consulting surgeon must be informed of this fact.

E. Arterial injury.
   1. Should be suspected whenever an injury is near an artery. Physical findings include a pale, cold, painful, pulseless limb. Sensory loss may be the only early finding. With penetrating trauma, vascular and neurological injury should be assumed.
   2. Detailed arteriography should be performed as soon as possible and a vascular surgeon consulted.

XI. **Laboratory and Diagnostic Procedures**
   A. All victims of significant trauma will require certain baseline laboratory studies, which should include the following:
      1. complete blood count and platelet count.
      2. coagulation studies.
      3. electrolytes, BUN, calcium, glucose.
      4. ethanol level.
      5. urine analysis.
      6. arterial blood for blood gas analysis.
      7. Type and screen unless patient is hypotensive or has evidence of significant hemorrhage, in which case type and cross for at least 6 units should be obtained.
      8. Toxicology screens as indicated.
      9. Pregnancy test in women of child-bearing age.
      10. Amylase, liver, bone, cardiac enzymes as indicated.
   B. Radiographs should be obtained as early as possible in the course of management of the trauma victim. These should include the following as indicated by the clinical situation:
      1. Lateral C-spine, obtained before any manipulation of the patient. Additional views should be obtained when patient is stable.
      2. AP chest, obtained with the patient semi-erect if possible.
      3. Pelvis.
      4. Flat plate of the abdomen.

5. Additional films as indicated, with life- and limb-threatening injuries receiving priority.

References

Asensio J, et al. American Family Physician, Sept. 1988, pp 97-112.

Mills J, *et al*, eds. <u>Current Emergency Diagnosis and Treatment</u>. Los Altos: Lange Medical Publications, 1985.

Rosen P, *et al*, eds. <u>Emergency Medicine: Concepts and Clinical Practice</u>. St. Louis: C.V. Mosby Company, 1988.

AIRWAY MANAGEMENT

I. **Overview**
   A. Airway control is the first, most important step in the management of critically ill patients. All critically ill patients should receive supplemental oxygen. Several techniques for maintaining an airway must be available to the practitioner to deal with various clinical situations. Options for definitive control of the airway include the nonsurgical techniques of direct orotracheal intubation, blind or visualized nasotracheal intubation and digital orotracheal intubation. Surgical options are cricothyrotomy and tracheostomy. An invasive but nonsurgical option is percutaneous transtracheal ventilation (PTV).

II. **Evaluation**
   A. History (When possible).
      1. Preceding symptoms and illnesses.
      2. Last meal.
      3. Medications, including potential overdoses.
      4. Pertinent past medical history (pulmonary disease, prior surgeries especially related to the airway, cardiac disease).
   B. Examination.
      1. Detailed rapid inspection--patient size, level of consciousness, evidence of trauma to head, face or neck, drooling, character of phonation, evidence of distress, inspection of thorax for evidence of trauma, inspiratory effort, rate and pattern.
      2. Laboratory--arterial blood gases.
      3. Radiographic--chest film to evaluate for intrathoracic processes. Consider soft tissue views of the airway if patient has drooling or altered phonation.

III. **Intervention** (Fig 1-7).

Airway Management

A. Indications: if patient is unable to maintain own airway patency or protect own airway, requires active regulation of ventilation.

```
┌─────────────────────────────┐      ┌─────────────────────────────┐
│ Initial Airway Assessment:  │      │ Supportive Oxygen:          │
│   Ventilation (RR, effort)  │      │   Continual reassessment    │
│   Oxygenation (cyanosis?)   │      │   to ensure adequate vents  │
│   Level of Consciousness?   │      │   with intact gag response. │
└─────────────────────────────┘      │ Is patient deteriorating?   │
                                     └─────────────────────────────┘
                          no ↑           yes │      no ↑
┌─────────────────────────────────────┐      │
│ Does patient meet                   │ ←────┘
│ Criteria for airway intervention?   │
│   Apneic                            │
│   Will require prolonged active ventil. │
│   At risk for aspiration (poor gag/ altered │
│     level of consciousness          │
│   Route for medication eg. code situation │
└─────────────────────────────────────┘
        yes - [bag mask ventilation until airway secured]
```

Is there neck trauma with obscured landmarks indicating tracheal or laryngeal laceration? — yes → Tracheostomy Emergent consult with Otolaryngologist

no

Is there a potential C-spine injury? — no → Endotracheal Intubation or visualized Nasotracheal Intubation (paralyze as needed)

yes
        yes →
Clinical situation allows for C-spine and x-rays. Do they clear a C-spine injury? → Blind Nasotracheal Intubation

no

Is severe maxillofacial trauma present? — no →
— Tactile Orotracheal Intubation
— Cricothyrotomy
— PTV (percutaneous trans-tracheal ventilation.)

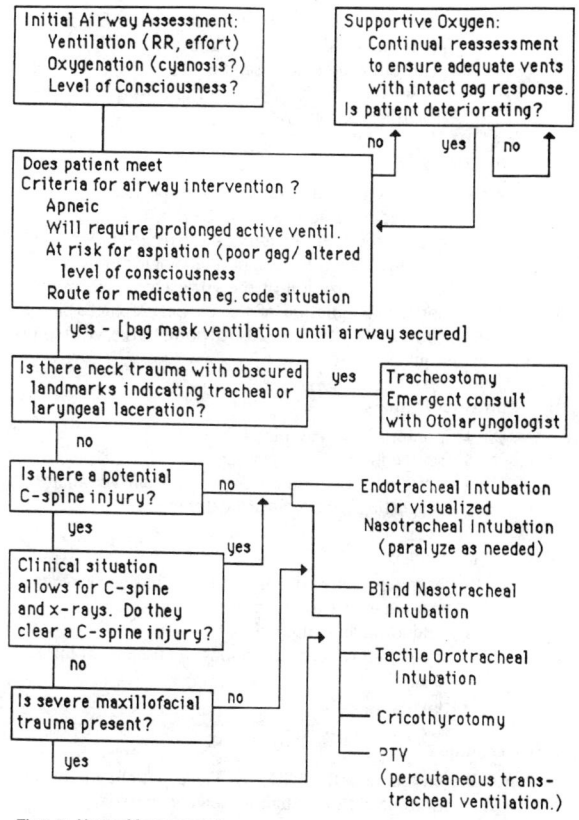

yes

Fig 1-7. Airway Management

B. Methods: techniques for intervention are described in the following sections.

OROTRACHEAL INTUBATION

I. **Advantages**
- definitive form of airway management. ET tube is placed under direct visualization.
- generally can be done rapidly.
- allows placement of a larger ET tube than does nasotracheal route.

II. **Disadvantages**
- requires adequate training and experience.
- may require interruption of CPR.
- requires either an unconscious patient or some amount of sedation or pharmacologic paralysis.
- direct visualization of the vocal cords will require some manipulation of the cervical spine, which is contraindicated in the case of potential cervical spine injury.

III. **Contraindications**
- potential cervical spine injury.
- severe maxillofacial trauma.
- anterior neck trauma with obscured surface anatomy suggesting laryngeal/tracheal fracture.

IV. **Complications**
- esophageal or piriform recess intubation.
- trauma to airway or oral structures.
- endobronchial intubation.
- hypoxia secondary to prolonged attempts at intubation.
- laryngospasm.

V. **Technique**
A. Preoxygenate with 100% O_2. Place patient in sniffing position (neck flexed slightly, head extended).

B. With left hand insert laryngoscope into the right hand corner of the mouth and advance, gently sweeping the tongue to the left as the blade is moved to the midline. When the epiglottis is visualized it is lifted anteriorly (with the blade tip in the vallecula for curved blades, behind the epiglottis for straight blades.) The line of force used with the laryngoscope is parallel to the axis of the handle, not a levering action.

C. When vocal cords are visualized the ET tube is inserted through the glottic opening far enough that the cuff is just past the vocal cords. (Direct visualization of the tip of the ET tube as it passes though the glottic opening is the best way to ensure proper placement).

D. Assess placement--auscultation of lung fields in the axillary regions bilaterally and the epigastrium, observation of symmetrical chest movement with ventilation, clouding of the ET tube with exhalation. Inflate cuff with just enough air to prevent leakage, secure in place. Obtain chest X-ray to confirm placement as soon as the clinical situation allows.

NASOTRACHEAL INTUBATION

I. **Advantages**
- blind technique can be performed if spontaneous respirations present to guide intubation without significant manipulation of the cervical spine.
- more comfortable and better tolerated by a conscious patient.

II. **Disadvantages**
- cannot be performed as quickly as direct orotracheal intubation, more difficult technique.
- generally requires smaller diameter ET tube.

III. **Contraindications**
- any significant facial trauma or head trauma suggesting the possibility of basilar skull fracture (attempts at nasotracheal intubation in this setting can result in insertion of the ET tube into the cranial vault).

- coagulopathies are a contraindication because of possible uncontrollable epistaxis.

IV. Complications
- same complications as with orotracheal intubation with the following additions:
- epistaxis.
- improper placement is more likely, especially with the blind technique.

V. Technique

A. Preoxygenate with 100% O_2. Leave patient's head and neck in neutral position. Anesthetize the nasal mucosa with cocaine or lidocaine jelly.

B. Gently advance well-lubricated ET tube (about one full size smaller than would be used for direct orotracheal technique) through the nares. It should not be advanced against resistance

C. Listen at the proximal end of the ET tube for sounds of patient respirations and advance tube through glottic opening when respiratory sounds are at a maximum. May pass through opening more easily if advanced during inspiration.

D. Direct visualization and advancement of the tube with Magill forceps will facilitate placement of the ET tube in the proper position. However, proper alignment of the cervical spine in the face of potential C-spine injury cannot be guaranteed with use of the laryngoscope, even with manual cervical traction.

E. Assess placement, inflate cuff, and secure as for orotracheal intubation.

TACTILE OROTRACHEAL INTUBATION

I. Advantages
- blind technique but can be performed very rapidly and without manipulation of the cervical spine.
- can be used in the unconscious patient with significant facial and head trauma, a situation where nasotracheal intubation should not be attempted be-

cause of potential basilar skull fracture and also where direct visualization with the laryngoscope is not desirable because of the potential for cervical spine injury.
- can be used with some facility in situations where acquiring an airway can be quite difficult--when vocal cords cannot be visualized because of blood, secretions or foreign matter, in patients with short obese necks.

II. Disadvantages

- can only be used in patients that are completely unconscious or paralyzed because of risk of bite injury to the physician.

III. Contraindications

- a conscious or semiconscious patient or evidence of tracheal or laryngeal fracture.

IV. Complications

- the major potential complication of this and other blind techniques is that of improper tube placement (esophageal or piriform recess intubation).

V. Technique

A. Preoxygenate with 100% O_2. Place an oral airway sideways in the left corner of the patient mouth to serve as a bite block.

B. Insert the index and long finger of your gloved left hand into patient's mouth, moving in the midline along the surface of the tongue. As the fingers are reaching into the oropharynx, allow your hand to move to the right hand corner of the patient's mouth--this allows those with short fingers to reach the epiglottis. The long finger will strike the epiglottis. Lift it anteriorly with the long finger.

C. Insert the ET tube (preferably with stylet in place and distal tip slightly flexed anteriorly) on the palmar side of your left hand. Insert it along the midline of the tongue, using the volar surface of the index finger and the radial side of the long finger as a guide.

D. As the distal tip goes behind the epiglottis, shift the long finger to the posterior surface of the tube alongside the index finger. Use both fingers to lift the tube anteriorly. With the ET tube in the midline and lifted anteriorly to a position above the glottic opening it can be easily passed through the vocal cords.

E. Carefully assess position, inflate cuff and secure the tube.

PERCUTANEOUS TRANSTRACHEAL VENTILATION

I. **Advantages**
- provides very rapid access to the airway, especially in settings where direct laryngoscopy and nasotracheal intubation are at least temporarily not advisable.
- does not interrupt CPR.

II. **Disadvantages**
- requires some specialized equipment, including a high pressure (50 psi or greater) oxygen source.
- does not protect the airway from aspiration.
- unless a specialized ventilator is used that can provide high-frequency positive-pressure ventilation (HFPPV) this method will result in CO_2 retention after 20 to 30 minutes.

III. **Contraindications**
- loss of landmarks due to swelling or severe trauma to the anterior neck.
- severe COPD is a relative contraindication as these patients may be unable to tolerate the high pressures and CO_2.

IV. **Complications**
- subcutaneous and mediastinal emphysema are probably the most common.
- hemorrhage may occur if the thyroid or vessels are punctured.

V. Technique

A. If time permits the skin over the cricothyroid membrane is prepared with betadine or alcohol. In a conscious or semi-conscious patient the area should be anesthetized with local infiltration of anesthetic.

B. An over-the-needle catheter (16 gauge or larger) with a 5- or 10-mL syringe attached is used to puncture the cricothyroid membrane. Needle is in the midline, directed downward and caudally at a 45 degree angle. Negative pressure is applied to the syringe during insertion. Air entering the syringe indicates the trachea has been cannulated. The catheter is advanced off the needle.

C. Distal end of the oxygen tubing is attached to the catheter. Adequate pressure must be used to result in expansion of the chest wall. Pressure is released as soon as this is observed and exhalation occurs passively. (Complete upper airway obstruction may prevent adequate deflation of the lungs and cricothyrotomy should be immediately performed.)

CRICOTHYROTOMY

I. Advantages

- provides a relatively simple and rapid surgical airway, especially useful in patients with complete upper airway obstruction that cannot be relieved by other means, in patients with potential cervical spine injury and basilar skull fracture, and in patients with severe laryngospasm preventing passage of an endotracheal tube.

II. Disadvantages

- cannot be in used in children less than 10 -12 years of age because of the narrow cricothyroid space and the fact that the cricoid is the narrowest part of the lumen in children.

III. Contraindications

- should not be used in children.

- loss of landmarks because of trauma, especially if tracheal or laryngeal laceration is suspected.
- overlying hematoma, tumor, or thyroid.

IV. **Complications**
- hemorrhage, false passage, esophageal injury, damage to the recurrent laryngeal nerve. Subglottic stenosis is not a common complication if the cricothyroid tube is replaced by another method of airway control in 24 to 48 hours.

V. **Technique**
A. Skin should be prepared with alcohol or other antiseptic solution if at all possible, and anesthetized as indicated by patient's level of consciousness and the urgency of the situation.
B. A horizontal incision is made in the skin overlying the crico-thyroid membrane and extended down through the membrane.
C. A mosquito or Kelly clamp may be used to open the incision in the membrane to allow passage of an ET or tracheostomy tube.
D. Assess placement by ventilating through the tube and observing and ascultating the chest. Inflate the cuff of the tube and secure the tube to the neck.

References

Jaffe A, *et al*, eds. Textbook of Advanced Cardiac Life Support. Dallas: American Heart Association, 1987.

Rosen P, *et al*, eds. Emergency Medicine: Concepts & Clinical Practice, 2nd edition. St. Louis: The C.V. Mosby Co., 1988.

RESPIRATORY DISTRESS

I. **Initial Evaluation**

   A. Assessment: rapid primary survey, done as O_2, monitor, IV started.

   1. General appearance: mental status (conscious, anxious), color.

   2. Respirations: rate, presence of stridor, retractions, character of phonation.

   3. Auscultation of chest: lungs (crackles, wheezes, diminished breath sounds), heart (gallop, rub).

   4. Arterial blood gas if time allows: essential for diagnosing respiratory failure and its acuteness. Chronic respiratory failure is not as immediately life-threatening.

II. **Intervention**

   A. Upper airway obstruction:

   1. Always an immediate life-threat. May occur from foreign body or airway narrowing from swelling due to infection or edema. Indicated by stridor (inspiratory and/or expiratory), cyanosis, ineffective respiratory effort as evidenced by retractions, dysphonia.

   2. Treatment:

      a. Heimlich maneuver.

      b. Finger sweep of the hypopharynx (not in conscious patient, child or suspected epiglottitis).

      c. Direct laryngoscopy (in emergency room this should be the first step if patient in extremis) to remove foreign body under direct visualization or pass ET tube if laryngeal edema. Should not be done if suspected epiglottitis.

      d. Cricothyrotomy.

   B. Pneumothorax.

   1. History of trauma is usually present but not necessarily. Diagnosis based upon physical findings of decreased breath sounds in one hemithorax. Tension

pneumothorax may also demonstrate hyperresonant hemithorax, shift of trachea, hypotension, distended neck veins. If time permits a chest X-ray confirms diagnosis.

   2. Treatment:
      a. If tension pneumothorax is present with hypotension, immediate needle thoracostomy should be performed as cardiovascular collapse can occur suddenly. This should be followed by tube thoracostomy.
      b. Tube thoracostomy should be performed as soon as possible in any patient with hemopneumothorax and respiratory distress.

C. Massive aspiration.
   1. Indicated by gurgling respirations, presence of food or vomitus in the oropharynx, cough.
   2. Treatment:
      a. Suctioning of oropharynx.
      b. Endotracheal intubation should be considered and is indicated if the patient has depressed level of consciousness.
      c. Consultation for possible flexible bronchoscopy for removal of particulate matter should be considered.

D. Pulmonary edema.
   1. Indicated by worsening of dyspnea with reclining, crackles present on auscultation, bilateral infiltrates on CXR.
   2. Treatment:
      a. May require endotracheal intubation if respiratory failure present.
      b. Intravenous morphine and diuretics (furosemide) will generally provide rapid improvement. Additional treatment will require careful monitoring and should be instituted after patient is in the intensive care unit.

E. Obstructive pulmonary disease.
    1. Asthma, COPD, cystic fibrosis are usually present in the history.
    2. Treatment: please see chapter 3.

Reference

Mills J. and Luce J. Dyspnea, Respiratory Distress, and Respiratory Failure. In <u>Current Emergency Diagnosis and Treatment</u>. Mills J, *et al*, eds. Los Altos: Lange Medical Publications, 1985.

SHOCK

Shock is a clinical syndrome characterized by inadequate tissue perfusion with resulting cellular dysfunction due to circulatory failure.

I. **Etiology**

   Shock can be classified into categories based upon the major pathophysiologic process involved.

   A. Hypovolemic shock: decreased intravascular volume from hemorrhage or loss of fluid and electrolytes.

   B. Distributive shock: an abnormal distribution of vascular volume due to altered vascular resistance and/or permeability resulting in circulatory failure. Anaphylactic and septic shock are the most common examples of this type of shock.

   C. Cardiogenic shock: inadequate cardiac function because of primary pump failure, arrhythmia, or valvular disease.

II. **Diagnosis**

   A. Hypotension--criteria should be based upon normals for age and take into consideration the individuals own "normal" range. Orthostatic vital signs should be obtained if blood pressure is borderline.

   B. Tachycardia will usually be present as part of the physiologic response to inadequate perfusion.

   C. Orthostatic changes in vital signs will be present (but of course are unnecessary and should not be measured in a patient that is hypotensive in the supine position). A decrease in systolic blood pressure of 10-20 mm Hg with an increase in pulse rate of 15 beats/minute or more after assuming an upright position from supine (with 2-3 minute interval to allow blood pressure to stabilize) suggests inadequate intravascular volume.

   D. Hypoperfusion may be evidenced in the peripheral circulation by cool, mottled extremities and weak pulses.

   E. Altered mental status may be present and demonstrated by restlessness, agitation, confusion, lethargy.

III. Clinical Severity

A. Mild: decreased perfusion of nonvital organs, with intact mentation, normal or slightly decreased urine output, and no metabolic acidosis.

B. Moderate: decreased perfusion of vital organs other than heart and brain, with relatively intact mentation, oliguria and mild metabolic acidosis.

C. Severe: inadequate perfusion of heart or brain with severe oliguria or anuria, metabolic acidosis, altered mentation, and possibly signs of cardiac compromise such as abnormal EKG.

IV. Management

A. Immediate:

1. Place patient in supine position. Keep warm.
2. Establish adequate airway and provide O_2, 5-10 L/minute via nasal prongs or mask.
3. Stop obvious external hemorrhage by direct pressure.
4. Obtain IV access, obtain blood samples for arterial blood gas analysis, type and cross if hemorrhage is contributing factor, electrolytes, CBC, renal function, cardiac enzymes as indicated.
5. Intravenous fluids, initially saline or Ringer's lactate. In cardiogenic shock due to left ventricular failure, fluid administration will be necessary only if there is also hypovolemia. Otherwise rapid fluid administration can be harmful. For other types of shock, 1-2 L of crystalloid should be infused over 30 minutes, with further administration of fluid guided by clinical response (urine output, pulse, blood pressure).
6. Cardiac monitoring.
7. Epinephrine for suspected anaphylactic shock.
8. Insert Foley catheter to monitor urine output.

B. Determination of cause and specific treatment:

1. Laryngeal edema, bronchospasm, urticaria, and history of recent insect sting or parenteral medications suggest anaphylaxis. Epinephrine is the drug of choice and can be given IM for mild or moderate anaphylaxis but should be given IV for severe shock.

Dose is 0.1-0.5 mg IM, repeated as necessary, or 0.1-0.2 mg IV over 3-4 minutes. For severe shock an infusion may be necessary and may be started at 1 microgram/minute and increased to 4 micrograms as needed. In addition, an antihistamine such as diphenhydramine 50 mg should be given IV or IM. 100-250 mg of hydrocortisone can be given IV and repeated every 1-4 hours as indicated. H-2 blockers can also be used such as cimetidine 300-600 mg/IV q6 hr.

2. History of trauma indicates the possibility of hemorrhage. Evidence of chest trauma suggests tension pneumothorax or cardiac tamponade as possible causes. In all cases of trauma with shock, blood pressure should be supported with crystalloid and appropriate studies begun as the patient is being stabilized. Immediate surgical consultation is advisable.

3. History of chest pain, hypertension, cardiac disease, and findings of jugular venous distension and cardiac gallops suggest cardiogenic shock. Modest fluid challenge can be given if hypovolemia is suspected. EKG should be obtained as soon as possible. Dopamine may be used to treat hypotension not responsive to fluid.

4. Fever, hypothermia, rigors, petechiae, or other rash indicate sepsis. Toxic shock syndrome must be considered (most cases occur in young women using tampons within 5 days of onset of menses). Dopamine may be required to support pressure. Cultures should be obtained and the patient started on empiric antibiotic treatment.

5. If none of the preceding signs or symptoms are present to suggest an etiology of the shock, unusual causes should be considered such as Addison's disease, pulmonary embolism.

Reference

Trunkey D. *et al*, Shock. In <u>Current Emergency Diagnosis and Treatment</u>, Mill J. *et al*, eds. Los Altos: Lange Medical Publications, 1985.

COMA

Coma is an altered mental state in which the patient demonstrates either inappropriate or no response to environmental stimuli and maintains eye closure throughout the stimulus.

I. **Overview**
   A. Coma has multiple causes. Initial evaluation and management must be rapidly directed toward those causes that are reversible and have significant risk of morbidity or mortality. Therapeutic measures aimed at correcting these reversible causes must be instituted simultaneously with diagnostic procedures.
   B. Etiologies.
      1. Traumatic: subdural hematoma, epidural hematoma, cerebral laceration or hemorrhage, brain contusion, concussion.
      2. Primary vascular disease: cerebrovascular accident, hypertensive encephalopathy, ruptured aneurysm, arteriovenous malformation, vasculitis.
      3. Infectious: abscess, encephalitis, meningitis.
      4. Neoplastic: primary CNS, metastatic.
      5. Seizure.
      6. Systemic disorders: hypoxia, metabolic derangements including hypoglycemia, DKA, uremia, hyponatremia, hyperosmolar coma, hyper- and hypocalcemia, intoxications including carbon monoxide, alcohol, sedatives such as barbiturates, opiates, tricyclics, phenothiazines and benzodiazepines, and hypo- and hyperthermia.

II. **Evaluation and Management**
   A. Primary survey.
      1. Establish unresponsiveness, check for respirations, pulse. Initiate CPR if indicated.
      2. If pulse present, secure airway and provide supplemental O_2. Obtain vital signs.

3. Confirm diagnosis of coma by evaluating for response to painful stimulus. Absent or abnormal response (such as mere grunting or posturing) confirms the diagnosis. (Avoid using maneuvers to produce painful stimulus that will leave bruises that may be mistaken for signs of trauma.)

B. Resuscitation.
1. Obtain IV access and blood for laboratory test. Rapid determination of glucose level in the emergency room via use of Glucometer, Accucheck, or similar device can be extremely valuable. Initial laboratory evaluation should include true glucose, CBC, electrolytes including calcium, hepatic and renal function tests. Arterial blood for blood gas determination and carboxyhemoglobin level should be obtained when possible. Intervention continues while labs are pending.
2. Glucose, 50ml of 50% dextrose(25g) IV over 3 to 4 minutes. Pediatric dose is 0.5 to 1.0 mg/kg. (If ischemic brain injury such as stroke or prolonged hypoxia is strongly suspected glucose should not be given as hyperglycemia may worsen ischemic damage. If initial estimation of blood sugar by portable glucometer is in the normal range, glucose should not be given.)
3. Naloxone (Narcan) 2 to 4 mg IV initially, then 2 mg every 5 minutes if no or only partial response. Pediatric dose is .01 mg/kg followed by 0.1 mg/kg, every 5 minutes as indicated. This dose of naloxone is higher than those initially recommended as several of the synthetic opiates require these higher doses and naloxone is quite safe. In addition, there is some evidence that these higher doses can partially reverse ethanol-induced coma and may protect against further CNS damage in cases of ischemic or traumatic injury.
4. Thiamine 100 mg IV to protect against the potential development of Wernicke-Korsakoff encephalopathy in patients with depleted thiamine who are given a glucose load. Routine administration to children is not recommended.

5. If patient demonstrates seizure activity, treatment of status epilepticus should be instituted after the above measures have been completed.

C. Secondary survey.

1. History as available. Should be acquired as soon as possible following initial stabilization. Must include information regarding chronic illnesses such as diabetes, hypertension, cancer, renal failure, seizures, and details regarding medications and possible substance abuse or intoxication.

2. Complete set of vital signs, including core temperature. Cardiac monitoring is essential for ruling out arrhythmias. Hyperthermia (temperature 41°C or higher) can rapidly cause irreversible brain damage and should be immediately corrected. Hypothermia is better tolerated and can be more deliberately corrected. An elevated blood pressure in association with relative bradycardia (in a patient without a history of HTN or on medication to account for these findings) suggests increased intracranial pressure (Cushing's reflex.)

3. Physical exam. Look specifically for evidence of trauma, meningeal irritation, and other findings that suggest a specific etiology for the altered mental status. Meningeal signs suggest meningitis or subarachnoid hemorrhage.

4. Detailed neurological exam. Observation of respiratory pattern, posture, spontaneous movements, and reaction to stimulus are helpful. These findings should be assigned to a rating scale (Table 1-2) so that serial exam can accurately detect significant change. Cranial nerves should be examined with particular attention to the pupils. Motor exam is performed with the intent of demonstrating hemiplegia (which may be evidenced by bilateral asymmetry of tone). Asymmetry of reflexes also suggests unilateral structural lesion.

5. Laboratory and radiological evaluation. Initial laboratory studies may need to be supplemented based upon findings on physical exam or upon response to initial resuscitative measures. Evidence

of meningeal irritation indicates the need for lumbar puncture unless physical findings suggest mass lesion (focal neurological deficits, papilledema).

Table 1-2. Glasgow Coma Scale

Parameter	Response	Score
Eye Opening	Spontaneous	4
	To voice	3
	To pain	2
	None	1
Verbal Response	Oriented	5
	Confused	4
	Inappropriate	3
	Incomprehensible sounds	2
	None	1
Motor Response	Localizes pain	5
	Withdraws to pain	4
	Flexion response to pain	3
	Extension response to pain	2
	None	1

Note: Coma score is most useful in triage and in following status. Initial score of <7 indicates a poor prognosis if a cause other than trauma cannot be found and corrected quickly. Assessment should be done frequently and recorded accurately on a flow sheet with times documented. See Reference Data section for pediatric coma scale.

Radiographic evaluation should include cervical spine films if there is any question of trauma to the head or neck. Chest x-ray is a necessary part of the general medical evaluation and is needed to check endotracheal tube placement if the patient has been intubated. CT scan of the head should be considered if a specific cause has not been demonstrated, or if there are focal findings suggesting mass lesion, hemorrhage or stroke.

III. **Disposition**

A. All comatose patients will require admission even if there is a prompt response to initial resuscitative measures. All of these patients should undergo serial examination to detect change in status and to detect any further findings that may suggest an etiology. Early consultation is essential if an etiology cannot be determined. The patient that remains comatose will usually require the extensive observation that is generally available only in an intensive care unit.

Reference

Simon R, Coma. In <u>Current Emergency Diagnosis and Treatment</u>, Mills J, *et al*, eds. Los Altos: Lange Medical Publications, 1985.

POISONING AND OVERDOSE

Poisoning is a leading cause of death in children, adolescents and young adults. Most poisonings are with agents that do not have a specific antidote and require decontamination and supportive care. The regional poison control center should be contacted as soon as possible whenever a poisoning occurs.

I. **Resuscitation and Initial Management**
   A. Airway.
      1. An adequate airway should be established immediately. If necessary ventilations should be assisted. O₂ should be provided. If the patient is comatose or has depressed mental status with absent gag reflex, intubation is indicated. (Nasotracheal intubation will be better tolerated by patients that are semiconscious and will allow better access to the oropharynx if gastric lavage is required.)
      2. Suction should be immediately available to assist in managing the airway.
   B. Circulation.
      1. IV access should be obtained as early as possible in patients with potentially serious poisoning. Hypotension should be treated initially with crystalloids. Pressor agents should be used if there is inadequate response to volume expansion.
      2. Cardiac monitoring should be instituted as soon as possible.
   C. Neurological status.
      1. Coma should be treated as soon as vital signs have been stabilized. (See page 41 on evaluation and treatment of coma.) Glucose should be given by IV bolus (50 ml of 50% solution). Naloxone should be given up to 2mg IV and repeated as necessary.
      2. Seizures can be treated with IV diazepam, 0.1-0.2 mg/kg. If this fails to eliminate seizures, phenytoin can be used 15-18 mg/kg infused at a rate of up to 50 mg/minute.

Poisoning and Overdose

II. **Diagnosis**

   A. History to determine the agent or agents ingested and the time of the ingestion must be obtained when patient is stable so that appropriate method for decontamination can be chosen.

III. **Decontamination**

   A. Emesis.
   1. May be induced if the ingestion is recent (less than 1 hour), or if there is reason to believe that significant amounts may still be in the stomach, such as large ingestions or medications that slow gastric emptying. Recent studies have suggested that most poisonings are more appropriately treated with early activated charcoal. without the delay that is caused by induced emesis. Emesis should not be induced if there is depressed mental status or absent gag reflex.
   2. Ipecac, 15 ml for children and 30 ml for adults, is given orally followed by large amounts of water. Physical agitation helps to induce vomiting (massage of the stomach or walking). Dose may be repeated if vomiting is not induced in 20-30 minutes.

   B. Gastric Lavage.
   1. Indicated if the ingestion has been recent (less than one hour) and if the patient is combative or has depressed gag reflex, in which case orotracheal intubation will precede lavage. The lavage tube must have a large diameter (at least 36 French) and an aspirate should be obtained before lavage commences--the sample confirms the placement of the tube and can be used for analysis.
   2. Lukewarm tap water or saline may be used in 150-200 ml increments. Lavage should be continued until fluid is clear of pill fragments. Contraindications to both induced emesis and lavage are ingestion of caustic agents and unprotected airway.

   C. Activated charcoal.
   1. Activated charcoal is the decontamination procedure of choice for most poisonings. Recent studies have shown that charcoal alone is the decontamination

procedure of choice with the exception of ingestion within an hour of arrival at the emergency room. For several medications, it is most effective when given in multiple doses. Standard dose for adults is 100 grams, with proportionally smaller doses for children.

2. Indications for multiple doses of charcoal:
- theophylline.
- tricyclics.
- digitalis preparations.
- phenobarbital.

IV. Toxindromes

A. There are several poisoning syndromes that are sufficiently characteristic as to allow specific diagnosis.

1. Cholinergic poisoning: may be caused by organophosphates, carbamates, certain mushrooms, pilocarpine and other cholinergic medications.
- characterized by diaphoresis, salivation, lacrimation, diarrhea, vomiting, urination, miosis, mental status changes ranging from confusion to coma. May induce bronchospasm.
- treatment is supportive as above with protection of airway and support of respirations and circulation. Atropine is a specific antidote for the cholinergic symptoms and can be given 0.5-1.0 mg IV and repeated as necessary. May require very large doses.

2. Anticholinergic poisoning: caused by atropine, scopolamine, belladonna, antihistamines, tricyclic antidepressants, and some plants including jimsonweed, night shade, and some mushrooms.
- characterized by mydriasis, dry mucosal membranes, urinary retention, cutaneous flush, and mental status changes ranging from delirium and hallucinations to frank psychosis.
- specific treatment is available in the form of physostigmine given 0.01-0.03 mg/kg slowly IV. However, this should be reserved for patients with severe symptoms such as hyperthermia or uncontrollable arrhythmias since physostigmine is quite toxic itself. Supportive therapy is all that is required for most cases.

3. Opiate poisoning: should be considered in any comatose or lethargic patient.

- characterized by sedation, hypotension, bradycardia, hypothermia, and respiratory depression. Pinpoint pupils are typical, although may not be present in cases of mixed overdoses.
- specific therapy in the form of naloxone is given IV or ET, 0.4-2.0 mg initially. This may need to be repeated frequently. Ventilatory support must be maintained.

V. **Specific Therapy**

A. Acetaminophen.

1. Primary concern is hepatic toxicity, which occurs 24-72 hours after ingestion due to accumulation of a toxic metabolite. Toxic dose is > 140 mg/kg.

2. Treatment: severity of ingestion can be estimated by obtaining a serum acetaminophen level. For toxic ingestions acetylcystein (Mucomyst) is used at a dose of 140 mg/kg orally or IV followed by 70 mg/kg every 4 hours until serum acetaminophen level is 0. Repeat doses if vomited within 1 hour. Effectiveness of this treatment depends upon early use of acetylcysteine; within 12-16 hours of ingestion. If activated charcoal is to be used, either for the acetaminophen or for other agents that may have been simultaneously ingested, the dose of acetylcystein must be increased by 25% as it is partially inactivated by charcoal.

B. Stimulants.

1. Manifest by euphoria, mydriasis, restlessness or agitation up to psychosis and seizures. May be hypertensive with either tachycardia or bradycardia, occasionally ventricular arrhythmias.

2. Treat agitated behavior with diazepam (2-5 mg IV, repeated q5 minutes as needed). Seizures should be treated with diazepam or phenytoin. Hypertension can be treated with nitroprusside if necessary. Tachyarrhythmias can be treated with IV propranolol (0.5-3 mg).

C. Beta Blockers.
   1. Toxicity is demonstrated by profound beta-blockade with bradycardia and hypotension.
   2. Treatment is with Glucagon, 5-10 mg IV bolus, followed by an IV infusion of 1-5 mg/hr titrated to response. (Glucagon is an inotropic and chronotropic agent via a receptor pathway separate from the beta receptors.)

D. Salicylates.
   1. The minimum acute toxic dose is 150 mg/kg, with severe toxicity occurring at doses of 300 mg/kg or more. Early signs of salicylate toxicity are tinnitus, nausea and vomiting, listlessness, and hyperventilation resulting in an initial respiratory alkalosis. This is followed by severe metabolic acidosis, hypokalemia, and hypoglycemia. Seizures, hyperpyrexia and coma indicate severe toxicity.
   2. Treatment consists of supportive care and decontamination as outlined above. In addition, dehydration should be corrected and the metabolic acidosis corrected with sodium bicarbonate, 1 meq/kg/hr. This will promote excretion of salicylates. Hemodialysis is recommended for critically ill patients. Salicylate levels should be obtained and followed.

E. Carbon monoxide.
   1. Symptoms of carbon monoxide intoxication correlate relatively well with levels of carboxyhemoglobin. The initial symptom is headache, followed by dyspnea on exertion, irritability, nausea, fatigue, lightheadedness, and malaise. At high levels, 50% or greater, coma and cardiopulmonary collapse occur.
   2. In addition to supportive care, treatment consists of 100% O_2. This provides oxygen to tissues that may be suffering from hypoxia, and dramatically reduces the half-life of carboxyhemoglobin (from about 6 hours on room air to 1-1.5 hours on 100% O_2). All symptomatic patients should receive oxygen therapy. Patients with levels above 30% or severe symptoms should be admitted to an intensive care unit for

F. Digoxin.
1. Intoxication is indicated by anorexia, nausea and vomiting, blurred vision and disturbance of color vision. Cardiac dysrhythmias can occur and are life-threatening. Third-degree A-V block, bradycardia, ventricular ectopy and paroxysmal atrial tachycardia with A-V block may occur. In chronic atrial fibrillation, toxicity may be evidenced by a regular ventricular rhythm. Hyperkalemia may occur with acute overdose.

monitoring. Patients with very high levels, evidence of myocardial ischemia, or coma should be treated in a hyperbaric oxygen chamber if available.

2. Treatment consists of correcting electrolyte abnormalities. Hyperkalemia should be treated but calcium should be avoided if possible as it may potentiate the effects of digoxin on the myocardium. Atropine may be used for symptomatic bradycardia. Phenytoin is effective for ventricular arrhythmias and is given as a 250 mg loading dose IV over 10 minutes. Subsequent doses of 100 mg each may be given every 5-10 minutes up to 15 mg/kg. Digoxin-specific antibody fragments are indicated for life-threatening arrhythmias that do not respond adequately to standard therapy (Vtach, Vfib, severe bradyarrhythmias) hyperkalemia of >5 or ingestion of >10 mg in adults and > 4 mg in children.

H. Tricyclics.
1. Intoxication with tricyclic antidepressants occurs with doses of about 5 mg/kg, with severe poisoning occurring with doses of 10 mg/kg or more. Symptoms and signs include mydriasis, dry mouth, tachycardia, and agitation. Seizures may occur. Cardiovascular effects are potentially life-threatening and may be demonstrated by widening of the QRS complex and prolonged QT or PR intervals. A-V block and ventricular tachycardia may occur.

2. Treatment includes supportive care as described above. Decontamination including emesis or lavage should be performed as these agents slow gastric emptying and may not leave the stomach for several

hours. Activated charcoal should be given in repeated doses. Ventricular arrhythmias may respond to sodium bicarbonate given as a bolus of 30-40 meq. Phenytoin has been recommended 15 mg/kg infused at a rate up to 50 mg/minute when QRS is widened to prevent ventricular arrhythmias.

3. All patients with known or suspected tricyclic overdose must be hospitalized for monitoring as toxic effects may not develop for several hours.

References

Epstein F, *et al*, Poisoning. In <u>Emergency Medicine: Concepts and Clinical Practice</u>, Rosen, *et al*, eds. St. Louis: C.V. Mosby Company, 1988.

Olson K, *et al*, Poisoning. In <u>Current Emergency Diagnosis and Treatment</u>, Mills J., *et al*, eds. Los Altos: Lange Medical Publications, 1985.

ENVIRONMENTAL ILLNESSES

I. **Heat-Related Illnesses**

   Heat-related illnesses occur when the body is unable to maintain a balance between heat load and heat loss. Several factors can contribute to the development of heat illness including dehydration, alcohol, anticholinergic drugs, fatigue, infection, old age, obesity, chronic debilitating disease and altered skin function as occurs in burns, scleroderma, and cystic fibrosis.

   A. Heat Edema.

      1. Caused by muscular and cutaneous vasodilatation and venous stasis in nonacclimatized individuals.

      2. Seen during the first few days of heat exposure. Core temperature remains normal.

      3. Self-limited, requires no therapy other than elevation of the affected parts.

   B. Heat syncope.

      1. Occurs because of hypotension due to cutaneous and muscular vasodilatation and peripheral venous pooling. Dehydration is not necessarily present. May occur following strenuous activity in the heat.

      2. Physical findings include transient hypotension with weak pulse, and normal or very mildly elevated core temperature.

      3. Responds promptly to rest in recumbent position and removal from the hot environment. Oral rehydration is generally adequate for those patients that are dehydrated.

   C. Heat Cramps/Tetany.

      1. Heat tetany may occur in patients with all degrees of heat illness, but generally does not occur in salt-depleted states. It is thought to be due to alkalosis from hyperventilation and usually occurs after brief periods of very intense heat stress. Carpopedal spasm is the most common manifestation--does not generally involve large, heavily-worked muscles as in heat cramp. No treatment is required.

2. Heat cramps are due to salt depletion and present as cramps of the most heavily worked muscles, usually occurring after heavy exertion during which the patient consumed large amounts of hypotonic fluid. Hemoconcentration and low-normal sodium levels may be present. Potassium is usually normal. Cramps can be relieved by stretching the involved muscle. (Truly rigid muscles that do not relax with stretching suggest neuroleptic malignant syndrome or malignant hyperthermia.) Treatment is with oral electrolyte solutions or normal saline intravenously.

D. Heat exhaustion.

1. Systemic response to heat exposure, generally occurring only after prolonged exposure. Caused by salt depletion and/or dehydration. Is a prodrome to heat stroke.
2. Presents as vague malaise, body ache, tachycardia, orthostatic hypotension, possibly overt clinical dehydration. Temperature may be elevated but generally not above 39°C. Mental status should be essentially normal or with slight confusion or irritability.
3. Laboratory studies should include CPK, LDH, SGOT, SGPT which may be mildly elevated (in heat stroke these are markedly elevated), hematocrit, BUN, and electrolytes to assess hydration and determine appropriate fluid therapy.
4. Treatment should include cooling of the body if temp is elevated with fans or moistening the skin. Rehydration may be oral if there is mild dehydration and no nausea. Initial fluid therapy for more severe dehydration may be with $D_5 0.45\%$ sodium chloride infused 1L over 30 minutes (if patient does not have underlying cardiovascular disease) with subsequent fluids based upon response and laboratory results. May require up to 4 liters of fluid. Patients will generally respond quickly and feel normal within a few hours.

E. Heat stroke.

1. Heat stroke is characterized by loss of normal thermoregulatory function with elevated core temperature (usually above 40°C) and altered mental status.

The loss of thermoregulation allows the body temperature to continue rising to the point of widespread cellular damage including renal, cerebral, myocardial and hepatic. Death results unless core temperature is quickly lowered to a more normal range.

2. Symptoms prior to collapse are those of heat exhaustion. Laboratory findings include hemoconcentration, altered potassium and sodium levels, respiratory alkalosis and/or metabolic acidosis, and elevated CPK, LDH, SGPT, SGOT (usually these are dramatically elevated).

3. Treatment must be prompt to prevent further exposure of vital organs to damaging temperatures. Respirations should be supported with supplemental O_2. Body temperature should be reduced by placing the victim on a cooling blanket and placing ice packs on the axillae, neck and inguinal region. Skin should be moistened and cool dry air blown across the patient if possible. Chlorpromazine may be used to control shivering (dose 10-25 mg slowly IV).

4. All patients with heat stroke should be admitted to an intensive care unit and monitored for anticipated complications including DIC, renal failure, hepatic failure, rhabdomyolysis and arrhythmias.

II. Cold-Related Illnesses

A. Peripheral cold injury:

1. Chilblain: a peripheral cold injury that does not involve freezing of tissue. Commonly occurs on the dorsum of hands and anterior portion of lower leg. Chilblains are pruritic, reddish-blue, swollen patches that may have associated blisters. Rewarming will cause increased itching and burning. Treatment consists of slow rewarming. Some authors recommend warm water immersion of the affected part while others prefer to allow gradual rewarming to room temperature. No permanent injury results, although the affected area may be more temperature sensitive in the future.

2. Immersion injury (trench foot, immersion foot): non-freezing injury that occurs from exposure to wet and cold. Initially the affected body part is cold and pale with decreased sensation and pulses. This is due to vasoconstriction. Hyperemia follows rewarming, causing the affected part to be warm, dry, erythematous, and quite painful. This may last up to 10 days and may result in blisters, ulceration with potential for serious infection. During the recovery period the affected part generally will have decreased sensation with increased sensitivity to cold, depigmentation, pain with weightbearing, and weakness. These may be permanent. Treatment consists of rewarming and elevation of the affected part until all ulcerations have healed. Physical therapy should be started early.

3. Frostbite: injury to tissue due to freezing. Classified in a similar fashion to burns:

- frost nip--cold injury without blistering, characterized by skin that blanches. Results in no tissue loss. Symptoms are numbness and pruritus. Rewarming produces a tingling sensation in the area and erythema that quickly resolves.
- superficial frostbite--freezing of skin and subcutaneous tissue. Characterized by pale skin that does not blanch. Underlying tissue is soft. Rewarming results in edema and erythema. Blisters develop and will take several days to resolve. Generally followed by eschar formation, which may take three to four weeks to resolve.
- deep frostbite--freezing injury of skin, subcutaneous tissue and underlying structures. The injured part will be hard, cold, mottled, and blue-gray even after rewarming. Blisters and blebs may not appear for weeks and will be present at the demarcation between healthy and dead tissue. The necrotic part will mummify and spontaneously amputate.

Treatment consists of rapid rewarming by immersion in water warmed to $38°$ to $42°C$. After rewarming the affected part should elevated and kept dry. Patient should be kept in protective isolation, blisters protected from rupture, and the affected part treated with whirlpool baths of warm water and mild disinfectant daily. Escharotomies may be necessary to prevent contractures and compartment syndrome. Smoking is not allowed because of the vasoconstriction it causes. Debridement should be delayed until spontaneous amputation of the affected soft tissue as the extent of injury is frequently overestimated.

B. Systemic cold injury (Hypothermia):
1. Hypothermia is defined as a core temperature less than 35°. Common predisposing factors are alcohol use, elderly age, debilitating disease such as stroke, hypothyroidism, use of sedative-hypnotic or antidepressant drugs.
2. Mild hypothermia, with core temperature above 33°, may present with weakness, fatigue, lethargy, ataxia and dysarthria. Blood pressure and pulse are usually in the normal range.
3. Moderate hypothermia, with core temperature of 28° to 32°, will demonstrate progressive mental status and cardiovascular depression. Coma is likely with temperatures less than 30°, and reflexes will be depressed. Shivering may no longer be present. EKG may show Osborne waves (deformed terminal portion of the QRS complex) and rate will be bradycardic. Atrial fibrillation is common.
4. Severe hypothermia, with core temperature of 27° or less, is characterized by coma with loss of all reflexes (including corneal), hypotension or pulselessness, significant bradycardia, ventricular fibrillation or asystole.
5. Treatment: basic principles for resuscitation of hypothermia are that irreversibility of cardiac arrest can only be determined after the patient has been rewarmed to 35°C, further heat loss must be prevented, core should be rewarmed before periphery, continuous monitoring of core temperature is essential, and all manipulations of the patient should be as gentle as possible because of myocardial instability and the risk of arrhythmias.
   a. CPR should be initiated only after careful evaluation has revealed the absence of a pulse. Even extreme bradycardia may provide suffi-

cient cardiac output in the setting of severely depressed body temperature. O_2 should be provided to all victims of hypothermia. Hyperventilation with resulting hypocapnia should be avoided as this will contribute to myocardial instability. If ventricular fibrillation occurs, some authors recommend attempting defibrillation once at 2 Joules/kg. If this does not succeed, CPR should be continued and further attempts at defibrillation delayed until core temperature is increased to 30°C. Antiarrythmics are also generally ineffective in the severely hypothermic patient, although bretylium has been reported to be effective in ventricular fibrillation.

   b. Laboratory analysis should include blood gases, electrolytes, glucose. Acidosis is likely (both respiratory and metabolic) and should be corrected slowly.

   c. Rewarming should be started as soon as possible.

- In mild hypothermia (where shivering is still present) passive external rewarming is sufficient. Dry blankets are used to prevent further heat loss and allow the process of thermogenesis to gradually increase body temperature.

- In moderate to severe hypothermia active rewarming is necessary. Most authors feel that active core rewarming should be used instead of active external rewarming which may result in core temperature afterdrop. Heated humidified oxygen provides an adequate rewarming rate, supplemental O_2, and avoids rewarming collapse from core temperature afterdrop. The gas should be heated to 40° to 45°C. This will generally provide a rate of rewarming between 1° to 2°C/hour. Other modalities of active internal rewarming should be used as adjunct to warmed humidified ventilation. Heated IV fluids alone will not provide an adequate rate of rewarming.

6. Disposition: all patients with moderate to severe hypothermia will require careful monitoring in an intensive care unit for complications.

References

Auerbach P. Disorders due to physical and environmental agents. In <u>Current Emergency Diagnosis and Treatment</u>. Mills J, *et al*, eds. Los Altos: Lange Medical Publications, 1985.

Callaham M. Heat Illness. In <u>Emergency Medicine: Concepts and Clinical Practice</u>, Rosen P, *et al*, eds. St. Louis: C.V. Mosby Company, 1988.

Danzel D. Accidental hypothermia. In <u>Emergency Medicine:Concepts and Clinical Practice</u>, Rosen, *et al*, eds. St. Louis: C. V. Mosby Company, 1988.

Shaw J. Frostbite. In <u>Emergency Medicine: Concepts and Clinical Practice</u>, Rosen, *et al*, eds. St. Louis: C.V. Mosby Company, 1988.

2/ CARDIOLOGY

John J. D'Amore, M.D., John E. Littler, M.D., and Timothy Momany, M.D.

ISCHEMIC HEART DISEASE

Angina: Symptomatic myocardial ischemia caused by imbalance between oxygen supply and demand.

I. **Etiology**: Almost invariably an underlying impairment in oxygen supply secondary to coronary artery disease and/or vasospasm. Further impairments in O_2 supply to (anemia, hypotension, arrhythmia) or an increase in O_2 demand (exercise, emotional stress, CHF, HTN, tachycardia, sepsis).

II. **Types**

   A. Stable: intensity, character and frequency of episodes occur predictably in response to a known amount of exercise or other stress.

   B. Unstable: intensity, frequency and/or duration of episodes no longer occurring in a predictable fashion (e.g., precipitated by less exercise or of longer duration). This includes angina at rest and new onset angina.

   C. Variant: Secondary to vasospasm of coronary arteries. May occur at rest. Most patients have spasm at the site of a fixed obstructing lesion. May be demonstrable during angiography with ergonovine challenge.

III. **Diagnosis**

   A. History: Classically described as substernal chest pressure or heaviness radiating to the left shoulder and arm, neck or jaw, associated with nausea, diaphoresis and shortness of breath, brought on and exacerbated by exercise and stress, alleviated with rest. Typically lasts 2-10 minutes and rarely > 30 minutes. Atypical presentations may include epigastric pain, indigestion, right arm pain, lightheadedness, nausea or shortness of breath alone.

   B. Physical exam: Generally will be normal. S4 gallop may be transiently present during an episode.

   C. Laboratory:

1. EKG: during an episode of pain will show ST segment depression, T wave inversion. May be normal. Coronary artery disease is suggested if there is evidence of an old MI.

2. Exercise treadmill (GTX): Approximately 90% specific but only 65% sensitive.

3. Thallium dipyridamole scan: useful for patients who cannot tolerate the physical demands of the GTX (arthritis, COPD).

4. MUGA.

5. Coronary angiography.

IV. Treatment

A. Medical; daily aspirin plus antianginal medication. May use two or three drug combination to maximize benefit while minimizing side effects. In general, either a beta-blocker or calcium channel blocker should be used as they protect against ischemic-induced arrhythmias.

1. Beta blockers: negative chronotropic and inotropic agents. Decrease O_2 demand. Examples are propranolol, 40-200 mg/day (either divided qid or as long-acting agent), atenolol 50-200 mg/day. The different beta-blockers vary as to cardioselectivity and side-effects. Asthma is a contraindication as is a history of CHF (due to the negative inotropism). Diabetes also relative contraindication since masks hypoglycemic symptoms.

2. Calcium channel blockers: effects include negative inotrope/chronotrope, peripheral vasodilatation (which reduces O_2 demand), coronary artery vasodilatation and decrease in coronary artery vasospasm. These are the drugs of choice for variant angina. Diltiazem 30-120 mg tid, nifedipine 10-40 mg qid, nicardipine 20-40 mg tid, verapamil 80-120 mg tid (also available in sustained release form).

3. Nitrates: effects include venous and arteriolar vasodilatation (which produces decreased demand for O_2), and coronary artery vasodilatation (which increases O_2 supply). Tolerance may develop and can be either overcome by increasing the dose or

prevented by providing an 8 hour nitrate-free interval each day. Isosorbide dinitrate 10-30 mg po qid, nitroglycerine ointment 2% topical 1/2"-2" qid, transdermal patch 5, 7.5, 10 one qD (remove for 8 hours/day).

    4. Sublingual nitroglycerin is used for acute episodes of angina, 0.3-0.4 mg S.L. prn, may repeat q5 minutes up to three total doses. Patient should be instructed to go to ER if not relieved after 3 nitro.

B. Revascularization.
   1. Coronary artery bypass grafting (CABG). Indicated for:
      a. left main coronary lesion.
      b. left main equivalent--proximal LAD and proximal left circumflex.
      c. 3 vessel CAD with ejection fraction (50%).
      d. medically refractory angina.
   2. Percutaneous transluminal coronary angioplasty (PTCA). Indicated for discrete proximal lesion.

Ischemic Heart Disease

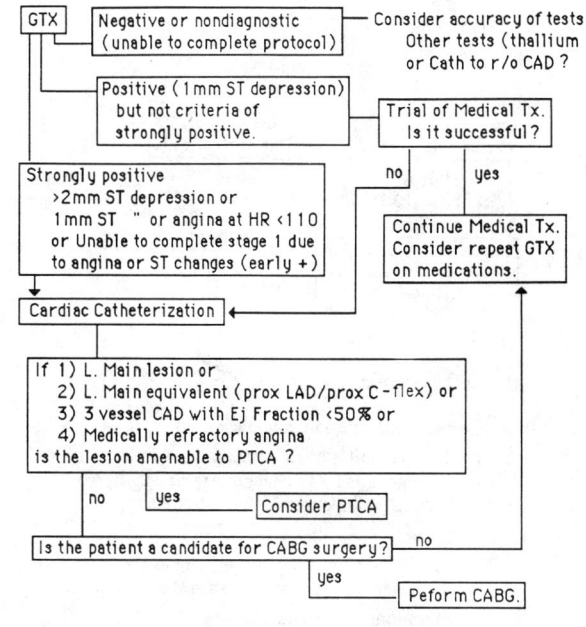

```
┌─────┐   ┌──────────────────────────────┐
│ GTX │───│ Negative or nondiagnostic    │──── Consider accuracy of tests
└─────┘   │ (unable to complete protocol)│     Other tests (thallium
   │      └──────────────────────────────┘     or Cath to r/o CAD ?
   │      ┌──────────────────────────────┐    ┌──────────────────────┐
   ├──────│ Positive (1mm ST depression) │────│ Trial of Medical Tx. │
   │      │ but not criteria of          │    │ Is it successful?    │
   │      │ strongly positive.           │    └──────────────────────┘
   │      └──────────────────────────────┘         no       yes
   │      ┌──────────────────────────────┐
   └──────│ Strongly positive            │
          │  >2mm ST depression or       │         ┌──────────────────────┐
          │  1mm ST " or angina at HR<110│         │ Continue Medical Tx. │
          │  or Unable to complete stage1│         │ Consider repeat GTX  │
          │  due to angina or ST changes │         │ on medications.      │
          │  (early +)                   │         └──────────────────────┘
          └──────────────────────────────┘
                      │
          ┌──────────────────────────┐
          │ Cardiac Catheterization  │◄────────
          └──────────────────────────┘

   If 1) L. Main lesion or
      2) L. Main equivalent (prox LAD/prox C-flex) or
      3) 3 vessel CAD with Ej Fraction <50% or
      4) Medically refractory angina
   is the lesion amenable to PTCA ?
          no       yes
                   └──── Consider PTCA

   Is the patient a candidate for CABG surgery? ── no
                   │
                  yes
                   └──── Perform CABG.
```

Fig 2-1. Stable angina

ISCHEMIC HEART DISEASE--INPATIENT

Inpatient treatment indicated for: (1) unstable angina, (2) prolonged anginal episode, rule out infarction, (3) myocardial infarction.

I. **Unstable Angina**
   A. Definition: angina that:
      1. is new onset.
      2. occurs at rest or with minimum exertion.
      3. is crescendo; occurring with increased frequency, duration, severity or with less exertion than in the past.
   B. Management: (Fig 2-2).

```
Admit to ICU/CCU
Labs to r/o MI (CPK q 8 x3, EKG q am x 3)
Increase anti-anginals. Is angina controlled?
   │
   ├── no (or needs IV nitroglycerin) ──┐
   │                                    │
   └── yes ──► Increase activity in the hospital
                Is angina controlled?
                   │
                   ├── no ──► Cardiac Catheterization
                   │          (see stable angina for
                   │           additional steps)
                   │
                   └── yes ──► GTX on medications
                               (see Stable Angina)
```

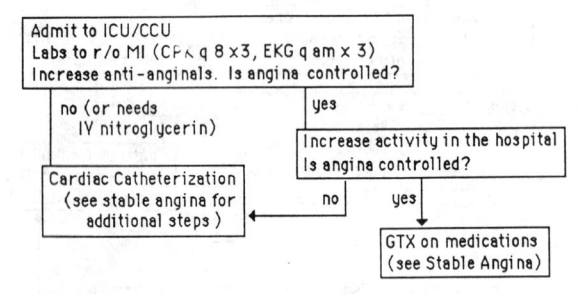

Fig 2-2. Unstable angina

II. **Prolonged Anginal Episode**, rule out MI.
   A. Decision to admit is based upon history (with or without EKG changes). If EKG changes are classic for MI or if enzymes are positive treat as MI (see below).
   B. Management:
      1. Admit to ICU; it is not appropriate to use first set of enzymes to decide if patient should be in ICU.
      2. Continuous cardiac monitoring.
      3. O_2 should be provided (2L per nasal prongs).

Ischemic Heart Disease--Inpatient

4. IV access should be assured.
5. Obtain screening labs, including CBC with diff, glucose, electrolytes if indicated (patient on medication that may affect electrolytes), and cardiac enzymes.
6. Obtain serial cardiac enzymes; a common protocol is CPK q 8 hr times 3, not counting the initial set. Obtain isoenzymes (MB bands) for any elevated values.
7. Serial EKG; ex. qAM times 2-3.
8. Bed rest, possibly bedside commode.
9. Sedation may be of some benefit in certain patients.
10. Pain relief with increased doses of antianginal agents; topical, oral or sublingual nitrates, calcium channel blockers, beta blockers. If IV nitroglycerin is required to control pain, consider cardiac catheterization.

C. Cardiac enzymes:(Table 2-1)

Table 2-1. Cardiac Enzymes

Enzyme	Rises	Peaks
CPK	6-8 hours	24 hours
SGOT	8-12 hours	18-36 hours
LDH	24-48 hours	3-6 days

D. Disposition:
   1. If enzymes become positive, treat as MI.
   2. If enzymes remain negative, treat as for unstable angina.

III. **Myocardial Infarction**
   A. Defined by EKG changes and/or serum enzyme changes.
      1. EKG patterns:
         a. Ischemia/injury: indicated by elevated ST segment, T wave inversion. (ST depression can indicate digitalis effect, non-Q wave infarct).
         b. Infarct: indicated by evolution of EKG changes with ST segment elevation followed by development of Q waves.
      2. Infarct location by EKG (Table 2-2).

Table 2-2. Infarct Location by EKG

EKG Changes	Location of Injury	Coronary Artery Involved
II, III, AVF	inferior wall (may be associated with right ventricle injury, consider right precordial leads)	right coronary artery
V_{1-3}	anteroseptal	left anterior descending
V_{3-5}	anterior wall	left anterior descending
V_6, I, AVL	lateral	marginal branch off circumflex or diagonal off LAD
reciprocal changes in V_{1-2} with large R wave, ST depressions, and Q wave in V_6	posterior	RCA

B. Management.
   1. Consider thrombolytic therapy (Fig 2-3). The intravenous administration of a thrombolytic agent (streptokinase or tissue plasminogen activator [tPA]), early in acute MI can dissolve an obstructing coronary artery thrombus leading to reperfusion of ischemic myocardium, thereby limiting infarct size. tPA is much more expensive than streptokinase but felt by some to be more successful in reperfusion.
   2. Stabilize with O_2, IV access. Treat complications as indicated in next section.
   3. Control pain.
      a. Sublingual nitroglycerine 0.3-0.4 mg, repeat q 5 minutes as needed. If pain persists after nitro x 3, consider nifedipine.
      b. Nifedipine, 10 mg capsule. Have patient bite capsule (or use needle to place a hole in it) and swallow the liquid contents and capsule. (Caution; nifedipine can produce significant hypotension, tachycardia.)
      c. Morphine may be used for pain unresponsive to sublingual nitro or nifedipine. 2 mg IV, repeat every 5 to 10 minutes as needed.

Ischemic Heart Disease--Inpatient 67

d. Consider IV nitroglycerin for pain not responsive to the above measures.

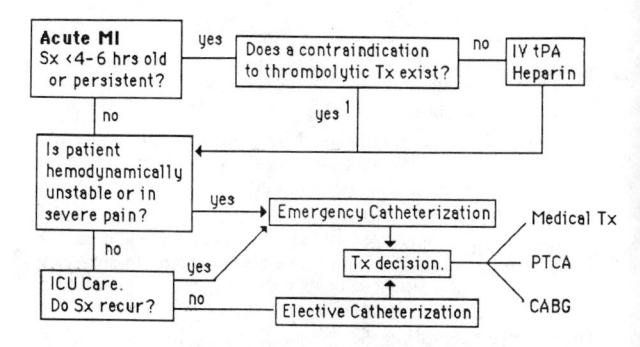

```
┌─────────────────┐  yes  ┌──────────────────────────┐  no   ┌──────────┐
│ Acute MI        │─────▶│ Does a contraindication  │─────▶│ IV tPA   │
│ Sx <4-6 hrs old │      │ to thrombolytic Tx exist?│      │ Heparin  │
│ or persistent?  │      └──────────────────────────┘      └──────────┘
└─────────────────┘                   │
         │ no                         │ yes¹
         ▼                            │
┌─────────────────┐                   │
│ Is patient      │◀──────────────────┘
│ hemodynamically │
│ unstable or in  │  yes   ┌──────────────────────────┐
│ severe pain?    │──────▶│ Emergency Catheterization│──┐        Medical Tx
└─────────────────┘       └──────────────────────────┘  │       ╱
         │ no                                            ▼      ╱
         ▼                                    ┌──────────────┐ ── PTCA
┌─────────────────┐  yes                      │ Tx decision. │
│ ICU Care.       │──────────────────────────▶└──────────────┘ ── CABG
│ Do Sx recur?    │                                   ▲        ╲
└─────────────────┘  no   ┌──────────────────────────┐│         ╲
         └──────────────▶│ Elective Catheterization │┘
                         └──────────────────────────┘
```

Fig 2-3. Thrombolytic therapy, Acute MI
Note: Consider immediate catheterization and PTCA if available for high risk patients.

COMPLICATIONS OF ACUTE MYOCARDIAL INFARCTION

I. **Hypotension**
   A. Causes:
      1. Vasodilatation from nitroglycerin, nifedipine, morphine.
      2. Right ventricular infarct (commonly associated with inferior wall MI).
      3. Decreased left ventricular function due to ischemia/infarct.
   B. Treatment:
      1. Consider hemodynamic monitoring with Swan-Ganz.
      2. Hold (or minimize) vasodilators.
      3. In the setting of right ventricular infarct, hypotension will generally respond to fluid bolus (250-500 cc of normal saline). Central venous pressures can be helpful in this setting.
      4. Dopamine 2-10 micrograms/kg/minute IV or dobutamine 2.5-10 micrograms/kg/minute IV.
      5. Balloon pump if available and not responding to above measures.

II. **Shock**
   A. Hypotension with decreased organ perfusion (decreased urine output, mental status changes). Treat as above for hypotension. If not responsive, consider other causes.
   B. Other causes of shock include arrhythmias, acute ventricular septal defect, papillary muscle ischemia/rupture with mitral regurgitation.
   C. Treatment consists of volume expansion, inotropes, antiarrhythmics as indicated. Consider emergent cardiac catheterization with aortic balloon pump or surgery if valvular etiology.

III. **Pulmonary Edema**
   A. Etiology: severe left ventricular dysfunction due to ischemia/ infarct, arrhythmia, valvular incompetence.

B. Treatment:
1. Increase FiO_2.
2. Elevate head.
3. Avoid exacerbating factors: beta blockers, calcium channel blockers (especially verapamil), fluid overload.
4. Nitrates sublingually.
5. Furosemide IV, dose dependent upon prior use of diuretics.
6. Morphine IV, 2-5 mg.
7. Consider dobutamine (and hemodynamic monitoring).
8. Digitalis has slow onset and is relatively ineffective in setting of MI so not indicated for acute treatment.

IV. **Arrhythmias**
  A. Ventricular tachycardia, ventricular fibrillation.
    1. Cause: reentrant arrhythmias, ventricular irritability or enhanced automaticity. Risk is highest in first 4 days following MI.
    2. Treatment: defibrillation for V-fib, lidocaine for stable V-tach. (See ACLS protocols for details.)
    3. Lidocaine prophylaxis has traditionally been recommended in setting of multiformed PVCs, triplets, R on T phenomenon, greater than 5-10 PVCs/minute. Caution should be used in the elderly as they are at increased risk of adverse effects (drowsiness, slurred speech, seizures). Also relatively contraindicated in the setting of shock, heart block, hepatic insufficiency.
  B. Bradyarrhythmmias.
    1. Cause: in setting of inferior wall MI, heart block (including high degree block) is usually due to increased parasympathetic tone. In setting of anterior wall MI, heart block is usually due to ischemic dysfunction of the Purkinje system.

2. Treatment:
   a. Heart block in setting of inferior wall MI is generally transient and responds to atropine. (Some consider the external pacer to be treatment of choice as there is no risk of inducing tachyarrhythmias as there is with atropine).
   b. Heart block in anterior wall MI may be permanent and often requires a pacemaker. Indications for pacemaker placement:

- type II second degree block.
- third degree block.
- new left bundle branch block.
- new right bundle branch block plus left anterior hemiblock or left posterior hemiblock.

CONGESTIVE HEART FAILURE

I. **Overview.** Congestive heart failure results when the heart is unable to provide adequate blood to tissues because of decreased cardiac output or increased metabolic demand. Compensatory mechanisms include increased renin, angiotensin, and aldosterone production; increased sympathetic activity. These lead to tachycardia, increased intravascular volume, and increased peripheral resistance. Hypertension is the most common contributing cause. CAD, valve disease, alcoholism are also common contributing factors.

II. **Evaluation**

   A. History: primary symptoms include fatigue, dyspnea on exertion, exercise intolerance, and orthopnea. Paroxysmal nocturnal dyspnea and nocturia may also be present. Possible precipitating causes of the acute exacerbation should be sought, including alcohol use, anemia, MI, increased salt intake.

   B. Physical exam: will generally reveal the findings consistent with fluid retention including peripheral edema, hepatojugular reflux, and crackles present in lung fields on auscultation. S3 gallop may be present.

   C. Laboratory exam: CXR will reveal congestion of the pulmonary vasculature, possibly cardiomegaly. Electrolytes, BUN/Cr, ABGs and CBC should be obtained. Digoxin levels also for those on chronic digoxin therapy.

III. **Treatment**

   A. Physical and dietary measures include bed rest with elevated legs (and usually head), salt and fluid restriction, compressive leg stockings to reduce risk of thrombosis (consider s.q. heparin).

   B. Diuretics: promote salt and fluid elimination and may have some vasodilatory effect. Overly vigorous diuresis may result in intravascular volume depletion (evidenced by tachycardia, increasing BUN, hypotension).

   1. Thiazide diuretics may be used in patients with normal renal function, but are not as effective in patients with low GFR (with the exception of metolazone).

2. Furosemide is effective even at low GFR and has vasodilatory effects. Furosemide and metolazone may be combined when inadequate diuresis occurs with furosemide alone.
3. Spironolactone has anti-aldosterone effects in addition to some diuretic effect. Hyperkalemia may result and K^+ should be monitored carefully. It may be particularly effective at mobilizing ascites.

C. Preload/afterload reducers: preload and afterload reduction can be used in CHF not completely controlled by diuretics. Cardiac output can be optimized by adjusting preload and/or afterload.

1. Nitrates primarily affect preload through venodilation. Isosorbide dinitrate is commonly used, dosed 5-20 mg p.o. q 6-8 hours. Nitrates also available sublingually, transdermally and IV.
2. Captopril, enalapril and lisinopril have been shown to reduce long term mortality of CHF. Function primarily as afterload reducers, but have some affect on preload. Initial dose should be very low and increased to a maintenance dose equivalent to captopril 12.5 - 25 mg q 8 hours.
3. Minoxidil and hydralazine primarily affect afterload through arterial dilatation. Both can cause hypotension, tachycardia, worsening of angina. Dose is hydralazine 50-100 mg q 6 hours, minoxidil 10-20mg q 12 hours.
4. Prazosin reduces both afterload and preload. Tends to reduce GFR which may result in tolerance to its effects. Dose is 1 mg initially at bedtime, increased as needed to 2-10 mg q 6 hours. Effective and relatively low toxicity.
5. Nifedipine is effective at reducing afterload, but its negative inotropic effects may actually cause decreased cardiac output. Most likely to occur in patients with severe CHF or hyponatremia. Dose is 10-30 mg q 6-8 hours.

D. Inotropic agents:
1. Digitalis: positive inotrope, can result in increased cardiac output and reflex fall in peripheral resistance.

Most effective in CHF due to HTN, valve disease, CAD (especially if atrial fibrillation is present). Not as effective in sinus rhythm. Effects are not immediate and it is not useful for acute treatment of pulmonary edema. Should not be used in patients with IHSS. Maintenance dose should be adjusted for renal function. Levels should be followed and checked after changes in dose or in other medications. See Formulary for dose recommendation.

2. Dobutamine is the parenteral inotropic agent of choice for acute severe CHF. Dose is 2 micrograms/kg/minute. Onset of effects is immediate and stop quickly with discontinuation of the infusion. Should not be used in patients with IHSS. May cause tachycardia, angina, ventricular arrhythmias.

IV. **Chronic Therapy**

A. Should include education regarding the importance of compliance with medications and dietary restrictions. Patients should be cautioned against exerting themselves in hot, humid weather. NSAIDs should be avoided, including OTC preparations.

B. Medical therapy should be minimized and will generally include diuretics. ACE inhibitors should be added when additional measures are required because of their proven benefit in terms of mortality. Digoxin is commonly used but should not be added until diuretics and perhaps ACE inhibitors have proven to be inadequate alone.

HYPERTENSION

I. **Overview.** Blood pressure is determined by a complex set of interrelated factors including the sympathetic nervous system, extracellular fluid volume, sodium balance, renin-angiotension mechanism, mineralocorticoids. These factors affect cardiac output and peripheral vascular resistance, which directly determine arterial blood pressure. The level above which blood pressure adversely affects morbidity varies with age. However, it has been demonstrated that adults with diastolic blood pressure above 90 mmHg will have reduced morbidity due to blood pressure if it is treated.

II. **Causes**
   A. Essential hypertension is the most common cause of hypertension. For all age groups with the exception of young children, it is the most common cause. The etiology of essential hypertension is not understood, but probably lies within the complex network of interrelated factors listed above.
   B. Secondary hypertension is the result of some identifiable pathological process, usually related to renal physiology. Causes of secondary hypertension include renal artery stenosis, renal parenchymal disease (glomerulonephritis, diabetic nephropathy, polycystic disease, obstructive uropathy), drugs (oral contraceptives, steroids), increased levels of catecholamines (pheochromocytoma), glucocorticoids (Cushing's), or mineralocorticoids.

III. **Evaluation**
   A. Initial evaluation of the patient with newly detected mild to moderately elevated blood pressure should include the following:
      1. Thorough history regarding diabetes, HTN, and cardiovascular disease in the family, personal history of cardiovascular symptoms, drug and alcohol use, level of physical activity, diet.
      2. Physical examination to include weight, fundiscopic exam for evidence of prolonged blood pressure

elevation, cardiac exam to estimate heart size, sounds and murmurs, auscultation of abdomen and neck for bruits, and palpation of kidneys.
3. Laboratory evaluation may be postponed until follow-up visits have determined the presence of HTN.
4. Recommend salt restriction, increased exercise, weight reduction if indicated, and follow-up in 2 to 4 weeks for blood pressure recheck.

B. Evaluation of the patient with documented blood pressure elevation on at least two or three office visits (i.e., diagnosis of HTN), should include:
1. Urine analysis and serum creatinine to evaluate for renal disease, EKG and CXR to establish baseline and detect evidence of end-organ damage, cholesterol and triglycerides to evaluate other risk factors, electrolytes and uric acid as baseline for determining appropriate medications, and serum glucose to evaluate for diabetes.
2. Other tests may be indicated by physical exam or laboratory results that suggest a cause of secondary hypertension. IVP, renal arteriography, urine for catecholamines. Routine use of these studies is not indicated unless additional factors indicate the presence of secondary cause.

IV. Treatment:

A. Education: All patients with HTN should be counseled regarding the nature of the disorder and the importance of long-term compliance with treatment regimen. Home blood pressure monitoring should be taught.

B. Life-style interventions: Exercise, salt restriction, and weight reduction as indicated are appropriate for all patients with HTN.

C. Medications: Numerous medications are available for pharmacologic treatment of HTN. The widely varying side-effects, costs, and dosing schedules allow tailoring of the medications to the particulars of each case. Pharmacologic intervention is indicated in the mild to moderately hypertensive individual when the above measures have not produced adequate control. A stepped care regimen has been advocated as the most appropriate approach to pharmacologic intervention because it begins with the least toxic medications and adds additional meds with different mechanisms of action, thereby allowing lower total doses of more potent agents. Some studies have suggested, however, that monotherapy with more potent agents may be as or more effective in preventing the cardiac sequelae of HTN.

1. Diuretics: thiazide diuretics, effective alone and useful in offsetting the fluid retention caused by other agents. Loop diuretics are more effective in patients with impaired renal function. Examples of thiazides are hydrochlorothiazide and chlorothiazide. Advantages: safe, inexpensive. Disadvantages: may result in hypokalemia, impair glucose tolerance, increase uric acid levels and contribute to gout, increase plasma lipids.

2. Beta blockers: reduce cardiac output (negative inotropic and chronotropic effect), may reduce peripheral resistance. Also used to treat angina, arrhythmias, and prophylaxis against migraines. Generally felt to be most effective in younger patients with "hyperdynamic" cardiovascular system as evidenced by elevated resting pulse (high normal or tachycardic) and excessive response of blood pressure to exercise. Advantages: many are relatively inexpensive, effective. Disadvantages: contraindicated in CHF, may cause significant bradycardia or A-V block, sedation, fatigue, bronchospasm in patients with asthma, erectile dysfunction, impaired glucose tolerance, possibly elevated uric acid and plasma lipids.

3. Central sympatholytics: includes methyldopa, clonidine, guanabenz and guanfacine. Sedation, fatigue may occur.

4. Alpha-receptor blockers: prazosin and terazosin. Severe orthostatic hypotension may occur with first dose. Fluid retention is commonly seen. Sedation and headache are commonly seen early, tend to diminish. May be of some benefit in CHF.

Hypertension

5. Arterial vasodilators: hydralazine and minoxidil. Both are potent vasodilators and may cause reflex tachycardia and fluid retention. Should be used only in conjunction with diuretic and sympathetic inhibitor (such as a beta blocker). Should not be used in patients with angina. Minoxidil usually reserved for severe hypertension. Lupus-like syndrome has been seen with hydralazine.
6. Calcium channel blockers: verapamil and diltiazem, and nicardipine are approved for use in HTN. Nifedipine is also effective in lowering BP and has been used for acute treatment of HTN, but its short-lived effects do not lend themselves to long-term treatment. Verapamil and diltiazem are available in sustained-release preparations for convenience. Both have some negative inotropic effects (especially verapamil) and peripheral vasodilatory effects. Neither will adversely affect glucose tolerance, plasma lipids. Both are relatively expensive but may be used as single agent.
7. ACE inhibitors (angiotensin-converting enzyme): captropril, enalapril, and lisinopril. All are effective for HTN and have been used in CHF. Captopril requires more frequent dosing. All may contribute to hyperkalemia, decreased renal function. Side-effects tend to be minimal with no significant sedation, fatigue, or exercise intolerance. Are relatively expensive but may be used as single agent.

D. Follow-up: Initially patients should be scheduled for frequent office visits until pressure is adequately controlled and potential side-effects evaluated. Thereafter, visits may be scheduled every 3 to 6 months. Laboratory evaluation should include those indicated by the medications they are using (such as K^+ level for those on diuretics).

SYNCOPE

I. Definition

A. Syncope is a sudden, brief loss of consciousness (LOC), and strictly speaking, is related to abrupt cerebral hypoperfusion.

B. Near syncope, a sense of impending LOC or weakness, occurs more frequently and provides valuable diagnostic clues since the patient usually has better recollection of the event.

C. Frequency of causes: 65% hypotension, 10% cardiac, 10% neurological, 5% metabolic, 10% unknown causes.

II. Causes of Syncope/Near Syncope

A. Cardiac/Circulatory.

1. Vasodepressor Syncope (vasovagal syncope)- MOST COMMON CAUSE. Occurs when susceptible persons are confronted with a stressful situation. Prodromal symptoms: restlessness, pallor, weakness, sighing, yawning, diaphoresis, nausea. Followed by lightheadedness, blurred vision, collapse and LOC. Occasionally mild clonic movements occur. Spells are brief in duration.

2. Orthostatic Hypotension - fall in BP with assuming upright position. Seen in a variety of settings:

   a. Hypovolemia (hemorrhage, vomiting, diarrhea, diuretics).

   b. Interference with normal reflexes (nitrates, vasodilators, calcium channel blockers, neuroleptics).

   c. Autonomic failure. Primary or secondary. Diabetes most common cause of secondary autonomic neuropathy.

   d. Venous pooling-late pregnancy, prolonged, immobile standing.

3. Outflow Obstruction-IHSS or aortic stenosis usually present with exertional syncope. Mechanical valve malfunction may also cause outflow obstruction.

4. Myocardial ischemia/infarction.

5. Arrhythmias.
    a. Bradyarrhythmias--sick sinus syndrome, A-V blocks, etc.
    b. Tachyarrhythmias--PSVT, Wolf Parkinson White, V Tach, etc.
6. Hypersensitive Carotid Sinus Reflex. May occur with shaving, wearing of a tight neck shirt.

B. Metabolic Causes. Episodes usually amplified by exertion, may occur while supine, onset and resolution usually prolonged.
   1. Hypoxia--such as shunting in congenital heart disease.
   2. Hyperventilation (hypocapnia). Results in cerebral vasoconstriction with symptoms of breathlessness, anxiety, circumoral tingling, parasthesias of hands/feet, carpopedal spasm.
   3. Hypoglycemia.
   4. Alcohol intoxication.

C. Neurological.
   1. Migraine. Second most common cause in adolescents. LOC is followed by headache.
   2. Seizure. Usually easily differentiated by aura, history of tonic/clonic movements, and post-ictal state.
   3. TIA/Drop Attacks.
   4. Abrupt rise of intracranial pressure.

D. Miscellaneous.
   1. Cough Syncope.
   2. Post Micturition Syncope.
   3. Hysteria.

III. Evaluation.

A. History. Most important part of evaluation. Witnesses, if available, should be interviewed:
   1. Precipitating circumstances?
   2. Prodromal symptoms?
   3. Time course of onset and recovery?
   4. Medication history.

5. Medical and family history.
- B. Physical Exam.
    1. BP and pulse supine and standing.
    2. Auscultation of subclavian and carotid arteries.
    3. Cardiac exam with attention to murmurs, extra heart sounds. Provocative maneuvers (Valsalva) as indicated.
    4. Careful neurological exam.
- C. Laboratory Studies. Should be directed by history and physical exam, not all inclusive! May include blood glucose, blood gases, electrolytes.
- D. EKG/Holter Ambulatory Monitoring
- E. Echocardiography. Useful in evaluating valvular and myocardial disease.
- F. EEG. Obtain if seizure disorder is suspected; however, may be falsely negative in 50% of cases. Nasopharyngeal leads, sleep deprivation, and hyperventilation may all increase yield.

IV. **Treatment**. Dependent on etiology.
- A. No Treatment--for vasodepressor syncope, cough syncope.
- B. Medical--antiepileptics, antiarrhythmics, mineralocorticoids (for chronic orthostatic hypotension), migraine prophylaxis.
- C. Surgical--for critical aortic stenosis, carotid artery disease, etc.

EVALUATION OF HEART SOUNDS AND MURMURS

I. **Heart Sounds:**

   A. S_1: produced by closure of the mitral and tricuspid valves and the associated change in blood flow in the ventricle. Generally is lower pitched than S_2 and of lesser intensity when auscultated at the base of the heart. Intensity of S_1 will vary in atrial fibrillation or with PVCs. The first heart sound may be slit, with two distinct components, in right bundle branch block, where delayed contraction of the right ventricle results in delayed closure of the tricuspid valve.

   B. S_2: Produced by closure of the aortic and pulmonic valves. Greatest intensity is heard at the base of the heart. S_2 is commonly split during inspiration, heard best at the pulmonic region. A widely split S_2 will occur with RBBB, pulmonary hypertension, or right ventricular volume overload. Paradoxical splitting, where splitting decreases or disappears with inspiration, is caused by delayed closure of the aortic valve due to LBBB, aortic stenosis, PDA.

   C. S_3: occurs shortly after S_2, is low pitched and heard best with bell at apex. May be heard in children and young adults and is called physiologic S_3. In older adults, S_3 is not normal and indicates volume overload of the left ventricle or myocardial dysfunction.

   D. S_4: occurs right before S_1, is low pitched and heard best at apex with bell. Result from increased compliance of the left ventricle (HTN) or from increased volume of filling in the left ventricle. Does not imply the presence of cardiac failure.

   E. Systolic sounds: ejection sounds (early) or clicks (late) may be heard during systole. The most common is a mid to late systolic click heard with mitral valve prolapse. Ejection sounds are heard in early systole at the time of the opening of the aortic and pulmonic valves. May indicate stenotic but mobile valve, aneurysm or coarctation of the aorta, hypertension (systemic and pulmonary).

II. Murmurs

A. Grading of murmurs:
   1. softest murmur, heard only in quiet conditions by careful and skilled auscultation.
   2. slightly louder, heard consistently by all examiners, heard immediately.
   3. intermediate intensity, no associated thrill.
   4. loud murmur with palpable thrill.
   5. loud murmur, heard with edge of stethoscope tipped off the skin.
   6. very loud murmur, heard with stethoscope lifted off the chest wall.

B. Systolic ejection murmurs: characterized by onset after S_1, cessation before S_2.
   1. Innocent: common. Seen in many normal children and young adults. Characterized by low intensity, grade 1 or 2/6, variable intensity (quieter while sitting than lying, quieter with inspiration). S_1 and S_2 are normal and there are no associated systolic ejection sounds or clicks. May be musical, does not radiate. If other findings are present (widely split S_2, diastolic murmur, ejection click), then CXR, EKG and echocardiogram are indicated.
   2. Functional: common. Seen in older patients, believed due to thickening and sclerosis of the aortic valve and aorta. Usually not associated with other abnormal cardiac sounds. Evaluation should include CXR, EKG and echocardiogram if there is evidence of hemodynamic compromise, or associated abnormal heart sounds.
   3. Pathologic: may be seen with aortic stenosis, pulmonic stenosis. Aortic stenosis heard best at base and commonly radiates into the neck. Classically crescendo-decrescendo. Altered heart sounds, such as an early systolic ejection sound, or diastolic murmur are often present and indicate need for evaluation. LVH on EKG is commonly present. Echocardiogram will accurately diagnose the presence of pathology but cardiac catheterization may be required to ac-

curately determine the hemodynamic significance of the stenosis.

C. Systolic regurgitant murmurs: characterized by onset with the first heart sound and cessation with or after S2. Mitral insufficiency, tricuspid insufficiency, and ventricular septal defect are causes. Mitral insufficiency is characterized as blowing, apical. Symptoms may include palpitations, fatigue, dyspnea on exertion. Murmur increases in intensity with sustained hand grip or squatting, decreases with deep inspiration, valsalva. Mitral valve prolapse will increase with standing and valsalva, decrease with squatting. Echocardiogram is indicated for physical findings suggesting hemodynamic compromise or mitral regurgitation.

D. Regurgitant diastolic murmurs:
  1. Aortic regurgitation can be produced by dissecting aortic aneurysm and should be suspected if sudden onset. Typically murmur is early diastolic, high pitched, decrescendo heard best along left sternal border. Volume overload of the left ventricle will occur with moderate to severe regurgitation and result in cardiomegaly from dilatation of the ventricle. Widened pulse pressure is often present. Early evaluation with EKG, CXR and echocardiogram is indicated and if regurgitation is found a cardiologist should be consulted. Ideally the valve is replaced before significant cardiac compromise occurs.
  2. Pulmonic regurgitation may be secondary to pulmonic hypertension and can produce a murmur similar to that of aortic regurgitation. However, it tends to be softer, not associated with widened pulse pressure or signs of left ventricular enlargement. If due to pulmonary hypertension, secondary to mitral valve disease, replacement of the mitral valve should be accompanied by replacement of the pulmonic valve.

E. Diastolic flow murmurs:
  1. Mitral stenosis: may be due to rheumatic heart disease. Stenosis can produce pulmonary hypertension and RVH. Symptoms may include dyspnea on exer-

tion, fatigue, palpitations. Murmur is diastolic, low pitched, often with opening snap. Heard best at apex. EKG and CXR are normal with mild to moderate disease, but will show right axis deviation and RVH, with evidence of left atrial enlargement as the disease progresses. Atrial fibrillation is related to the degree of dilatation of the left atrium.

2. Other causes of diastolic flow murmurs include ASD, VSD, and tricuspid stenosis. Echocardiogram will establish the cause.

III. **Maneuvers to Differentiate Murmurs**: (Table 2-3)

Maneuver	AS	IHSS	MR	MVP
isometric	↓	↓	↑	-
valsalva	↓	↑	↓	↑
squatting	-	↓	↑	↓
standing	↑	↑	↓	↑

Adapted from: Driscoll CE, et al, eds. Handbook of Family Practice. Chicago: Year Book Medical Publishers, 1986.

DYSLIPIDEMIAS

The dyslipidemias represent a heterogeneous group of lipid disorders manifest with various elevations of serum cholesterol (chol), in its various forms, triglycerides (TG), and chylomicrons.

I. **Introduction**
   A. Many of the dyslipidemias are associated with atherosclerotic vasculature disease and coronary artery disease, the leading causes of death in industrialized Western nations.
   B. Coronary artery disease risk varies on a continuum by five-fold over the range of cholesterol.
   C. Lipid hypothesis--favorable alteration of plasma lipoproteins can reduce atherosclerotic vasculature disease risk.

II. **Lipid Metabolism.**
   A. Five principle classes of lipoproteins: 1. chylomicrons, 2. very low density lipoproteins (VLDL), 3. intermediate density lipoproteins (IDL), 4. low density lipoproteins (LDL), 5. high density lipoproteins (HDL). #'s 1 and 2 are rich in TG, #'s 4 and 5 are rich in chol.
   B. Dietary fat is transported in blood as chylomicrons, endogenous (hepatic) TG as VLDL.
   C. Chylomicrons and VLDL are converted to IDL by lipoprotein lipase in various tissues.
   D. IDL is metabolized in the liver to LDL which is taken up by tissue or secreted in the bile. LDL is ATHEROGENIC.
   E. HDL can be formed from any of the other lipoproteins, is responsible for transport of chol. from tissues to the liver for catabolism or excretion. Serves a protective function.

III. **Classification.**
   A. May be grouped on the basis of phenotype, based on serum lipid concentrations and electrophoretic patterns, genotype, or by pathophysiology (see Table 2-4).

Table 2-4. Classification of Lipoprotein Disorders by Phenotypes and Genotypes and Corresponding Clinical Manifestations

Phenotype	Plasma Lipid Levels Cholesterol/Triglyceride	Lipoprotein in Excess	Genotype	Xanthomas	Other Clinical Manifestations
I	Normal or ↑ / ↑ Lipemia	Chylomicrons	Familial lipoprotein lipase deficiency, Apo C-II deficiency	Eruptive, tuberoeruptive	Recurrent abdominal pain, other gastrointestinal symptoms, hepatosplenomegaly
IIA	Normal	LDL	Familial hypercholesterolemia Familial combined hyperlipidemia, Polygenic and sporadic hypercholesterolemia	Tendinous, xanthelasma, tuberous; planar (homozygous)	Premature CAD, arcus corneae, aortic stenosis (homozygous FHC), arthritic symptoms
IIB	↑ / ↑	LDL + VLDL	Familial combined hyperlipidemia, familial hypercholesterolemia		
III	↑ / ↑	VLDL, IDL	Familial dysbetalipoproteinemia	Planar (especially palmar), tuberous	Premature CAD and peripheral vascular disease, male > female, obesity, abnormal glucose tolerance, hyperuricemia, aggravated by hypothyroidism, good response to therapy
IV	Normal or ↑ / ↑	VLDL	Familial hypertriglyceridemia, familial combined hyperlipidemia, sporadic hypertriglyceridemia	Usually none; rarely eruptive, or tuberoeruptive	CAD and peripheral vascular disease, obesity, abnormal glucose tolerance, hyperuricemia, arthritic symptoms, gallbladder disease
V	Normal or ↑ / ↑	Chylomicrons + VLDL	Homozygous familial hypertriglyceridemia	Eruptive, tuberoeruptive	Recurrent abdominal pain, other gastrointestinal symptoms, hepatosplenomegaly, peripheral pares

B. May also be classified as primary or secondary.
C. Secondary causes include:
  1. Endogenous - alcohol, oral contraceptives, estrogens, androgens, corticosteroids, diuretics (thiazides), beta blockers, obesity, high cholesterol diet.
  2. Endocrine/Metabolic - diabetes, hypothyroidism, Cushing's or Addison's diseases, hepatic disease, nephrotic syndrome.
  3. Miscellaneous - pregnancy, pancreatitis, SLE.

IV. Evaluation and Initial Therapy.

A. Initial Classification Based on Total Cholesterol.
   - < 200 desirable, repeat every five years.
   - 200-240 borderline.
   - 240 high
B. If on repeat testing chol > 240 OR 200-240 and CHD or two CHD risk factors from the following: 1. male sex, 2. FHx of premature CHD, 3. smoker, 4. hypertension, 5. HDL < 35, 6. diabetes, 7. obesity, 8. history of cerebral or peripheral vasculature disease, THEN obtain full lipid profile after a 12-14 hour fast.
C. If total chol borderline and < 2 risk factors, initiate Step I diet.
D. Classify other than IV c above on the basis of LDL. Calculate LDL:
   - LDL = Total Chol - TG/5 - HDL.
   - < 130 desirable, repeat every five years.
   - 130-160 and no CHD or < 2 risk factors, Step I diet.
   - 130-160 and CHD or > 2 risk factors, treat as high LDL (> 160).
E. If high LDL, evaluate for secondary causes. If none identified, set goal of LDL < 160 (total chol < 240) if no CHD or < 2 risk factors; OR LDL < 130 (total chol < 200) if CHD or > 2 risk factors.
  1. Initiate Step I diet:
     a. Reduce total fat to < 30%, saturated fat to < 10% calories.
     b. Reduce chol to < 300 mg/day.

2. Check chol in 6 weeks and 3 months. If no improvement, refer to dietitian for retrial of Step I diet, or advance to Step II diet:
   a. Reduce saturated fat to < 7%.
   b. Reduce chol to < 200 mg/day.
3. Exercise, weight loss, smoking cessation should also be part of program.
4. Administer above for a minimum of 6 month trial. If no improvement, consider pharmacologic therapy.

F. Consideration for pharmacologic intervention.
   1. LDL 160-190 and no CHD or < 2 risk factors--maximize nonpharmacologic therapy and repeat lipid profile every year.
   2. LDL > 190; OR 160-190 and CHD or > 2 risk factors--begin drug therapy and recheck profile in 6 weeks and 3 months. If goal not achieved, change drug or add second agent.

G. Increased Triglycerides.
   1. Must evaluate for increased cholesterol as well.
   2. TG < 250--no treatment needed.
   3. TG 250-500--weight loss, low fat diet (<10% fat), exercise, smoking cessation, reduced alcohol consumption.
   4. TG > 500--risk of pancreatitis. If TG remains >500 after management as per G 3, consider pharmacologic therapy.

V. Pharmacologic Therapy.

A. Hypercholesterolemia--first line therapy includes the use of cholestyramine or niacin.
   1. Cholestyramine: bile acid binding resin which decreases LDL by 20-40%. Start at 4 gm BID, increase to 16-24 gms/day. Side effects: GI--bloating, constipation, unpalatable and gritty.
   2. Niacin: decreases hepatic VLDL production leading to decreased LDL. Decreases LDL by 20% and VLDL by 40%. Increases HDL by 20-30%. Start at 100 mg BID-TID, increase to 3 gms/day divided TID. Flushing is common and can be reduced with aspirin,

325 mg every AM or with the use of sustained release niacin. Side effects: increased liver function tests, glucose, uric acid.

B. Hypercholestolemia--Second line agents include lovastatin and gemfibrozil.

1. Lovastatin: HMG-CoA reductase inhibitor (decreases hepatic chol synthesis). Decreases LDL by 40%. May see slight decrease in VLDL and slight increase in HDL. Start at 20 mg daily and increase to 20-40 mg BID. Side effects: increased liver function tests, myositis.

2. Gemfibrozil: complex pharmacology. Decreases LDL 10-20%, Dose as 600 mg BID. Side effects: myositis, cholesterol gallstones, GI upset, leukopenia, impotence.

C. Hypertrilglyceridemia, isolated.

1. Niacin is drug of choice.

2. Gemfibrozil also good choice.

D. Combined dyslipidemia (increased VLDL and LDL).

1. Niacin is drug of choice.

2. Combination resin and gemfibrozil.

References

Barker LR, Burton JR, and Zieve PD, eds. <u>Principles of Ambulatory Medicine, 2nd edition</u>. Baltimore: Williams & Wilkins, 1986.

Driscoll CE, *et al*, eds. <u>Handbook of Family Practice</u>. Chicago: Year Book Medical Publishers, 1986.

Holvey DN and Talbott JH, eds. <u>The Merck Manual of Diagnosis and Therapy, 12th edition</u>. New Jersey: Merck & Company, Inc., 1972.

Orland M, *et al*, eds. <u>Manual of Medical Therapeutics, 25th edition</u>. Boston:Little Brown and Company, 1986.

Rakel RE and Conn HF, eds. <u>Textbook of Family Practice, Third edition</u>. Philadelphia: W.B. Saunders Company, 1984.

3/ PULMONARY MEDICINE

Shelley A. Breyen, M.D.

PULMONARY FUNCTION TESTS

I. **Lung Volumes and Capacities**
   A. Diagram (Fig 3-1).

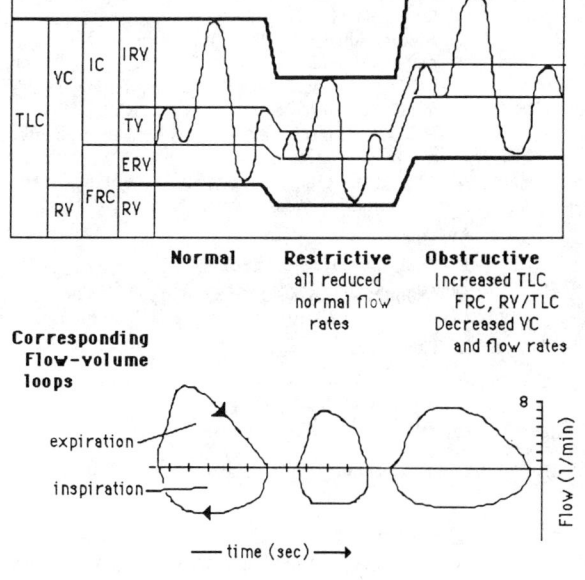

Fig 3-1. Pulmonary function tests

- Normal: values may vary +/- 20% predicted, values will change with position, age, sex, height, and altitude.
- Restrictive: most all volumes are proportionately decreased, flow rates are normal.

- Obstructive: Increase in TLC, FRC, RV/TLC, decrease in VC, flow rates.

B. Definitions.
- TV: Tidal Volume, volume inspired and expired during normal respirations.
- IRV: Inspiratory Reserve Volume, volume inspired in addition to normal inspiratory volume.
- IC: Inspiratory Capacity, maximum volume inspired from normal expiratory level (IRV + TV).
- ERV: Expiratory Reserve Volume, maximum volume expired from the end of a resting expiration (app. 25% of VC).
- RV: Residual Volume, volume in lungs after maximal expiration.
- FRC: Functional Residual Capacity, volume in lungs at normal expiratory level (ERV + RV).
- VC: Vital Capacity, maximum volume expired after maximal inspiration.
- TLC: Total Lung Capacity, volume in lungs at the end of maximum inspiration.

C. Average Values.
1. Vital Capacity (predicted).
- Women = (21.78 -[0.101 x age in years]) x ht in cm.
- Men = (27.63 -[0.112 x age in years]) x ht in cm.
2. Tidal Volume.
- Child: 7.5 ml/kg.
- Adult female: 6.6 ml/kg.
- Adult male: 7.8 ml/kg.

II. Pulmonary Mechanics (Spirometry)

A. Diagram (Fig 3-2).
B. Definitions.
- FVC: Forced Vital Capacity, maximum volume gas expired forcefully after maximum inspiration.
- FEV 1 : Forced Expired Volume, volume of gas expired at one second during a FVC maneuver.

III. Interpretations

A. Patterns of Abnormal Pulmonary Function Tests.

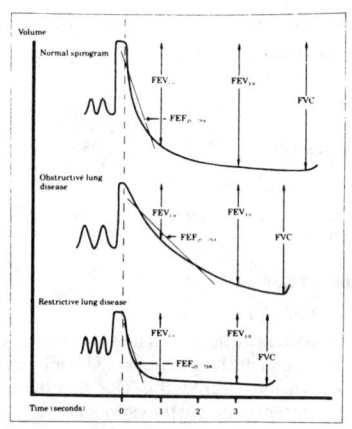

Fig 3-2. Spirometry

1. Obstructive Disorders: emphysema, chronic bronchitis, asthma.
2. Restrictive Disorders:
    a. Interstitial Lung Disorders: sarcoidosis, environmental disease, interstitial pneumonias, connective tissue disorders, pulmonary vascular diseases.
    b. Bellows Disorders: obesity, kyphoscoliosis, post-surgery, paralysis, ascites, pleuritis, pleural effusion. (Table 3-1)

Table 3-1.

PFT/ Lung Volumes	Obstructive	Restrictive/ Interstitial	Bellows
VC	N-D	DD	D
RV	I	DD	N-I
TLC	N-II	DD	D
mechanics			
FVC	D	DD	D
FEV 1	D	N-D	N-D

N = normal, D = decreased, DD = markedly decreased, I = increased, II = markedly increased

B. Assessment of Severity of Obstructive and Restrictive Diseases (Table 3-2).

Table 3-2.

Obstructive Diseases	Mild	Moderate	Severe
VC (%pred)	70-80%	50-70%	<50%
FEV 1/FVC (% pred)	65-80%	50-65%	<50%
RV/TLC	0.3-0.45	0.45-0.6	>0.6
Restrictive Diseases			
VC (% pred)	65-80%	50-65%	<50%
TLC (% pred)	70-80%	50-70%	<50%

IV. Ventilation/Perfusion Tests

A. Ventilation (V) Studies.

Radioexenon Lung Scan: determines how rapidly and evenly gas is distributed in the lungs. Xenon 133 is mixed with air and inhaled via closed spirometry. The scintillation camera records the concentrations at the various periods listed below.

1. Single breath scan: initial breath taken to total vital capacity.
2. Wash-in phase: tidal breathing.
3. Equilibration phase: the concentration of radioactivity is equilibrized between patient's lung and the spirometer.
4. Wash-out phase: the patient resumes breathing room air. The recordings made late in this phase are the most sensitive for detecting ventilation abnormalities.

B. Perfusion (Q) Studies.

1. Perfusion Scintiphotography: reveals area(s) of absent or diminished perfusion. Technetium 99 is labeled to macroaggregated albumin and injected. The microspheres lodge in approximately 0.1% of the pulmonary capillaries. Scintiphotography records their distribution. Areas of decreased uptake correlate with hypoperfusion (a normal Q scan rules out pulmonary emboli, a high probability scan for pulmonary emboli must have segmental or multiple subsegmental defects). The microspheres disintegrate and are cleared within eight hours.

2. Pulmonary Angiography: provides a qualitative analysis of lung perfusion, only perfused vessels are imaged. It is the gold standard for diagnosing pulmonary embolus. However, multiple microemboli may be missed.
C. Interpretation.
 1. Mismatched Defects (decrease in Q with normal V). Pulmonary emboli, vasculitis, unilateral agenesis of a pulmonary artery.
 2. Matched Defects (decreased Q and decreased V). Pulmonary parenchymal disease: pneumonia, COPD (may see delayed clearance in washout phase), asthma.

VENTILATORS AND OXYGEN THERAPY

I. **Overview**

   Respiratory failure results from failure of the lung to provide adequate gas exchange or the failure of the heart to adequately supply blood to be oxygenated. Acute respiratory failure is a medical emergency requiring prompt diagnosis and management and should be suspected when a patient breathing room air has a PO_2 < 60 mm Hg or a PCO_2 > 50 mm Hg with a pH < 7.3.

II. **Oxygen Therapy**

   A. Oxygen delivery systems (Table 3-3).

   B. Complications of oxygen therapy.

   1. Pulmonary oxygen toxicity including: mucosal drying, mucociliary dysfunction, atelectasis, interstitial and alveolar edema, and alveolar hemorrhage.

   2. Carbon dioxide retention in patients with chronic hypoxemia and altered respiratory regulation resulting in a decreased respiratory drive.

   3. Retrolental fibroplasia in neonates of low birth weight or gestational age < 34 weeks.

   4. Bronchopulmonary dysplasia in infants who required mechanical ventilation after birth.

   5. Risk of fire and explosion.

III. **Ventilators**

   A. Indications: Apnea, respiratory failure or impending respiratory failure, inadequate oxygenation.

   B. Intubation (see Airway Management).

   C. Modes of mechanical ventilation.

   1. Controlled Ventilation. The ventilator is initiating all breaths at a preselected rate and volume. There are few indications for this use.

   2. Assist-Control (AC). A minimum rate and volume is delivered by the machine. Each of the patient's spontaneous breaths are assisted with the selected volume by the ventilator. This mode allows the patient to adjust to changing metabolic status. It is the mode most

Ventilators and Oxygen Therapy

Table 3-3. Oxygen Delivery Systems

Type	Liter Flow	%O_2 Delivered	Comments
Low Flow System - does not meet total patient O_2 demand			
1. Nasal Cannula	1-8 L/min	25-50%	1. Delivers approximately 4%/L, however true FIO_2 uncertain 2. Comfortable, but limited to low flow rate <4 L/min 3. Nasal mucosa drying common
2. Simple Mask	5-8 L/min	40-50%	1. Delivers approximately 4%/L 2. Less comfortable, hot, skin irritation 3. Not low enough FIO_2 for COPD 4. O_2 rates must be at least 5 L/min to clear CO_2 5. Offers little over nasal cannula
3. Reservoir Masks			
a. Non-rebreathing	6-10 L/min	70-100%	1. High FIO_2 delivered; reservoir fills during expiration which provides increased volume of O_2 2. Flow must be sufficient to keep reservoir bag from deflating upon inspiration
b. Partial rebreathing	6-10 L/min	55-70%	
High Flow System-meets total inspirational demand of patient			
1. Venturi Mask	variable	24-50%	1. Exact FIO_2 can be delivered 2. Poor humidification 3. Uncomfortable
2. Nebulizer with:			
a. aerosol mask, face tent	0-12 L/min	30-100%	1. Used to deliver precise FIO_2 and/or aerosol 2. Can provide con-

Table 3-3 (continued)

Type	Liter Flow	%O$_2$ Delivered	Comments
			trolled temperture of gas 3. May need 2-3 setups to meet inspirational flows for FIO$_2$ > .5 4. Aerosol may induce bronchospasm, fluid overload, overmobilization of secretions or contamination.
b. T-tube	0-12 L/min	30-100%	1. For spontaneous breathing through endotracheal tube 2. Flow rates should be 2-3 times minute ventilation

commonly used.

    3. Intermittent Mandatory Ventilation (IMV). The patient's spontaneous breathing is combined with ventilator breaths. Ventilator breaths are either intermittent (IMV) or synchronized (SIMV) to the patient's spontaneous breaths. This can be used as a weaning method, allowing the patient to gradually assume more of the work of breathing.

    4. Continuous Positive Airway Pressure (CPAP). The ventilator supplies a continuous source of positive airway pressure and oxygen. The patient ventilates on his own.

D. Ventilator Management.

    1. Minute ventilation. This is the product of tidal volume and rate. Generally it is approximately 5-10 l/min or 100 ml/kg/min.

    2. Tidal volume (Vt). Initial volume is 10-12 cc/kg. A large Vt improves gas exchange and prevents atelectasis. However, it may decrease venous return which may require a smaller volume with PEEP.

3. Rate. After choosing Vt, rate can be determined by: Rate = Minute Ventilation/Tidal Volume. Generally a slower rate and larger tidal volume will reduce intrathoracic pressures and improve compliance.

4. FIO_2. The goal is to maintain PO_2 60-100 mm Hg (50-60 in COPDer's) with an FIO_2 < 0.6, as toxicity is seen earlier when the FIO_2 > 0.6. Start with a high FIO_2 and adjust in 5-10% increments approximately every 30 minutes following ABGs.

5. Positive End Expiratory Pressure (PEEP). It increases compliance, FRC and PO_2; it decreases the work of breathing, atelectasis and shunting. It is usually begun at 3-5 cm H_2O and increased in small increments. High levels, >8 cm H_2O may result in decreased venous return, overventilation and barotrauma. Cardiac output should be measured with each increment of PEEP over 10 cm H_2O.

6. Peak airway pressure. This reflects the pressure required to overcome airway resistance and is the peak pressure during the inspiratory cycle. The alarm limit should be set 10 cm H_2O above this. If the peak airway pressure increases, you need to consider obstruction in the tube, bronchospasm or decreased lung compliance.

7. Sedation and neuromuscular paralysis.

    a. Sedation allows better patient compliance with the ventilator, rest and anxiety control. Initial therapy includes: midazolam 1-2 mg IV titrating up in 1 mg increments, or diazepam in similar dosages. Dosages should be titrated to desired affect monitoring hemodynamic and respiratory status.

    b. Neuromuscular paralysis is occasionally necessary if sedation fails. Monitoring alarms must be functioning as ventilator malfunction is rapidly fatal. Short term paralysis (3-7 minutes) can be achieved with succinylcholine 1 mg/kg IV. For long-term paralysis use pancuronium bromide. Initial dose 0.08 mg/kg IV, followed by maintenance dose 0.01-0.04 mg/kg IV as needed. Tachycardia may follow the use of pancuronium.

If necessary a neostigmine-atropine combination can be used to reverse its effects. Sedation should be provided for paralyzed patients.

E. Withdrawal of mechanical ventilation.
   1. Guidelines for withdrawal of mechanical ventilation.
      a. An awake alert patient.
      b. $PO_2 > 60$ mm Hg, with an $FIO_2 < 0.5$.
      c. PEEP < 5 cm H_2O.
      d. PCO_2 acceptable, with pH in the normal range.
      e. Vital capacity > 10 ml/kg.
      f. Minute ventilation < 10 l/min, respiratory rate < 25/min.
      g. Patient is able to generate maximum voluntary ventilation more than twice minute ventilation.
      h. Patient is able to generate a peak negative inspiratory pressure less than 25 cm H_2O.
   2. Weaning from the ventilator.
      a. Explain to the patient and encourage cooperation.
      b. Begin during the daytime, allow the patient to rest at night.
      c. Place patient in upright position.
      d. Discontinue weaning if:
   - pH < 7.3, $PCO_2 > 55$ mm Hg, $PO_2 < 60$ mm H.g
   - Heart rate > 120 or < 60 or increases > 20 beats/min.
   - Blood pressure changes by 20 mm Hg systolic or 10 mm Hg diastolic.
   - Respiratory rate > 30/min.
   - Patient becomes anxious, fatigued or demonstrates increasing respiratory distress or develops significant arrhythmias.
      e. T-tube method. Place the patient on a T-tube with humidified oxygen. If patient tolerates this for 1-4 hours as demonstrated by above parameters, discontinue ventilation. If patient fails attempt, resume ventilation and consider IMV method.

f. IMV method. Gradually decrease the number of assisted respirations in 1-2 breath increments over 30-90 minute intervals. Monitor ABGs and vital signs. When an assisted rate of < 4 breaths/min. is achieved, consider a brief T-tube trial. If patient remains stable, discontinue ventilation. If the trial fails, increase assisted rate until patient stabilizes. Repeat attempt the following day with a more gradual decrease in the rate of assisted breaths.

VIRAL UPPER RESPIRATORY TRACT INFECTIONS

I. **Overview**

Approximately 80% of acute respiratory illnesses result from viral infections. These are usually self-limited syndromes caused by a variety of viruses: rhinovirus, adenovirus, echovirus, coxsackie virus, influenza and parainfluenza. Occasionally pneumonia may complicate these infections, either primary viral or secondary bacterial. In the compromised host less common pathogens: varicella, measles, cytomegalovirus, and herpes simplex can result in life threatening infections.

II. **The Common Cold**

A. Etiology: rhinovirus, adenovirus, echovirus and coxsackie virus

B. Clinical Presentation.

Chief complaints include: congestion, sneezing, clear to mucopurulent nasal discharge, dry sore throat, low grade fever and cough. Physical examination reveals erythematous nasal and oropharyngeal mucosa, normal chest exam.

C. Management.

Treatment is primarily symptomatic. Rest, hydration, decongestants for comfort, acetaminophen for analgesia and fever should be recommended.

III. **Influenza**

A. Overview.

Influenza is a systemic illness resulting from infection with orthomyxovirus types A, B, or rarely C. These viruses can change their envelope proteins as their host population develops immunity, thereby maintaining their ability to cause recurrent infection in a single host population. Influenza vaccinations for the predicted virulent strains are available in the fall months.

B. Clinical Presentation.

There is usually an abrupt onset of high fever, chills, dry cough, headache, myalgia and prostration. Physical exam is usually unremarkable with the exception of an occasional finding of basilar crackles on chest examination. Chest x-ray is usually normal, occasionally, perihilar prominence and increased markings can be present. The development of infiltrates suggests a complicating pneumonia.

C. Management.

The illness is usually self limiting lasting 4-7 days. Rest, hydration, and acetaminophen are recommended. For influenza type A, Amantadine hydrochloride 100 mg PO bid for 10 days given early in the course can reduce symptoms, and be used for prophylaxis in compromised close contacts of infected individuals.

PNEUMONIA

I. Overview

A. Pneumonia is an inflammatory process of the lung's air spaces. It may involve an entire lobe (lobar pneumonia) or the conducting airways and their surrounding parenchyma (bronchopneumonia).

B. Possible etiologies include: aspiration, bacterial, hypersensitivity, Legionnaires, Mycoplasma, Pneumocystis carinii, TB and viral pathogens.

C. Common causes differ with age, respiratory and immune status (Table 3-4).

II. Neonates

A. Presentation.
- Fever, poor feeding, irritability, jaundice and apneic spells are common.
- Meningitis should be considered in this setting.

B. Evaluation.
1. Obtain cultures for bacteria and viruses from blood, pharyngeal secretions, urine and CSF.
2. CBC, electrolytes, urine for latex agglutination (Group B strep, E. coli).
3. Chest X-ray.

C. Management.
1. Support respiratory status.
2. Begin empiric antibiotic therapy pending identification of the organism. Ampicillin 100 mg/kg/dose q 12h IV and gentamicin or tobramycin 2.5 mg/kg/dose q 12 h IV. A parenteral third generation cephalosporin may be substituted for the aminoglycoside.
3. Hospitalize in the NICU.

III. Infants and Children (1 month - 5 years)

A. Presentation.
1. Tachypnea out of proportion to fever is common. Grunting respirations suggest pneumonia.

Table 3-4. Causative Agents of Pneumonia According to Type of Patient

Type of Patient	Common Pathogens	Less Common Pathogens of High Virulence
Neonate (<1 month)	Escherichia coli Group B streptococci Cytomegalovirus Herpes Simplex Virus Rubella virus	Listeria monocytogenes Staphylococcus aureus
Infant or young child (1 months to 5 years)	Respiratory Syncytial & Parainfluenza viruses Chlamydia trachomatis Mycoplasma pneumoniae	S. Aureus Haemophilus influenzae Streptococcus pneumonia
Child (5-14 years)	M. pneumoniae S. Pneumoniae Influenza viruses adenoviruses	S. aureus (especially after influenza) H. influenzae M. tuberculosis Group A Streptococcus Mixed Aerobic-anaerobic infection*
Adult	M. pneumonia S. pneumoniae H. influenzae Mixed Aerobic-anaerobic infection*	Klebsiella pneumoniae or other gram neg. bacilli Legionella pneumophila M. tuberculosis
Immunocompromised Patient	Aerobic Gram-negative bacilli S pneumoniae H influenzae S. aureus Pneumocystis carinii	M tuberculosis Nocardia Cytomegalovirus

* mixed infection with oropharyngeal flora (aerobic and anaerobic streptococci, Bacteroides and Fusobacterium species) following aspiration of oropharyngeal secretions.

Adapted from: Mills J, et al. Current Emergency Diagnosis and Treatment, 2nd edition. Los Altos:Lange 1985.

2. Chlamydia trachomatis pneumonia typically occurs at 4-12 weeks of life, presenting without fever, a staccato cough, hyperaeration of the lungs and eosinophilia.
3. Bronchiolitis secondary to RSV or parainfluenza virus occurs at 2-8 months and is most common between December and April. It presents with wheezing, hyperaeration of the lungs without signs of consolidation or pulmonary infiltrates.
4. Rales and decreased breath sounds may be absent until after one year of age.

B. Evaluation. Obtain:
 1. CBC (WBC > 15,000 suggests bacterial pneumonia).
 2. Oxygen saturation or ABG if respiratory distress is present.
 3. Electrolytes, BUN to assess hydration status.
 4. Chest x-ray may reveal lobar infiltrates (S. pneumonae), pneumatoceles (S. aureus), or pleural effusions (S. aureus, H. influenzae).
 5. Blood cultures.
 6. Sputum for gram stain and culture if possible.

C. Management.
 1. History and presentation, positive x-ray findings and/or sputum gram stain with predominate organism indicate antibiotic therapy. Empiric antibiotic therapy includes:
    - Ampicillin 100 mg/kg/dose q 12 h IV for S. pneumoniae, H. influenzae, Group A Strep.
    - Penicillin G 100,000-200,000 units/kg/day IM or IV div q 6 h for S. pneumoniae, Group A Strep.
    - Oxacillin, methicillin or nafcillin [1-2 gm IM/IV for S. Aureus).
    - Cefuroxime 75-100 mg/kg/day IV div q8 h for all the above pathogens.
 2. Chlamydia infections should be treated with Erythromycin 50 mg/kg/day oral or IV div q 6 h.
 3. Antibiotic therapy may be withheld in patients who are stable and demonstrate only hyperaeration or atelectasis on x-ray.

4. Hospitalize if there is evidence of respiratory distress, hyperthermia, PO_2 <70 mm Hg on room air or dehydration.
5. If clinically stable and viral diagnosis is made, observe as an outpatient with followup at 24 hour intervals until recovery is underway.

IV. Children 5-14 Years of Age

A. Presentation
 1. M. pneumoniae presents with insidious onset of malaise, nonproductive cough, hoarseness, sore throat, possible chest pain. Physical examination may reveal fine crackles, wheezes, or dullness especially over lower lobes; pharyngeal erythema; bullous myringitis (rare, erythematous TMs are more common); maculopapular rashes are common.
 2. S. pneumoniae, H. influenzae, S. aureus often follow a viral respiratory infection, or present with an abrupt onset of fever, chills, tachypnea, and cough. Auscultation may demonstrate fine crackles and/or decreased breath sound.

B. Evaluation.
 1. WBC > 15,000 suggests bacterial etiology. Mycoplasma infections may have normal WBC.
 2. Chest x-ray:
 - Mycoplasma infection: scattered segmental infiltrates, atelectasis, interstitial disease, rarely lobar consolidation.
 - Other bacteria: patchy infiltrates, increased bronchovascular markings, lobar consolidation, cavitary infiltrates, pleural effusions or empyema.
 3. Blood cultures.
 4. Sputum for gram stain and culture.
 5. If severely ill obtain nasotracheal aspiration, transtracheal aspiration and pleurocentisis for culture.
 6. A positive cold agglutination test strongly suggests a Mycoplasma infection. Bedside Agglutination test: add 3 drops of blood to the liquid anticoagulant in a

small blue topped tube. Immerse in ice bath for 15 secs. Rotate the tube slowly in the horizontal position, examine for hemagglutination that disappears as the tube rewarms.

C. Management.
1. Antibiotic therapy as directed by evaluation (see III. C. for details).
2. If mildly ill and unable to produce sputum, begin Erythromycin (50 mg/kg/day PO div q 6 h) for suspected M. pneumoniae, or S. pneumoniae with close follow-up until recovery is underway.
3. Hospitalize if severely ill.

V. **Ages 15 Years and Older**
A. Presentation is similar to children ages 5-14 with M. pneumoniae being the most common cause. Abrupt onset of fever, productive cough, pleuritic chest pain and signs of consolidation on chest exam signal other bacterial pathogens.
1. Elderly or debilitated patients may manifest fever and obtundation with S. pneumoniae the most common organism.
2. Aspiration pneumonia due to mixed aerobic-anaerobic flora is common in persons with depressed consciousness, poor dentition and foul smelling sputum. Involvement of dependant parts of the lung is common.
3. Alcoholics may develop severe pneumonia due to Klebsiella or other gram negative bacilli.
4. Patients with chronic lung disease are at risk for H. influenzae infections.
5. Legionella may cause community acquired pneumonia in middle-aged adults. Spiking fevers, diarrhea and delirium are common symptoms.
6. Immunocompromised patients are at risk for a wide range of pneumonial infections.

B. Evaluation.
   1. WBC may be normal in Mycoplasma infections, but is elevated for other bacterial pneumonias. The elderly may demonstrate leukopenia with a left shift.
   2. Chest x-ray findings are similar to those described in children. Bilateral pneumonia suggests a severe or atypical pneumonia (viral, septic emboli).
   3. Sputum for gram stain and culture should be obtained for causitive organism; leukocytes without significant bacteria suggests a Legionella or Mycoplasma infection.
   4. Pleurocentesis should be done for all significant effusions (see Pleural Effusions for diagnostic workup).
   5. Blood cultures should be obtained on severely ill patients.
   6. ABGs if respiratory compromise is suspected.
   7. Cold agglutination test if Mycoplasma is suspected (see IV.C.6 for details).
   8. Electrolytes, BUN, Cr may help in assessing the degree of dehydration in the elderly.
   9. Hyponatremia, hypophosphatemia and elevated liver enzymes are common in Legionella infections.
C. Management.
   1. Hospitalization is indicated for moderate to severely ill patients, elderly patients with pre-existing lung disease and all patients with bilateral pneumonia. Those with mild involvement may be treated on an outpatient basis with 24 hour follow-up until recovery is in progress.
   2. Antibiotic therapy depends upon the infecting organism, pre-existing lung disease and community versus hospital acquired disease (Table 3-5).

Table 3-5. Antibiotic Therapy for Adult Pneumonias

Type of Pneumonia	Etiology	Antibiotic
Community Acquired, no underlying lung	S. Pneumoniae Group A Strep	Pen G 600,000 units IM with Pen VK PO 250-500mg qid Ampicillin 250-500mg PO qid Erythromycin 250-500mg PO qid 1st Generation Cephalosporin
	M. pneumonia Chlamydia	Erythromycin 500mg PO qid Tetracycline 500mg PO qid
	Legionella	Erythromycin 500mg PO qid *if not improving 4gm/d IV add Rifampin 600mg PO bid
1. Community Acquired with underlying lung disease, or diabetes mellitus, or alcoholism 2. Hospital Acquired 3. Nursing home patients	S. pneumonia Group A Strep	Amoxicillin Clavulanate 500mg PO tid Ampicillin 500mg PO qid
	H. influenzae Klebsiella other Gram-negative bacilli	Ampicillin, Trimethoprim-sulfamethoxazole 3rd Gen. Cephalosporin Aminoglycoside & 1st or 2nd Gen. Cephalosporin Imipenem
	S. aureus	Vancomycin until methicillin resistance is ruled out, then Nafcillin, Oxacillin or Methicillin
	M. pneumoniae Legionella	Erythromycin 500mg PO qid, for Legionella as above* Tetracycline 500mg PO qid
Community Acquired and Immunosuppressed HIV and/or AIDS	Pneumocystis carinii Legionella M. Tuberculosis Candida Sp. Herpesvirus Cytomegalovirus	Trimethroprim-sulfamethoxazole & Erythromycin
Aspiration Pneumonia	Bacteroides sp. Peptostreptococci Fusobacterium sp.	Clindamycin Cefoxitin Pen G 2 million units IV

Table 3-5 (continued)

Type of Pneumonia	Etiology	Antibiotic
		divided q4-6 hours
Hospital acquired with: 1.Tracheostomy, broad-spectrum antibiotics or azotemia	Pseudomonas sp. Klebsiella Enterobacter Serratia sp. Proteus Providencia S. aureus	APAG* & AP Pen# APAG* & 3rd Gen Cephalosporin Imipenem-cilastatin
2.Immunosupression	all the above plus: Legionella M. Tuberculosis Candida sp. Aspergillus sp. Nocardia Pneumocystis carinii	Nafcillin & APAG* & AP Pen# or 3rd Gen. Cephaolosporin & Trimethroprim-sulfamethoxazole & erythromycin

*APAG = Antipseudomonal aminoglycoside: amikacin, gentamicin, netilmicin and tobramycin.

#AP Pen = Antipseudomonal beta lactamase susceptible penicillins: carbenicillin, ticarcillin, mezlocillin, azlocillin, and piperacillin.

Adapted from: Sanford J, Guide to Antimicrobial Therapy, 1988.

Asthma

I. **Overview**

Asthma is episodic reversible airway obstruction brought on by bronchospasm. Affects approximately 4% of the population. Episodes may become severe, prolonged and relatively resistant to therapy: status asthmaticus, a medical emergency.

   A. Etiology.

   Precipitating factors vary between individuals. There is an increased reactivity to various stimuli, resulting in bronchial smooth muscle contraction and obstruction. Typical stimuli include: irritants (dust, pollen, air pollutants, animal dander); infections (especially viral respiratory infections); exercise; drugs (aspirin, food colorings); and physical factors (cold and humidity).

   B. Differential Diagnosis: Croup, epiglottitis, bronchitis, emphysema, pulmonary embolism, pulmonary effusion, airway foreign body, angioedema, pulmonary aspiration, cystic fibrosis and psychogenic illness.

II. **Evaluation**

   A. History.

   On initial attack, a patient will complain of the sudden onset of progressive dyspnea. They may be able to relate an inciting event, exposure to irritant, exercise or aspirin. In young children the history may be less obvious; croup, epiglottitis, and bronchiolitis must also be considered. If it is a recurrent attack, patients are often aware of the precipitating factors and often have already attempted medical intervention.

   B. Physical Examination.

   Most patients will demonstrate some level of respiratory distress and anxiety. Observe for signs of respiratory failure: cyanosis, nasal flaring or use of accessory muscles. In severe respiratory distress, patients may appear comfortable secondary to CO_2 retention; this is an ominous finding. Chest examination reveals prolonged expiratory phase with wheezing and ronchi. In severe bronchospasm a patient may sound "tight" with decreased breath sounds secondary to decreased airflow. Tachycardia is usually present. Pulsus paradoxus greater than 10 mm Hg is indication of a severe attack.

C. Laboratory.

1. Chest x-ray.

   Most commonly the chest x-ray will be normal. However, classical findings of asthma are hyperaeration and peribronchial cuffing. May also demonstrate complications of asthma: pneumothorax, atelectasis or underlying pneumonia. Because of the frequency with which asthmatic attacks can occur, chest x-ray should not be routinely done unless there are clinical indications such as evidence of pneumonia (after bronchospasm has cleared).

2. ABGs

   These should be obtained on anyone in severe distress who does not respond quickly to initial management. Otherwise, pulse oximetry should be used to evaluate oxygenation. All patients will demonstrate some degree of hypoxemia. Most patients should be hypocapnic secondary to hyperventilation. A normal PCO_2 indicates impending respiratory failure.

3. Spirometry.

   A bedside peak flow meter is adequate for emergent evaluation, and is of value in monitoring response to therapy. Patients in acute distress and the young may be unable to cooperate. A minimum adult peak flow of 300 L/min should be obtained prior to discharge from the emergency room.

4. CBC.

   This will generally show leukocytosis as a result of demargination. Without evidence of a left shift, it alone is a poor indicator of infection.

5. Sputum examination is indicated if respiratory infection is suspected.

6. Electrolyte, BUN, Cr maybe helpful if dehydration and hypokalemia are suspected.

7. EKG is indicated in those patients with decreased cardiac function, monitoring for arrhythmias and signs of ischemia.

D. Clinical assessment of severity of the attack (Table 3-6).

Table 3-6. Clinical Asthma Severity Score

	1	2	3
PaO_2 mmHg	70-100 in room air	<70 in room air	<70 on 40% O_2
Inspiratory breath sounds	normal	unequal	decreased-absent
Accessory muscle use	none	moderate	maximum
Expiratory wheeze	none	moderated	marked
Cerebral function	normal	depressed or agitated	coma

1. A score of 5 or more indicates impending respiratory failure; obtain ABGs and prepare to intubate.

2. A score of 6 may require transfer to the ICU.

3. A score of 7 or more with a $PaCO_2$ >65 mm Hg indicates respiratory failure.

E. Other Factors Associated with Severe Attacks.

1. Duration of more than 1 week.

2. Persistance or progression of symptoms despite therapy.

3. Recent withdrawal of corticosteroid medication.

4. History of respiratory failure.

5. Complications (atelectasis, pneumothorax).

III. **Management**

A. Mild Asthma Attack.

1. Give inhalational sympathomimetics (see below).

2. Give parenteral sympathomimetics if failure to respond to inhalational agents.

3. Oral rehydration as indicated.

4. Obtain theophylline level and adjust dosage if necessary. (There is little benefit but significant risk of toxicity to increasing the theophylline level if it is already at or above 15.)

5. Monitor for improvement in respiratory status (improvement in peak expiratory flow). If stable, may discharge to home with close follow-up. If not improving with therapy, proceed with management for moderate attack, consider hospitalization.

B. Moderate to Severe Attacks. Most patients will require hospitalization.
   1. Maintain ventilation.
      a. For initial PaO_2 < 70 mm Hg on room air begin O_2 at 2-3 L/min per nasal cannula.
      b. For initial PaO_2 < 60 mm Hg on room air begin O_2, obtain ABGs, repeat in 20-30 minutes. For patients with normal or elevated PCO_2 repeat in 10 minutes.
      c. Endotracheal intubation is rarely indicated except for marked obtundation with severe hypercapnia (PCO_2 > 55 mm Hg) or progressively worsening ABGs despite therapy.
   2. Establish IV with D5W at 150 ml/hr for adults; maintenance fluids for children.
   3. Pharmacotherapy for bronchospasm.
      a. Inhalational therapy. Begin nebulized albuterol 2.5-5 mg in 2-3 cc saline. May repeat 2 times every 10-20 minutes, or Metaproterenol 15 mg in 2.2 ml saline repeated every 30-60 minutes.
      b. Parenteral therapy. Terbutaline (1 mg/ml) 0.01 mg/kg to total of 0.3 mg SQ (in children: 3.5-5 mcg/kg SQ) or Epinephrine (1 mg/ml): in children 0.01 mg/kg not to exceed 0.5 mg/dose SQ, for adults 0.3-0.5 mg SQ. May repeat in 10-20 minutes if dyspnea persists. Decreased dosages are necessary in the elderly and those with history of coronary arter disease or tachyarrhythmias.
      c. Corticosteroid therapy. Begin therapy early as they take approximately 12 hours to work.
   - Methylprednisolone: Adults; 1-2 mg/kg IV/IM loading dose then 0.5-1 mg/kg q 6 hr IV, children; 0.03-0.2 mg/kd IM.

- Prednisone: 10 mg PO bid for infants < 1 year; 20 mg PO bid for ages 1-2.0 years; 30 mg PO bid for ages 3-12 years; 50 mg PO bid for ages > 12 years.

  d. Theophylline therapy. Obtain stat theophylline level. Therapeutic range is 10-20 mcg/ml. Begin IV therapy if indicated. If the patient has not been on theophylline before, give initial loading dose and begin constant infusion. Dosages must be reduced for the elderly, patients with heart disease, liver disease, taking cimetidine, propranolol or erythromycin. Aminophylline contains 85% theophylline by weight and is the most commonly available parenteral form (Table 3-7).

Table 3-7. Aminophylline Dosing

<u>Loading Dosage:</u>

Initial therapy: 6 mg/kg IV over 30 minutes

Previous therapy: 0.6 mg/kg for each 1 mcg/ml < 10 mcg/ml serum concentration

<u>Maintenance Infusion:</u>

Group	Age	Aminophylline Infusion
Neonate	< 24 days	1.3 mg/kg/12 hr
	> 24 days	1.9 mg/kg/12 hr
Infants	6 weeks to 1 year	(0.08)(age in weeks) + 21 = mg/kg/hr
Children	1-9 years	1.0 mg/kg/hr
	9-12 years	0.9 mg/kg/hr
Adolescents (cigarette or marijuana smokers'	12-16 years 12-16 years	0.9 mg/kg/hr
Adolescents (non-smokers)	16-50 years > 16 years	0.6 mg/kg/hr
Adults (healthy cigarette or marijuana smoker)	> 16 years	0.6 mg/kg/hr
Adults (healthy non-smoker)		0.5 mg/kg/hr
Cardiac or liver disease		0.3 mg/kg/hr

Adapted from: Driscoll CE, et al. Handbook of Family Practice. Year Book Medical Publishers, Inc., Chicago: 1986.

  e. Pulmonary toilet. Rehydrate as indicated by oral or intravenous route.

CHRONIC OBSTRUCTIVE PULMONARY DISEASE (COPD)

I. **Overview**

COPD refers to generalized expiratory airway obstruction most often due to two separate diseases, chronic bronchitis and emphysema. While separate entities, clinically they usually coexist. Therefore patients with chronic expiratory obstruction are classified under the label of Chronic Obstructive Pulmonary Disease, COPD. Currently it is the fifth leading cause of death in the USA.

A. Chronic Bronchitis (Blue Bloater).

Defined as the presence of cough with excessive mucous production occurring on most days for at least three months in each of the past two years. It is the result of chronic irritation (smoking, pollutants), infections or hereditary factors.

B. Emphysema (Pink Puffer).

Defined as destruction of lung parenchyma beyond the terminal bronchiole with resultant coalescence of alveoli. There are two types:

1. Panlobular: involves alveoli, alveolar ducts and sacs. It is the result of a constitutional defect of alpha-1 antitrypsin defect or idiopathic causes.

2. Centrilobular: involves respiratory bronchioles. It is the result of chronic bronchitis (smoking, air pollution, infections, dusts).

C. Clinical Comparison (Table 3-8).

Table 3-8. Comparison of Clinical Manifestations

Characteristic	Emphysema	Chronic Bronchitis
Inspection		
Body	thin	stocky or obese (bloater)
Chest	hyperinflation (barrel chest)	normal
	Hypertrophy of accessory muscles	increased use of accessory muscles

Table 3-8 (continued)

Characteristic	Emphysema	Chronic Bronchitis
Breathing pattern	progressive dyspnea	variable
	labored (puffer)	normal
	retractions	normal
	decreased chest movements	normal
	decreased I/E ratio	decreased I/E ratio
Posture	orthopnea	variable
Cough	little	considerable
Sputum	little-mucoid	large-purulent
Color	normal (pink)	cyanosis (blue)
Palpation	normal to decreased fremitus	normal to decreased fremitus
Percussion	hyper-resonance	dull
Auscultation		
Breath Sounds	decreased	normal to decreased
Ronchi	little	episodic
Blood Gases		
P_{O_2} resting	slight decrease	moderate to severe decrease
P_{O_2} exercise	falls	stable
PCO_2	normal	increased
PCO_3	normal	increased
PFT's		
Spirometry	obstructive pattern	obstructive pattern
RV and TLC	increased	normal to decreased
Diffusion capacity	decreased	normal
Compliance	increased	normal
Hematocrit	<55%	55%
X-Ray		
Bronchovascular markings	decreased	increased
Hyperinflation	yes	no
Bullae/blebs	yes	no

Table 3-8 (continued)

Characteristics	Emphysema	Chronic Bronchitis
Past History	normal	frequent respiratory infections
Life Span	normal (60-80 yrs)	decreased (40-60 yrs)
Cor Pulmonale	uncommon	Common

Adapted from: Oakes DF, Clinical Practitioners Pocket Guide to Respiratory Care. Old Town:Health Educator Publications, 1988.

II. **Evaluation**

   A. History.

   1. Define present symptoms as to duration and relative severity. An acute exacerbation of chronic bronchitis will present with increased volume and purulent sputum. Fever is rare and should raise the suspicion of pneumonia. Emphysema presents with chronic progressive dyspnea

   2. Identify current medications, including home O_2.

   3. Review previous pulmonary history, severity and treatment.

   4. Review smoking habits.

   B. Physical Exam.

   1. Assess degree of distress.

   2. Obtain vital signs observing for tachypnea and tachycardia.

   3. Cardiopulmonary exam observing for prolongation of expiration, CHF, consolidation or pneumothorax.

   C. Laboratory.

   1. Arterial blood gases generally reveal hypoxemia. Chronic bronchitis is also likely to demonstrate CO_2 retention, emphysema most often will not. Hypercapnea and resultant respiratory acidosis is often compensated with bicarbonate retention to maintain a

normal pH. The presence of acidemia and hypercapnea suggests a recent increase in CO_2 retention.

2. CBC with differential may show leukocytosis secondary to corticosteriod or sympathomimetic drug use. Increased hematocrit (>55%) may suggest the need for phlebotomy.
3. Chest X-ray used to rule out pneumonia, pneumothorax and heart failure.
4. EKG may reveal atrial hypertrophy, right axis deviation and right ventricular hypertrophy. Evaluate for evidence of myocardial ischemia and arrhythmias.
5. Examine sputum by gram stain and culture.
6. Spirometry (see section on PFTs). Alternatively a bedside peak flow meter will give a good estimate of airflow and should be >120 L/min.

III. Management

A. Respiratory Failure.
1. Maintain Oxygenation. Begin O_2 at 2 L/min by nasal cannula for a pulse oximetry of < 88% or a PO_2 < 55 mm Hg, or if the patient is in clinical respiratory distress. Increasing FIO_2 should be done cautiously monitoring for hypercapnea and apnea. Intubation and mechanical ventilation may be required if there is progressive fall in oxygenation, increasing hypercapnea, persistent acidosis or obtundation.
2. Arterial Blood Gas Monitoring. Check ABG's after 20-30 minutes of O_2 therapy. Monitor for an increase in PCO_2 (if initially hypercapnic it should be no greater than 5-8 mm Hg) and an improved PO_2 (60-70 mm Hg is ideal).
3. Bronchodilator Therapy. While response may be limited in some, bronchodilator therapy and corticosteriods should be initiated (see section on Asthma for details).
4. Provide Adequate Hydration. Patients will require approximately 2500 ml of fluids per day.
5. Chest Physiotherapy and postural drainage is helpful only if patients are unable to cough.

Chronic Obstructive Pulmonary Disease (COPD)

B. Infection. Most exacerbations are accompanied by increased production of yellow or green sputum. Sputum gram stain may be helpful. Most common organisms are Hemophilus sp., S. pneumoniae and Branhamella catarrhalis. Recommended antibiotics include: Amoxicillin 500 mg po tid or Amoxicillin/ Clavulanate 500 mg po tid; Trimethoprim (80 mg); Sulfamethoxazole (400 mg) 2 tabs po bid; or tetracycline 500 mg po qid all for 10 days.

C. Indications for Hospitalization.
   1. Persistent respiratory distress: respiratory rate >24/min; tachycardia; deteriorating ABG's; peak flow < 120 L/min.
   2. Presence of coexisting disorder: CHF, pneumonia, pneumothorax, thromboembolism, etc.

D. Outpatient Management.
   1. Improve Ventilation
      a. Increase clearance of excessive secretions by maintaining adequate hydration and encourage deep breathing and coughing.
      b. Increase airway diameter by decreasing edema and relieving bronchospasm. Beta agonists, theophylline compounds and corticosteriods may be beneficial (see section on Asthma for details on administration).
      c. Supplemental home O_2 if necessary.
   2. Smoking Cessation.
   3. Environmental Factors: avoidance of air pollutants, altitude and extremes of humidity and temperature.
   4. Monitoring for potential complications: weight loss, respiratory infections, CHF, depression and sexual dysfunction.

PULMONARY EMBOLISM

I. Overview

Pulmonary embolus (PE) affects 500,000 persons per year in the U.S., resulting in 50,000 deaths per year. The diagnosis is often made by clinical history and ventilation/perfusion studies as physical examination and chest x-ray are nonspecific.

A. Predisposing Factors.

1. 95% of pulmonary emboli result from deep venous thrombi (DVT) of the lower extremities. Therefore, the diagnosis of PE often relies on the diagnosis of DVT's. Predisposing factors for venous thrombus include: immobility, post-operative states, pregnancy and postpartum states, oral contraception use, CHF, obesity, malignancy and coagulopathies.

2. Septic emboli occasionally arise from right sided endocarditis. In addition to signs of PE, these patients usually present with high fever, rigors and chest x-ray reveals multiple infiltrates. Therapy consists of respiratory support and treatment of the underlying cause. These patients should not be anticoagulated.

B. Differential diagnosis includes: myocardial infarction, pleurisy, pneumonia, pulmonary edema, pleural effusion and asthma.

II. Evaluation

A. History.

The patient usually presents with abrupt onset of dyspnea, anxiety, hypoxia and occasionally chest pain. Less often hemoptysis, fever, cough, wheezing and syncope occur. Frequently an underlying predisposing condition can be found.

B. Physical Examination.

This generally reveals an anxious patient. Tachypnea and tachycardia are common. Chest auscultation is generally normal. A pleural friction rub and signs of consolidation may be present if infarction has occurred. Signs of a DVT may be present. With massive PE severe chest pain, hypoxia, syncope and evidence of cardiovascular shock are present.

C. Laboratory.
   1. Chest x-ray is generally normal. However, the presence of a pulmonary infiltrate with ipsilateral elevation of the hemidiaphragm should raise the suspicion of PE. If infarction has occurred, atelectasis, effusion and infiltrates may be present.
   2. EKG generally reveals tachycardia. With massive PE right axis deviation, peaked P waves, right ventricular strain with ST-T wave changes may be present.
   3. ABGs generally reveal the nonspecific findings of hypoxia and hypocapnia secondary to reflexive hyperventilation. However, if hypercapnia is present, respiratory failure may be eminent and repeat ABGs in 15-20 minutes is indicated. A normal PO_2 can occur and should not be used as a basis for therapeutic decisions.
   4. Radionucleotide lung scan is necessary for diagnosis.
      a. Perfusion scan: a sensitive screen, however is nonspecific if abnormal. A normal scan generally rules out a PE.
      b. Ventilation-perfusion scan: increases specificity of perfusion scan alone. A normal ventilation scan over areas with decreased perfusion is highly specific for PE. Defects which are matched (poor perfusion and poor ventilation) are suggestive of other pulmonary disease such as COPD, pneumonia and asthma.
      c. Pulmonary angiography: considered the gold standard for the diagnosis of PE. However, it is invasive and should be used in those situations in which other studies are inconclusive and/or anticoagulation therapy is high risk.

III. **Management**
   A. Maintain respiratory status, begin O_2 at 5-10 L/min by mask. Follow for evidence of hypercapnia.
   B. Provide cardiovascular support if necessary. Dopamine 2-5 mcg/kg/h IV may be started prior to thrombolytic therapy if shock is present. Fluid resuscitation should be

done cautiously unless central venous pressure is monitored.
C. Treat pain if necessary, begin with morphine 1-2 mg IV.
D. Because of the lack of specific physical findings for PE, diagnosis is often made on clinical suspicions. If there are no contraindications to anticoagulation therapy, heparin should be started as soon as PE is sufficiently suspected unless thrombolytic therapy is contemplated.
   1. Check initial coagulation studies: PT, PTT, platelets.
   2. Begin heparin bolus 5,000 units followed by a constant infusion of approximately 1,000 units/hour.
   3. Monitor PTT, adjusting heparin infusion to maintain level 1.5-2 times normal.
   4. Monitor platelet count watching for a rapid decrease secondary to a hypersensitivity reaction, White Clot Syndrome.
E. Thrombolytic therapy should be reserved for patients with massive PE as evidenced by hemodynamic compromise or shock. Thrombolytic agents should not be given simultaneously with heparin. If heparin has been instituted, discontinue therapy. Thrombolytic therapy can be started when the PTT is less than 2 times baseline. Central venous catheters should be avoided. If necessary for hemodynamic monitoring, they should be placed peripherally and advanced retrograde into a central vein.
   1. Streptokinase therapy: 250,000 units loading dose IV over 20 minutes followed by 100,000 units/hour for 24 hours. Hydrocortisone 100 mg should be given before streptokinase to prevent allergic reaction.
   2. Urokinase therapy: 4400 units/kg over 10 minutes loading dose with IV infusion of the same dose every hour for 12 hours.
   3. Coagulation studies should be followed adjusting dose to keep them 1.5-2 times baseline.
   4. Begin heparinization after thrombolytic therapy.

al anticoagulation therapy should be begun after the ient is stable. Warfarin does not achieve an effective ithrombotic state until the PT has been in therapeutic ge for 3-5 days. Therefore, it should be started promptly and heparin not withdrawn until its full effect is achieved. Anticoagulation therapy should be continued for 2-3 months. Underlying factors may necessitate life long therapy.

G. Re-embolization. Heparin therapy does not resolve clot already present. Therefore, the patient is at risk for re-embolization until the clot has dissolved or become organized. If the patient re-embolizes or has sustained a massive PE, inferior vena cava interruption should be considered.

H. All patients with suspected PE should be hospitalized.

PLEURAL EFFUSION (HYDROTHORAX)

I. Overview

Pleural effusion is an abnormal accumulation of fluid in the pleural space secondary to a pathologic process. Effusions can be divided into transudates or exudates.

- A. Transudates result from plasma seeping from blood vessels into the pleural space, due to an increased hydrostatic pressure or decreased oncotic pressure within the vessel.
- B. Exudates are inflammatory effusions resulting from capillary damage or lymphatic blockage.
- C. Differential Diagnosis
   1. Transudate: cardiac, renal or hepatic failure; hyponatremia; superior vena cava obstruction.
   2. Exudate: rheumatoid arthritis, SLE, sarcoidosis, TB, pancreatitis, esophageal rupture.
   3. Either: trauma, neoplasms, infections, pulmonary emboli, idiopathic

II. Evaluation

- A. History. May present with an abrupt onset or gradually worsening dyspnea, tachypnea or orthopnea. Symptoms primarily dependent upon underlying disease.
- B. Physical Examination. Effusions greater than 300 ml per hemithorax should be detectable through physical examination with decreased breath sounds, decreased fremitus and dullness to percussion.
- C. Laboratory.
   1. X-ray examination may reveal radiopacity of the involved cavity, obliteration of the costophrenic angle, and interlobar fissure fluid collection. Mediastinal shift is also possible. If costophrenic angle blunting is present, obtain a lateral decubitus x-ray. If > 1 cm of fluid can be seen, pleurocentesis is possible.
   2. Pleurocentesis for diagnostic examination should include: specific gravity, pH, glucose, cell count and differential, amylase, total protein (serum also), LDH

Pleural Effusion (Hydrothorax) 127

(serum also), culture, gram stain, acid-fast stain, cytologic examination, CEA for tumor (Table 3-9).

Table 3-9. Differentiation of Transudate from Exudate

Characteristics	Transudate	Exudate
Specific Gravity	<1.016	≥1.016
Protein	<3 gm/dl	≥3 gm/dl
Pleural Fluid Protein		
Serum Protein	<0.5	≥0.5
Pleural Fluid LDH		
Serum LDH	<0.6	≥0.6

Adapted from: Bakserman S, A,B,C,'s of Interpretive Laboratory Date 2nd edition. New Bern, N.C.: Interpretive Laboratory Data Inc. Griffin & Tilghman Printers, 1984.

III. **Management**

A. Clinical findings suggest pleural effusion; perform pleurocentesis, determine if fluid is:

1. Gross blood, pus, chyle: drain fluid, treat underlying disease. For empyema evaluate pH. If:

    a. < 7.1; requires chest tube drainage.
    b. 7.1-7.2; drain only if purulent.
    c. 7.2-7.3; observe, drain if not resolving.
    d. 7.3; drainage not necessary.

2. Transudate: no further tests on effusion unless strong clinical reason. Treat underlying disease.

3. Exudate. Consider further evaluation for:

    a. Cancer: pleural fluid for cytology and CEA.
    b. Infection: pleural fluid for culture.
    c. SLE: LE prep, ANA.
    d. Rheumatoid Arthritis: Rheumatoid factor, ANA.
    e. T.B.: pleural fluid for cultures and acid-fast stain.

    If testing is non-diagnostic, consider chest CT. If CT shows,

    a. Parenchymal disease: fiberoptic bronchoscopy.

- b. Pleural-based mass: consider pleural biopsy, thoracosopy, or pleuroscopy.
- c. Normal except for the effusion:
- consider lymphoma, obtain abdominal CT.
- consider chest tube drainage or periodic thoracentesis.

B. If drainage is indicated, fluid should be drained cautiously (no more than 1 liter at a time). Because of the effusion, V/Q mismatching may be present. With rapid removal of the effusion further mismatching may occur. Obtain a post-drainage chest x-ray to rule out iatrogenic pneumothorax.

HEMOPTYSIS

I. **Overview**

   Hemoptysis is the coughing of blood. The quantity of blood can range from blood streaked sputum to frank bleeding. However, the differential diagnosis is essentially the same and can be divided into intrapulmonary and extrapulmonary disorders.

   A. Intrapulmonary Disorders: bronchitis, bronchiectasis, bronchogenic carcinoma, tuberculosis, fungal infections, pneumonia, pulmonary infarction, arteriovenous malformation, trauma, endotracheal foreign body, pulmonary vasculitis, Goodpasture's Syndrome.

   B. Extrapulmonary Disorders: coagulopathies, heart failure, mitral stenosis, hematemesis, oronasopharyngeal lesions.

II. **Evaluation**

   A. History.
      1. Differentiate hemoptysis from hematemesis: frothy blood versus brown blood, associated with coughing versus vomiting. (Note: Occult blood may be found in the gastrointestinal tract from sputum which has been coughed up and swallowed).
      2. Review pulmonary, cardiac, laryngeal, oropharyngeal and systemic symptoms which may localize bleeding source.

   B. Physical Examination.
      1. Ensure adequate airway.
      2. Check vital signs, evaluate for orthostatic changes.
      3. Respiratory examination with emphasis on detecting rubs or decreased breath sounds.
      4. Thorough examination of the oropharynx and larynx including laryngoscopy.

   C. Laboratory Examination.
      1. Sputum examination: gross, gram stain and culture.
      2. CBC with differential.
      3. Type and cross match if anemic or hypotensive.

4. Prothrombin time, partial thromboplastin time and platelet count.
5. Arterial blood gas.
6. Chest x-ray.
7. Tuberculin skin test.

III. Management

A. Massive Hemoptysis (> 100 ml/hour).
   1. Begin oxygen at 5-10 L/min
   2. Maintain slight Trendelenberg with dependent positioning of bleeding hemithorax, so as to prevent further aspiration.
   3. Maintain airway.
      a. Vigorous suctioning.
      b. Endotracheal intubation if necessary.
   4. Establish large bore intravenous catheter
   5. Treat shock with IV fluids.
   6. Obtain history as possible.
   7. Pursue laboratory evaluation.
   8. Obtain surgical consult.

B. Moderate Hemoptysis (< 20 ml/ 24 hours).
   1. Maintain ventilation.
      a. Begin oxygen at 2-10 L/min, adjust as indicated.
      b. Assist with pulmonary toilet as needed; do not suppress cough.
   2. Maintain circulation.
   3. Treat underlying etiology.
      a. Hospitalize if evaluation reveals disorders necessitating prompt medical attention.
      b. Follow-up with specialist for bronchoscopy within 1 week.

C. Minimal Hemoptysis (small amounts of blood tinged sputum).
   1. Evaluate and treat underlying etiology.

2. If stable patient should be referred for further evaluation within one week. In general, minimal hemoptysis requires the same evaluation as moderate hemoptysis.

References

Bakerman S, eds. <u>A. B. C's of Interpretive Laboratory Data, 2nd edition</u>. New Bern, NC: Griffin and Tilghman Printers, Inc., 1984.

Bertka KR and Wunderink RG: Outpatient management of COPD. <u>American Family Physician</u> 37(3):265, 1988.

Bordow RA and Moser KM eds. <u>Manual of Clinical Problems in Pulmonary Medicine, 2nd edition</u>. Boston:Little Brown and Company, 1985.

Driscoll CE, *et al*, eds. <u>Handbook of Family Practice</u>. Chicago: Year Book Medical Publishers, 1986.

Feinsilver SH, *et al*: Effusions: fast-track management. <u>Patient Care</u>, pp. 30-54, November 30, 1988.

Jay S: Pleural effusions 2. Definitive evaluation of the exudate. <u>Postgraduate Medicine</u> 80(5):181, October 1986.

Mills J, *et al*, eds. <u>Current Emergency Diagnosis and Treatment, 2nd edition</u>. Los Altos:Lange, 1985.

Oakes DF, ed. <u>Clinical Practitioners Pocket Guide to Respiratory Care</u>. Old Town:Health Educator Publications, 1988.

Orland M, *et al*, eds. <u>Manual of Medical Therapeutics, 25th edition</u>. Boston: Little Brown and Company, 1986.

Petersdorf RG, *et al*, eds. <u>Harrison's Principles of Internal Medicine, 10th edition</u>. New York: McGraw Hill, 1983.

Petty PL: Exacerbation of COPD. <u>Primary Care Emergency Decisions</u> 4(9):25, 1988.

Rakel RE and Conn HF, eds. <u>Textbook of Family Practice, Third edition</u>. Philadelphia: W.B. Saunders Company, 1984.

Sanford J: <u>Guide to Antimicrobial Therapy</u>, 1988.

4/ GASTROENTEROLOGY

Blaise P. Vitale, M.D., and John E. Littler, M.D.

GASTROINTESTINAL BLEEDING

I. **Types**
   A. Hematemesis - vomiting of blood.
      1. May be bright red or resemble coffee grounds.
      2. Implies bleeding source proximal to ligament of Treitz.
      3. Usually secondary to peptic ulcer disease, erosive gastritis, esophageal varices, Mallory Weiss tear, or swallowed blood from the upper respiratory tract.
   B. Melena.
      1. Passage of black tarry stools secondary to internal bleeding with time for metabolism of hemoglobin.
      2. Can be upper or lower in origin.
      3. Stools can be black from sources besides blood (e.g. iron, bismuth, licorice).
   C. Hematochezia; bright red blood per rectum usually secondary to anorectal disease or colonic disease.

II. **Etiology** (Table 4-1)

Category	Upper GI bleed	Lower GI bleed
Inflammatory	Peptic Ulcer Esophagitis Gastritis Stress Ulcer	Ulcerative colitis Crohn's Disease Diverticulitis Enterocolitis
Mechanical	Mallory Weiss tear Hiatal Hernia	Anal Fissure Diverticulosis
Vascular	Esophageal Varices	Hemorrhoids/ Hemorrhoids/ A-V malformations Angiodysplasia
Neoplastic	Carcinoma	Carcinoma/polyps
Systemic	Blood Dyscrasias	Blood Dyscrasias

III. Diagnosis and Treatment

A. Rapid bleeding will produce hemodynamic changes. In many cases, treatment must be started before the diagnosis can be made. Treatment is directed towards correcting the underlying disorder or to stabilizing the patient and stopping the bleeding.

B. See algorithms for managing upper and lower GI bleeds (Fig 4-1 and 4-2).

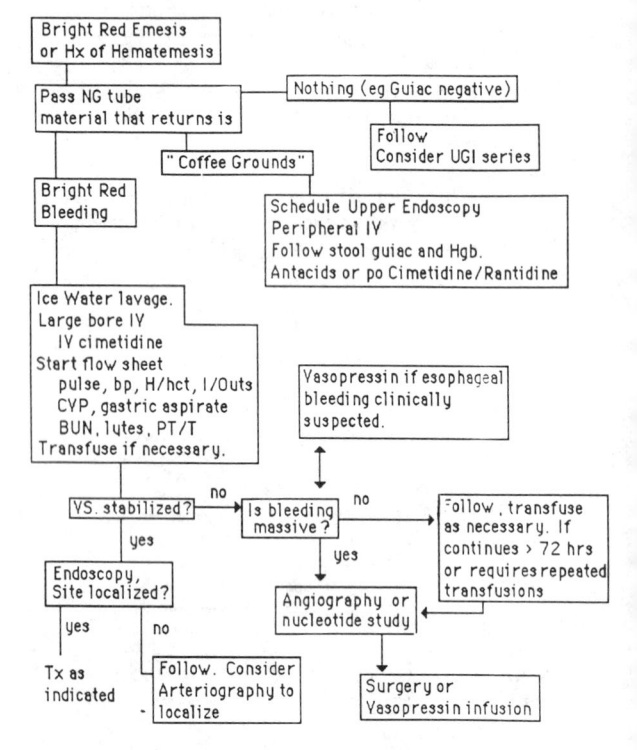

Fig 4-1. Upper GI Bleeding

Gastrointestinal Bleeding

Melena or **Bright Red Blood**

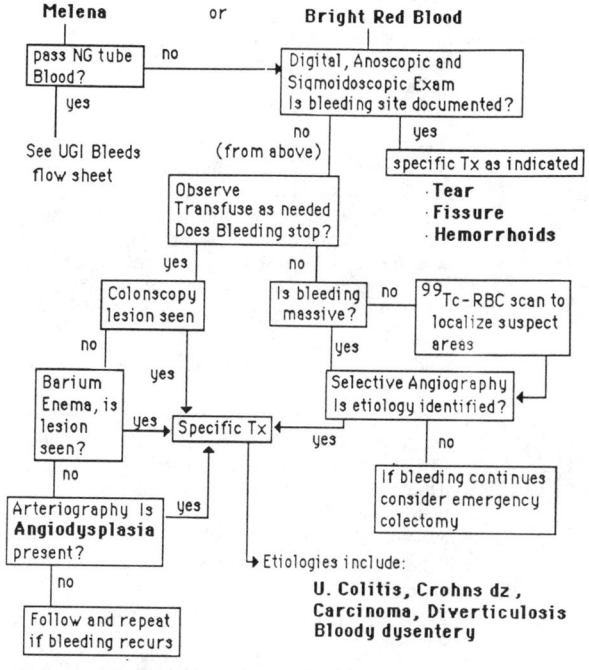

```
Melena                              Bright Red Blood
pass NG tube   no →   Digital, Anoscopic and
Blood?                 Sigmoidoscopic Exam
   ↓                   Is bleeding site documented?
  yes                        ↓              ↓
                             no            yes
See UGI Bleeds           (from above)       ↓
flow sheet                              specific Tx as indicated
                                          · Tear
                                          · Fissure
                                          · Hemorrhoids

              Observe
              Transfuse as needed
              Does Bleeding stop?
                ↓           ↓
               yes          no
                ↓           ↓
           Colonoscopy    Is bleeding    no →  99Tc-RBC scan to
           lesion seen    massive?             localize suspect
             ↓              ↓                  areas
             no            yes
             ↓              ↓
           Barium      Selective Angiography
           Enema, is   Is etiology identified?
           lesion       ↓           ↓
           seen?       yes          no
             ↓          ↓           ↓
            yes →  Specific Tx   If bleeding continues
             ↓          ↑        consider emergency
             no         |        colectomy
             ↓          |
         Arteriography Is  yes
         Angiodysplasia ───┘
         present?
             ↓
             no
             ↓
         Follow and repeat
         if bleeding recurs
```

→ Etiologies include:

U. Colitis, Crohns dz, Carcinoma, Diverticulosis Bloody dysentery

Fig 4-2. Lower GI Bleeding

Reference

Petersdorf RG, *et al*, eds. <u>Harrison's Principles of Internal Medicine, 10th edition</u>. New York: McGraw Hill, 1983.

DYSPEPSIA/PEPTIC ULCER DISEASE

I. **Overview**: Spectrum of clinical disease ranging from superficial erosions of the gastric or duodenal mucosa to ulceration through to muscularis to perforation. Predisposing factors include alcohol use, tobacco use, aspirin or other NSAID use. Acute physiologic stress (ICU setting, trauma, burns, neurosurgical problems) predispose to acute stress ulcers. Initial evaluation and treatment are similar in the entire clinical spectrum of disease with the exception of the acute complications of hemorrhage and perforation.

II. **Duodenal Ulcer**
   A. Clinical presentation;
      1. History will usually include midepigastric gnawing or burning pain that is worse several hours after meals, improved by eating. Symptoms have often been present for some time before patient presents for evaluation and the patient frequently will have found that various factors aggravate or alleviate the pain. Antacids have usually been used to some extent.
      2. Physical exam will generally reveal midepigastric tenderness. Rectal exam should be performed to evaluate for occult blood.
      3. Laboratory and x-ray: if patient has symptoms suggestive of anemia or has had black tarry stools, obtain CBC. Diagnostic studies are generally required only if the patient fails 4-8 week trial of medical treatment. Options include UGI and endoscopy. If endoscopy is available, it may be preferred as it allows the option of biopsy for suspicious lesions.
   B. Treatment:
      1. Eliminate use of tobacco, alcohol, caffeine, NSAIDs if possible.
      2. Liberal use of antacids. Alternating use of magnesium-containing antacids with aluminum-containing antacids can balance side effects of diarrhea and constipation. Regimen for possible PUD should be 30 ml po 1 and 3 hours after meals and at bed time, plus prn.

Dyspepsia/Peptic Ulcer Disease 137

3. H2 blockers: very effective, safe, convenient. Four preparations are currently available and all can be dosed qhs or bid. Cimetidine may have more side effects and potential drug interactions.

   a. Cimetidine: 800 mg qhs or divided bid. Maintenance is 400 mg qhs.
   b. Ranitidine: 300 mg qhs or divided bid. Maintenance is 150 mg qhs.
   c. Famotidine: 40 mg qhs or divided bid. Maintenance is 20 mg qhs.
   d. Nizatidine: 300 mg qhs or divided bid. Maintenance is 150 mg qhs. Treatment should be at full dose for minimum of four weeks. Maintenance dose will reduce risk of recurrence and is indicated in patients that have had a recurrence.

4. Sucralfate, dosed 1 gram prior to meals and at bed time, produces physical barrier over the ulcer. Requires acidic medium; should not be taken with or after antacids.

C. Treatment failure: indication for evaluation by UGI or endoscopy.

D. Surgery: indicated for intractable pain, significant hemorrhage, perforation, gastric outlet obstruction.

III. **Gastric Ulcer**

A. Clinical presentation is similar to duodenal ulcer. Patients tend to be somewhat older, and pain often occurs sooner after eating than with duodenal ulcers.

B. Evaluation: if empiric treatment failed to eliminate symptoms and evaluation by UGI or endoscopy reveals gastric ulcer, biopsies should be obtained. If biopsies are negative a 6-8 week trial of maximal medical therapy may be tried with repeat endoscopy to document healing.

C. Treatment is identical to that for duodenal ulcers.

D. Surgery is indicated for absence of complete healing, obstruction, perforation, hemorrhage.

ESOPHAGEAL DISEASES

Dysphagia, the subjective sensation of difficulty swallowing due to food "getting stuck on the way down," is a common presenting symptom of esophageal disorders.

I. **Causes of Dysphagia:**
   A. Achalasia.
   B. Zenker's diverticulum.
   C. Diffuse esophageal spasm.
   D. Scleroderma.
   E. G-E reflux.
   F. Other: cricopharyngeal incoordination, malignancy, radiation changes.

II. **Evaluation**
   A. Barium swallow: provides excellent information on anatomy, some on function.
   B. Esophagoscopy: can demonstrate tumor (and provide tissue diagnosis with biopsy), chronic changes from irradiation, or inflammation.
   C. Manometry: demonstrates function of the esophagus.

III. **Achalasia**: motility disorder in which lower esophageal sphincter does not relax with swallowing and peristalsis of lower esophagus is abnormal due to absence of Auerbach's neural plexus.
   A. Diagnosis: barium swallow will generally demonstrate achalasia by narrowing of the distal esophagus ("bird beaking") and dilatation of the proximal portion. On manometry, LES pressure will be elevated.
   B. Treatment: myotomy may be required.

IV. **Zenker's Diverticulum**: generally presents after age 60, may be preceded by years of symptoms from cricopharyngeal incoordination. Regurgitation of undigested food is classic.
   A. Diagnosis is by barium swallow.
   B. Treatment is diverticulectomy.

Esophageal Diseases

V. **Diffuse Esophageal Spasm**: Motor disorder with large amplitude, long duration, repetitive contractions of smooth muscle with absence of coordinated peristalsis. May present with chest pain, dysphagia.
   A. Diagnosis: barium swallow may reveal evidence of diffuse spasm. Manometry will show normal LES pressure and uncoordinated contractions.
   B. Treatment is small soft meals, nitroglycerin or nifedipine, and anticholinergic medications.

VI. **Scleroderma**; atrophy of smooth muscle portion of esophagus. Presents with dysphagia to solids and heartburn.
   A. Diagnosis: Barium swallow shows dilatation of lower esophagus with poor sphincter function. Manometry may show low pressures throughout.
   B. Treatment is directed toward symptomatic relief (generally from reflux symptoms--see below).

VII. **G-E Reflux & Esophagitis**; reflux of gastric contents into esophagus which may result in mucosal damage. May be asymptomatic or present with heartburn, dysphagia.
   A. Predisposing factors:
      1. Increased gastric volume (after meals, pyloric obstruction) or pressure (obesity, pregnancy, ascites, girdles).
      2. Hiatal hernia.
      3. Smoking.
   B. Diagnosis is frequently possible from the history alone. Barium swallow may demonstrate the presence of reflux. Esophagoscopy will reveal the presence of esophagitis. Manometry will show LES pressure to be low.
   C. Treatment should include elimination of causative agents, elevation of head of bed during sleep, liberal use of antacids, possibly H2 blockers, sucralfate. Surgery may be necessary for intractable pain or evidence of complication.
   D. Complications can include Barrett's esophagus with predisposition to carcinoma, stricture formation.

Reference

Petersdorf RG, *et al*, eds. Harrison's Principles of Internal Medicine, 10th edition. New York: McGraw Hill, 1983.

ACUTE PANCREATITIS

Abnormal activation of pancreatic zymogens producing autodigestion.

I. **Etiology**
   A. Alcohol (acute and chronic) ingestion.
   B. Biliary tract disease.
   C. Others include: post-op, post-ERCP, trauma, metabolic disorders (hypertriglyceridemia, hypercalcemia, renal failure), infections (viral, coxsackie, ascariasis, mycoplasma) drug-associated (diuretics, sulfonamides, tetracycline, azathiaprine, valproic acid, estrogens), connective tissue disorders/vasculitis, penetrating peptic ulcer, pancreas divisum, idiopathic.

II. **Clinical Features**
   A. Abdominal pain (often radiating to back), nausea, vomiting, low grade fever, tachycardia, hypotension.

III. **Diagnosis**
   A. Increased serum amylase (2-3 times normal).

IV. **Prognosis** - based on Ranson's criteria
   - On Admission.
   - Age > 55 years.
   - WBC > 16,000.
   - Blood glucose > 200 mg per dl.
   - LDH > 700 iu/dl.
   - SGOT > 250 units per dl.

During Initial 48 Hours
   - Fall in hct of > 10%.
   - Rise in BUN of > 5 mg per dl.
   - Serum Ca < 8 mg per dl.
   - Arterial PO2 < 60 mm Hg.
   - Base deficit > 4 ug/L.
   - Fluid sequestration > 6 L.

A combination of 3 or more factors has been associated with > 60% mortality. With 7 or more signs, mortality approaches 100%.

V. **Management**
   A. Analgesia, generally requires narcotics.
   B. IV fluids.
   C. NPO with nasogastric suction.
   D. H2 blockers.
   E. Antibiotics for documented infection.

VI. **Complications**; Abscess, pseudocyst formation, pancreatic ascites, pleural effusion, respiratory failure, infection, hypotension, DIC, GI hemorrhage, renal failure, diabetes.

Reference

Ranson JHC, *et al*, eds. Surg Gynecol Obstet 138:69, 1974.

CHRONIC PANCREATITIS

Several episodes of acute pancreatitis superimposed on previously injured pancreas

I. **Etiology**
   A. Similar to acute pancreatitis except increased prevalence of alcoholism as cause, decreased prevalence of biliary tract disease.

II. **Clinical features**; similar to acute pancreatitis but also often presents with weight loss, malabsorption, diarrhea, chronic pain.

III. **Diagnosis**
   A. Appropriate history.
   B. Amylases are often not helpful.
   C. Triad present in approximately 1/3 patients: Pancreatic calcification, steatorrhea, and diabetes.

IV. **Complications**
   A. Diarrhea, malabsorption, B12 deficiency, impaired glucose tolerance, pleural/peritoneal/pericardial effusions, icterus, and narcotic addiction.

V. **Management**
   A. Manage exacerbations as acute pancreatitis.
   B. Avoid alcohol and foods with high fat content.
   C. Pancreatic enzyme replacement.
   D. Manage diabetes.
   E. ERCP.
   F. Surgery.

Reference

Petersdorf RG, *et al*, eds. <u>Harrison's Principles of Internal Medicine, 10th edition</u>. New York: McGraw Hill, 1983.

LIVER DISEASE

I. **Hepatitis**
   A. Etiology.
      1. Viral: Hepatitis A, B, Delta, NonA-NonB, EBV, CMV.
      2. Drugs/Toxins: carbon tetrachloride, acetaminophen, halothane, INH, oral contraceptives, alphamethyldopa, alcohol
   B. Clinical Features.
      1. Usually systemic and variable symptoms.
      2. Can include jaundice, dark urine, ascites, RUQ pain, pruritis, anorexia, nausea, vomiting.
   C. Diagnosis; Test for viral antigens/antibodies.
   D. Laboratory features.
      1. Variable increases in liver enzymes.
      2. Prognosis worse for increased PT/PTT, bilirubin; decreased albumin, glucose.

Table 4-2. Comparisons of type A, type B, and non-A, non-B hepatitis

Feature	Hepatitis A	Hepatitis B	Non-A, non-B hepatitis
Incubation	15-45 days (mean 30)	30-180 days (mean 60-90)	15-160 (mean 50)
Onset	Acute	Often insidious	Insidious
Age preference	Children, young adults	Any age	Any age but more common in adults
Transmission route:			
Fecal-oral	+++	-	Unknown
Other nonpercutaneous	+/-	++	++
Percutaneous	+/-	+++	+++
Severity	Mild	Often severe	Moderate
Prognosis	Generally good	Worse with age, debility	Moderate
Progression to chronicity	None	Occasional (5-10%)	Occasional (10-50%)

Table 4-2 (continued)

Feature	Hepatitis A	Hepatitis B	Non-A, non-B hepatitis
Prophylaxis	IG	Standard IG (not documented) HBIG, hepatitis B vaccine	?
Carrier	None	0.1-30%	Exists but prevalence unknown

- E. Complications: Fulminant hepatitis, chronic hepatitis, hepatoma.
- F. Management.
    1. Discontinue hepatotoxic drugs.
    2. Supportive care (especially nutrition).
    3. Limit protein intake.
    4. Cholestyramine for pruritis.
    5. Enteric precautions (HepA).
    6. Blood/body fluid precautions (HepB, Delta, NonA-NonB).
    7. Immunization/prophylaxis for close contacts.
    8. Steroid for chronic hepatitis.

II. **Alcoholic Liver Disease**; includes fatty liver, alcoholic hepatitis, cirrhosis
   A. Etiology: Chronic alcohol ingestion, familial risk.
   B. Clinical features.
      1. Fatty liver: symptoms usually minimal. Hepatomegaly usually only sign.
      2. Hepatitis.
         a. Resembles viral hepatitis.
         b. Tender hepatomegaly is common.
      3. Cirrhosis.
         a. May be clinically silent.
         b. Symptoms include weight loss, malnutrition, fatigue, easy bruising, progressive jaundice, GI bleeding, ascites, encephalopathy.

C. Other clinical features of alcoholic liver disease: firm nodular liver which may be large or small, jaundice, palmar erythema, spider angiomas, parotid/lacrimal enlargement, clubbing, splenomegaly, muscle wasting, ascites, gynecomastia, female escutcheon, testicular atrophy, Dupuytren's contractures, asterixis.

D. Prognosis; worse with continued alcohol usage, ascites, encephalopathy, malnutrition, esophageal varices.

E. Treatment.
   1. Total abstention from alcohol.
   2. Alcoholic rehabilitation.
   3. Supportive care for liver disease.
   4. Avoid hepatically-metabolized drugs.

Reference

Petersdorf RG, *et al*, eds. Harrison's Principles of Internal Medicine, 10th edition. New York: McGraw Hill, 1983.

ACUTE DIARRHEA

I. **Definition**
   A. Abnormally increased frequency or decreased consistency of stools of less than 2-3 weeks duration.
   B. Usually secretory or exudative diarrhea.
   C. Large quantities of watery stool passed frequently suggests osmotic or secretory diarrhea.
   D. Frequent passage of small, solid stools admixed with gas suggest motility disorder or irritable bowel disease.
   E. Frequent tenesmus with passage of small blood-tinged feces suggests inflammatory diarrhea.

II. **Noninvasive** (Minimal or absent constitutional symptoms)
   A. Often present with cramping/bloating/periumbilical pain with large watery stools.
   B. Fecal blood and leukocytes usually negative.
   C. Etiology.
      1. Viruses (esp. Rotavirus, Norwalk agent).
      2. Campylobacter Enterotoxigenic E. coli, Giardia, Entamoeba histolytica, Cholera, Food poisonings.
      3. Pseudomembranous colitis.
      4. Drugs (esp. laxative/sorbitol usage).
      5. Psychogenic stress.

III. **Invasive** (Dysentery)
   A. Constitutional symptoms often present with fever, lower abdominal pain, tenesmus, bloody stools, fecal blood or leukocytes usually present.
   B. Etiology.
      1. Shigella, Salmonella, Yersinia, enteroinvasive E. coli.
      2. Acute proctocolitis (esp. with ulcerative colitis).
      3. Diverticulosis.

IV. **Diagnosis**
   A. Stool for leukocytes (>5/HPF implies invasive disease).
   B. Cultures for suspected invasive disease.

C. Sigmoidoscopy especially for:
   1. Pseudomembranous (yellow/grey plaques).
   2. Ulcerative (friable edematous mucosa).
D. Stool for C. difficile titer (especially if history of antibiotic usage).
E. Ova and parasites (Giardia/Amebiasis).
F. Small bowel aspiration or string test (Giardia).

V. Treatment/Supportive Measures

1. Rehydration.
   a. Oral (clear liquids, sodium + glucose containing solutions).
   b. Intravenous (especially if severely dehydrated or with intractable vomiting).
2. Binding agents (e.g., Kaopectate).
3. Antisecretory agents (e.g., bismuth).
4. Antiperistaltics.
   a. Lomotil: combination of diphenoxylate (chemically related to the narcotic meperidine) and atropine, available in tablets (2.5 mg of diphenoxylate) and liquid (2.5 mg of diphenoxylate/5 ml). Initial dose for adults is two tablets four times daily (20 mg/day). For children the dose is 0.1 mg/kg per dose, four times daily. The dose is tapered to maintenance as diarrhea improves. It is not indicated for diarrhea from pseudomembranous colitis or enterotoxin-producing or invasive bacteria. Should not be used in ulcerative colitis or in children less than 2 years of age.
   b. Imodium: loperamide, available in 2 mg capsules and 1 mg/5ml liquid. Dose is 4 mg initially, followed by 2 mg after each diarrhea stool, not to exceed 16 mg in one 24 hour period for adults. In children the dose is based upon age with 2-5 year old children receiving 1 mg tid, 6-8 year olds receiving 2 mg bid and 9-12 year olds receiving 2 mg tid on the first day of treatment. Thereafter, 0.1mg/kg is administered after each

diarrhea stool, not to exceed the total daily dose recommended for the first day of therapy.

5. Antibiotics: Not needed for most diarrheas, should be directed at known or strongly suggested pathogens

References

Petersdorf RG, *et al*, eds. Harrison's Principles of Internal Medicine, 10th edition. New York: McGraw Hill, 1983.

Rakel RE and Conn HF, eds. Textbook of Family Practice, Third edition. Philadelphia: W.B. Saunders Company, 1984.

CHRONIC DIARRHEA

I. Definition
   A. Diarrhea persisting from weeks to months.
   B. Often can be intermittent and functional in etiology but must look for manifestations of systemic disease.

II. Etiology
   A. Diarrhea with inflammatory symptoms.
      1. Crohn's Disease.
      2. Ulcerative Colitis.
      3. Amebiasis.
      4. Diverticulitis.
      5. AIDS.
   B. Diarrhea without inflammatory symptoms.
      1. Inadequate digestion: primary liver or biliary tract disease, pancreatic disease (chronic pancreatitis, alcoholism, cystic fibrosis).
      2. Infections (amebiasis, giardiasis).
      3. Endocrine Disorders: Thyrotoxicosis, diabetes, adrenal insufficiency, hypoparathyroidism, Zollinger-Ellison syndrome.
      4. Inadequate surface area, short bowel syndrome, fistulas.
      5. Inflammatory bowel disease (Crohn's Disease).
      6. Motility disorders, irritable bowel syndrome.
      7. Functional: psychogenic stress.
      8. Fecal impaction.

III. Evaluation - examine for abdominal tenderness, weight loss, anemia, impaction

IV. Diagnosis
   A. Identify class of diarrhea and most likely etiology.
   B. Stool for fat to identify malabsorption.
   C. Radiologic studies (identify ulcers, fistula, abnormal mucosa).

- D. Small intestinal biopsy (useful for Whipple's, Sprue, regional enteritis, parasites).
- E. D-xylose absorption (decreased in disorders of proximal small intestine).
- F. Breath hydrogen test for lactase deficiency.
- G. Labs - Calcium, albumin, cholesterol, magnesium, iron, vitamin B12 carotene, PT, PTT (often abnormal with malabsorption)

V. **Treatment**
- A. Treat underlying cause.
- B. Limit dietary intake of inciting agent (lactose, fat, gluten, alcohol).
- C. Pancreatic enzyme supplements for pancreatic exocrine deficiency.
- D. Increase dietary or supplemental fiber.
- E. Antiperistaltic agents may be useful in certain patients.

References

Petersdorf RG, *et al*, eds. Harrison's Principles of Internal Medicine, 10th edition. New York: McGraw Hill, 1983.

Rakel RE and Conn HF, eds. Textbook of Family Practice, Third edition. Philadelphia: W.B. Saunders Company, 1984.

CONSTIPATION

I. **Definition:** Increased consistency or decreased frequency of bowel movements

II. **Etiology**
   A. Drugs (esp. analgesics, antacids, anticholinergics, antidepressants, barium, bismuth, diuretics, iron).
   B. Dietary (inadequate fluid or fiber intake).
   C. Large bowel disease: anal fissure, diverticular disease, irritable bowel syndrome, rectal prolapse, scleroderma, strictures, tumor.
   D. Metabolic (esp. amyloidosis, diabetes, hypothyroidism, hypercalcemia, hypokalemia, porphyria, pregnancy, uremia).
   E. Neurogenic (esp. s/p CVA's, Hirschsprung's disease, multiple sclerosis, Parkinson's disease, Shy-Drager syndrome).

III. **Treatment** - Stepwise after evaluating underlying etiology
   A. Increase dietary fiber and fluids.
   B. Use supplemental fiber (e.g. psyllium, methylcellulose).
   C. Stool softeners (e.g., mineral oil, Docusate).
   D. Nonabsorbable carbohydrates (e.g., lactulose, sorbitol).
   E. Stimulant laxatives (bisacodyl, castor oil, phenolphthalein, senna, casanthrol, cascara).

IV. **Complications of Constipation/Treatment**
   A. Damage to bowel structure or function: diverticular disease, hemorrhoids, fecal impaction, rectal incontinence, rectal ulcer or fissure, melanosis coli (with laxative abuse), diarrhea (esp. with stimulant laxatives).
   B. Electrolyte abnormalities (esp. with ionic or stimulant laxatives).
   C. Lipoid pneumonia (with aspiration of mineral oil).

References

Petersdorf RG, *et al*, eds. Harrison's Principles of Internal Medicine, 10th edition. New York: McGraw Hill, 1983.

Rakel RE and Conn HF, eds. Textbook of Family Practice, Third edition. Philadelphia: W.B. Saunders Company, 1984.

COLORECTAL TUMORS

I. **Epidemiology**

   3rd most common site of cancer (exceeded by skin and lung). Two-thirds of people over age 60 will have adenomas. Five percent of all adults will eventually develop cancer of colon or rectum.

   A. Predisposing factors.
      1. Personal or family history.
      2. Environmental toxins.
      3. High fat, low fiber diet.
      4. Preexisting adenomas.
      5. Inflammatory bowel disease.
      6. Gardner's Syndrome (familial polyposis, osteomas and soft tissue tumors).
      7. Familial polyposis.
      8. Peutz-Jeghers syndrome (GI hamartomas with mucocutaneous pigmentation).
      9. Malignant tumors are thought to arise from benign colonic polyps.

   B. Types of polyps.
      1. Villous adenomas (largest, highest malignant potential).
      2. Tubular adenomas.
      3. Hyperplastic polyps (smallest, questionable malignant potential, most common).
      4. Juvenile polyps (hamartomas arising in childhood).
      5. Inflammatory polyps.

II. **Clinical Manifestations**

   A. Rectal bleeding (gross or occult).
   B. Anemia (iron deficiency anemia in male or postmenopausal woman should raise suspicion of cancer).
   C. Abdominal pain (vague, poorly localized).
   D. Change in bowel habits (decrease in caliber of stools, increasing laxative usage, tenesmus).

Colorectal Tumors

- E. Palpable mass (esp. cecal CA).
- F. Large bowel obstruction.
- G. Asymptomatic (majority of cases).

III. **Diagnosis and Screening Measures** (American Cancer Society)

    A. Screening.
1. Digital.
2. Fecal occult.
   a. False positives can be produced by red meat, horseradish, ASA, NSAID.
   b. False negatives can be produced by Vitamin C.

    B. Diagnosis: evaluation of patient with positive screening test or other clinical indication (see above).
1. Flexible sigmoidoscopy: if any polyp is found, patient will require barium enema and colonoscopy to evaluate rest of colon.
2. Barium enema - complementary exam with sigmoidoscopy, useful to evaluate areas of colon unable to be directly visualized. Will miss smaller lesions, increased yield with air contrast.
3. Colonoscopy; best test to evaluate small proximal lesions and as screening in patient with known carcinoma (synchronous lesions or distal polyps).

IV. **Prognosis** - best with low stage lesions.

    A. Duke's Classification.
1. Stage A - Cancer in mucosa.
2. Stage B - Cancer in muscularis.
3. Stage C - Cancer in regional lymph nodes.
4. Stage D - Distant metastases.

References

Petersdorf RG, *et al*, eds. <u>Harrison's Principles of Internal Medicine, 10th edition</u>. New York: McGraw Hill, 1983.

Rakel RE and Conn HF, eds. <u>Textbook of Family Practice, Third edition</u>. Philadelphia: W.B. Saunders Company, 1984.

ANORECTAL DISEASES

I. Hemorrhoids

A. Definition; dilated normal anal veins.

B. Etiology - Increased abdominal pressure secondary to constipation, cirrhosis, pregnancy.

C. Classification - External vs. internal - arising below or above pectinate line.

   1. Grade 1 - Smallest; no prolapse.
   2. Grade 2 - Prolapse with spontaneous reduction.
   3. Grade 3 - Prolapse with manual reduction.
   4. Grade 4 - Permanently prolapsed.

D. Symptoms.

   1. Bright red bleeding with defecation.
   2. External protrusion.
   3. Tenderness.
   4. Itching.
   5. Mucous staining of perineum.

E. Complication: Thrombosis - tender swollen hemorrhoidal clot.

F. Treatment.

   1. Avoidance of constipation (dietary fiber, stool softeners).
   2. Reduce inflammation (Sitz baths, ice packs, steroid/anesthetic ointments).
   3. Fixation procedures (rubber band ligation, cryotherapy, injection).
   4. Thrombus enucleation.
   5. Surgical hemorrhoidectomy.

II. Fissures

A. Definition - elliptical ulcerations in anus, usually posteriorly in midline.

B. Etiology.

   1. Trauma (constipation).
   2. Internal sphincter spasm.

C. Classification.
   1. Acute vs. chronic.
   2. Primary (idiopathic) vs. secondary (Trauma - constipation, foreign body, childbirth, Crohn's Disease, Leukemia).
D. Symptoms.
   1. Pain with defecation (can persist for hours).
   2. Bleeding.
   3. Pruritis.
E. Diagnosis.
   1. Inspection/Anoscopy.
   2. Classic triad - sentinel pile, fissure at anal verge, hypertrophied anal papilla proximal to fissure.
F. Treatment.
   1. Acute:
   - Sitz baths.
   - Stool softeners.
   - Topical anesthetics.
   2. Chronic:
   - Internal sphincterotomy.

III. **Anorectal Abscess**
   A. Etiology - bacterial invasion of perirectal spaces, usually from an anal crypt. Generally a mixed bacterial infection.
   B. Diagnosis:
   1. Symptoms may include pain, swelling, redness for superficial abscesses, but deeper abscesses may present only with toxic symptoms.
   2. Exam will reveal area of inflammation for superficial infections, tenderness on digital rectal exam for deeper infections.
   C. Treatment: Incision and drainage is necessary. Antibiotics will be of limited benefit. Complication resulting from such treatment can be fistula formation.

Reference

Rakel RE and Conn HF, eds. <u>Textbook of Family Practice, Third edition</u>. Philadelphia: W.B. Saunders Company, 1984.

5/ HEMATOLOGIC, ELECTROLYTE, AND METABOLIC DISORDERS

J. Matthew Johnson, M.D., Becky Leidal, M.D., and John E. Littler, M.D.

BLEEDING DISORDERS

I. **Differential Diagnosis**
   A. Qualitative Platelet Disorders.
      1. Defective adhesion.
         a. Von Willebrand's disease. Autosomal dominant disease, abnormal synthesis of glycoprotein polymer necessary for platelet adhesion to site of vascular injury. Also a decrease in factor VIII pro-coagulant.
         b. Acquired secondary to semi-synthetic penicillin and cephalosporins.
      2. Defective activation and secretion
         a. Non-steroidal anti-inflammatory drugs.
         b. Dipyridamole.
         c. Cardiopulmonary bypass.
   B. Quantitative Platelet Defects.
      1. Thrombocytosis, occurs in myeloproliferative disease. Can lead to bleeding problems.
      2. Increased destruction. Immunologic, occurs with drugs such as quinidine, methyldopa, sulfa, phenytoin, barbiturates, and with lupus, viral infection, ITP.
      3. Decreased production.
         a. Marrow failure. Associated with pancytopenia, but certain drugs (chlorothiazides, tolbutamide, ethanol) may cause only thrombocytopenia. Marrow failure may be due to a myelophthisic process.
      4. Increased pooling. Occurs with splenomegaly.

C. Defects of the Intrinsic Pathway
   1. Hemophilia A. Deficiency of factor VIII, X-linked recessive.
   2. Hemophilia B. Deficiency of factor IX, X-linked recessive.
   3. Factor XI deficiency. Autosomal recessive disease, occurs primarily in Ashkenazi Jews.
D. Defects of the Extrinsic Pathway.
   1. Hepatocellular insufficiency.
   2. Cholestasis. Absorption of lipid soluble vitamin K is impaired.
   3. Poor dietary intake of vitamin K.
   4. Broad spectrum antibiotics.
   5. Coumarin anticoagulants.
E. Vascular defects.
   1. Senile purpura. Petechiae in elderly secondary to atrophy of connective and fatty tissue.
   2. Cushing's syndrome. Bleeding secondary to atrophy of connective tissue.
   3. Scurvy. Collagen synthesis is defective.
   4. Purpura simplex. Mild condition which occurs in healthy women, and is probably associated with NSAID'S.
   5. Hereditary Connective Tissue Disorders: Ehlers-Danlos syndrome, Marfan's syndrome, Osler-Weber-Rendu syndrome.
   6. Drug induced vascular purpura. Caused by a variety of drugs including procaine penicillin, thiazides, quinine, iodides, sulfas, coumarins.
   7. Paraproteinemias: cryoglobulinemia, macroglobulinemia, myeloma.
   8. Miscellaneous: SLE, rhematoid arthritis, Sjogrens syndrome, amyloidosis.
F. Mixed Defects: seen in chronic renal failure, chronic liver disease, and DIC.

II. Clinical Presentation

A. History. Bleeding from multiple sites, spontaneous bleeding, ecchymosis greater than three centimeters in diameter, prolonged bleeding after surgical procedures suggest diathesis.

1. Assess for volume depletion (orthostatic symptoms, dry mouth, thirst, reduced urine output).
2. History suggesting platelet dysfunction; petechiae, purpura, limited to mucosal membranes, bleeding that is immediate and transient.
3. History suggesting coagulation defects; spontaneous bleeding, bleeding into joints of soft tissues, hemorrhage into GI or GU tracts.
4. Onset of bleeding problem in childhood suggests hereditary disorder.
5. Medication usage, specifically semi-synthetic penicillins, cephalosporins, dipyridamole, thiazide, alcohol, quinidine, methyldopa, sulfa, phenytoin, barbiturates, coumarin.

B. Physical Examination.

1. Vital signs. Orthostatic changes signify significant volume loss.
2. General appearance (Cushingoid, Marfan-like).
3. Petechiae (less than 3mm), ecchymosis (greater than 3mm) are suggestive of thrombocytopenia, qualitative platelet defects, and vascular defects.
4. Telangiectasias suggest Osler-Weber-Rendu syndrome.
5. Check mucous membranes for petechiae, which would suggest a platelet disorder.
6. Hemarthrosis suggests a clotting factor problem.
7. Look for hepatomegaly and splenomegaly.
8. Do a rectal exam for evidence of GI bleeding.

C. Lab Studies.

1. PT to assess extrinsic system.
2. PTT to assess intrinsic system (85% of hereditary coagulation disorders will have elevated PTT).
3. Platelet count.

162 Hematologic, Electrolyte, and Metabolic Disorders

4. Bleeding time.

III. Management

A. Thrombocytopenia.
   1. General Considerations.
      a. Platelet counts of 50,000 or greater not associated with significant bleeding.
      b. Spontaneous bleeding occurs with counts less than 20,000.
      c. Patients with thrombocytopenia should be instructed to avoid trauma and to seek early treatment following trauma.
      d. Platelet transfusions are reserved for patients with serious hemorrhage or before surgery.
   2. ITP.
      a. For the acute, self-limited form which occurs in children after viral infections, only symptomatic therapy is required. 90% will recover in three to six months.
      b. For chronic ITP: Because thrombocytopenia may be the initial manifestation of SLE or a primary hematologic disorder, all patients should have a bone marrow examination and ANA. Prednisone at a dose of 1-2 mg/kg/day until the platelet count is greater than 100,000 is recommended. For patients who are not responsive to steroids, splenectomy is recommended.
   3. TTP.
      a. Presents with thrombocytopenia, microangiopathic hemolytic anemia, and fluctuating neurologic abnormalities often with fever and renal dysfunction.
      b. Medical emergency. Treatment involves:
   - Plasma infusion 2 units IV q 6h.
   - Plasmaphoresis.
   - Aspirin 325 mg po qd.
   - Methylprednisolone 1 mg/kg IV.
   - Dipyridamole 75 mg po q 6h.

B. Coagulation Factor Deficiencies.

Bleeding Disorders

1. Factor replacement therapy.
   a. Fresh frozen plasma. Contains all of the coagulation factors in nearly normal concentrations. This is useful for patients with liver disease with multiple factor deficiency who require infrequent therapy.
   b. Cryoprecipitate. Contains factor VIII, VWF, and fibrinogen. This is treatment of choice for von Willebrand's disease.
   c. Factor VIII concentrate. Contains a high concentration of factor VIII, and variable amount of von Willebrand's factor. Greater transmission of hepatitis and HIV virus.
   d. Prothrombin complex concentration. Contains 500-1000 IU of prothrombin, factor X, and factor IX.
2. Hemophilia.
   a. Factor VIII deficiency.
- Minor cuts and abrasions, superficial ecchymosis, and non-traumatic hematuria require no therapy.
- Uncomplicated hemarthrosis, non-critical hematomas, and traumatic hematuria are treated with cryoprecipitate to achieve a factor VIII level of 50%.
- Life threatening hemorrhage and hematomas in critical locations require cryoprecipitate to achieve a factor VIII level of 100%.
   b. Factor IX deficiency.
- Minimal bleeding can be treated with FFP.
- Major hemorrhage is treated with prothrombin complex concentrate.
   c. Treatment of hemarthrosis.
- Immediate factor replacement.
- Immobilize joint for 2-3 days.
3. Von Willebrand's disease. Treatment involves cryoprecipitate infusion to achieve factor levels of 30-50%. A single infusion is enough to control mild bleeding. If bleeding persists, repeat the infusion every 12 hours.

164 Hematologic, Electrolyte, and Metabolic Disorders

   4. Vitamin K deficiency.
      a. Vitamin K is needed for carboxylation of factors II, VII, IX, X, protein C, and protein S.
      b. For serious hemorrhage, infuse FFP 15mg/kg IV, then 5-8mg/kg IV q8-12 hours.
      c. Mild Vitamin K deficiencies can be treated with 10-15mg IV or SQ qd for 1-3 days.
   5. Liver disease.
      a. Fresh frozen plasma.
      b. Vitamin K 10-15 mg IV or SQ for three days.
   6. Disseminated Intravascular Coagulation.
      a. Treat underlying disorder.
      b. Unless serious hemorrhage or thrombosis appear, therapy specific for DIC should be withheld.
      c. For bleeding complications, FFP and cryoprecipitate may be used.
      d. For thrombotic complications, low dose heparin at a dose of 500 units per hour by continuous IV infusion may be used.

References

Goroll AH, *et al*, eds. Primary Care Medicine: Office Evaluation and Management of the Adult Patient. Philadelphia: J.B. Lippincott Co., 1987.

Petersdorf RG, *et al*, eds. Harrison's Principles of Internal Medicine, 10th edition. New York: McGraw Hill, 1983.

Spivak JL and Barnes HV. Manual of Clinical Problems in Internal Medicine, 3rd edition. Boston/Toronto: Little, Brown & Company, 1983.

ANEMIA

(See also Pediatric section, Anemia)

I. **Microcytic Anemias**
   A. Iron deficiency:
      1. Etiology: Increased requirements (i.e., infancy, adolescence, pregnancy), inadequate intake, decreased absorption, (gastrectomy, achlorhydria, chronic diarrhea), blood loss, (women-menses, men-GI).
      2. Exam: skin may show pallor, nails may be dry and brittle with ridges, cardiovascular exam may reveal tachycardia and flow murmur. HEENT exam may demonstrate stomatitis or glossitis.
      3. Lab: CBC will show microcytic, hypochromic cells. Iron studies will show low serum ferritin, increased TIBC, low serum iron. FEP will be mildly elevated.
      4. Treatment: Ferrous sulfate 325 mg po tid on an empty stomach. Calcium and magnesium may impair Fe absorption. Better absorbed if administered between meals on an empty stomach, but less GI upset if taken with meals. Treat for six months to replace body stores.
   B. Sideroblastic anemia.
      1. Etiology: Hereditary, acquired (drugs and toxins--alcohol, lead, INH, chloramphenicol), neoplasia and inflammation (rheumatoid arthritis, carcinoma, lymphoma, leukemia), malnutrition (folate deficiency), idiopathic.
      2. Lab: CBC may show normochromic or hypochromic cells. Anisocytosis and poikilocytosis are pronounced. Sideroblasts may or may not be present. Iron studies will show increased serum iron, increased transferrin saturation, decreased TIBC.
      3. Treatment.
         a. Withdraw offending agent.
         b. Pyridoxine 200 mg qd x 2-3 months.
         c. Androgens may be of benefit.

166 Metabolic, Hematologic, and Electrolyte Disorders

C. Anemia of chronic disease.
 1. Etiology: chronic infections (SBE, osteomyelitis, TB), chronic medical disorders (RA, SLE, sarcoidosis, renal failure), neoplasms.
 2. Lab: Hemoglobin generally between 9 and 11 mg/dl. Cells may be normocytic or microcytic. Retic count usually less than 3%. Serum ferritin will be increased, TIBC and serum iron will be decreased.
 3. Treatment: Treat underlying disease. Transfuse only as needed for symptoms.

D. Sickle-cell anemia.
 1. Etiology: Abnormal substitution of saline for glutamate in position 6 of the beta chain.
 2. Diagnosis: hemoglobin electrophoresis. CBC/smear may show normochromic normocytic/microcytic anemia, sickled cells.

E. Thalassemias.
 1. Group of disorders in which there is a defect in the synthesis of one of the subunits of hemoglobin. The abnormality is quantitative rather than qualitative (i.e., in beta thalassemias the beta chain is normal in structure but produced in reduced or undetectable amounts).
 2. Alpha thalassemia:
    a. Silent carrier state. One of the four genes is deleted. No hematologic abnormalities.
    b. Alpha thalassemia trait. Either have homozygous alpha thalassemia 2(a-,a-) or heterozygous alpha thalassemia 1(--,aa). RBC's are microcytic, hypochromic. No significant anemia. Hemoglobin shows a decrease in Hgb A2.
    c. Hemoglobin H disease. Four beta chains.
 3. Beta Thalassemia Minor:
    a. Clinical Presentation. Symptoms of anemia (weakness, fatigue, lassitude, palpitations, lightheadedness), splenomegaly, icterus. Cells are microcytic. Examination of peripheral

smear shows target cells, cigar-shaped cells and basophilic stippling.
  b. Diagnosis. Hemoglobin electrophoresis shows increased Hgb A2 and possibly an increase of hemoglobin F.
  c. Treatment. None. Genetic Counseling is necessary.
4. Beta Thalassemia Major (Cooley's anemia):
  a. Clinical presentation. Manifestations begin approximately 4-6 months of life. Usually present with severe anemia (Hct less than 20%). There is marked wasting, slow growth and development, and delayed onset of secondary sex features. The patient will have skeletal abnormalities secondary to bone marrow expansion.
  b. Diagnosis. Hemoglobin electrophoresis shows large amounts of Hgb F with variable amounts of Hgb A.
  c. Treatment. Transfusion, splenectomy, desferoxamine, folic acid supplementation.

II. Normochromic-Normocytic Anemias

A. Hemolytic anemias: manifestations include fever, chills, tachycardia, tachypnea, backache, hemoglobinuria. Can progress to renal failure. Laboratory evaluation will show normochromic-normocytic anemia, elevated indirect bilirubin with normal direct bilirubin. Haptoglobin will be decreased.

  1. Antibody-induced hemolytic anemia:
     a. warm antibodies:
  - May be primary or occur secondary to underlying disease affecting the immune system (i.e., CLL, non-Hodgkins lymphoma, SLE). Commonly occurs with drugs (penicillin, alpha methyl dopa, INH, sulfonamides). May present with only positive direct Coombs test.
  - No therapy required if disease is mild. With significant hemolysis, prednisone at dose of 1mg/kg/d, transfusions, splenectomy, and cytotoxic agents

(Cytoxan, Immuran) all have been used with some success.

b. cold antibodies:

- These antibodies agglutinate RBC's by IgM cold agglutinins at cold temperatures. Seen with mycoplasma pneumoniae, infectious mononucleosis, and lymphoid neoplasms.
- Maintain patient in warm environment. Chlorambucil and cyclophosphamide are the most commonly employed agents in those patients in whom therapy is indicated.

2. Trauma in the circulation:
   a. Abnormalities of the vessel wall: seen in malignant hypertension, eclampsia, TTP.
   b. Diagnosis. Hemolytic anemia, fragmented and nucleated RBC's, thrombocytopenia, fever, neurologic dysfunction, and renal dysfunction.
   c. Therapy. Corticosteroids, plasma exchange, splenectomy, and anti-platelet drugs.
3. Hemolytic Uremic syndrome.
4. Disseminated Intravascular Coagulation.
5. Membrane abnormalities.
   a. Acquired.

- Spur cell anemia. Occurs in patients with severe hepatocellular disease. Clinical manifestations include a hematocrit between 16 and 30 per cent. splenomegaly, jaundice, hepatitis, encephalopathy, and prolonged prothrombin time. Diagnosis is made by demonstrating an elevated reticulocyte count, elevated bilirubin, and characteristic spur cells on peripheral smear. Treatment is splenectomy.
- Paroxysmal Nocturnal Hemoglobinuria. This disease is caused by an increased sensitivity to complement. It is manifested by anemia of varying degrees, intermittent hemoglobinuria, hemosiderinuria, low leukocyte alkaline phosphatase, a positive acid or sucrose hemolysis test, and venous thrombosis. Transfusions androgens, and iron supplementations are the mainstay of treatment.

b. Congenital: Hereditary spherocytosis, hereditary elliptocytosis, hereditary stomatocytosis. Diagnosis is made by demonstrating the characteristic morphology. Treatment is splenectomy.

B. Aplastic Anemia

1. Etiology: Congenital, drugs and toxins, (anti-neoplastic drugs, immunosuppresive drugs, ionizing radiation, benzene derivative, chloramphenicol), infectious hepatitis.

2. Clinical Manifestations: Weakness and fatigue from anemia, bleeding from thrombocytopenia. Course may be mild or severe.

3. Diagnosis: CBC will show pancytopenia with normochromic-normocytic anemia. Retic count will be very low. Bone marrow will show hypocellularity. Serum iron will be elevated with normal TIBC.

4. Therapy: supportive care, transfusions as needed. Androgens may stimulate marrow. Immunosuppressants.

C. Other causes of normocytic-normochromic anemias:

1. Anemia of Chronic Renal Failure.

   a. Pathophysiology: decreased production of erythropoietin.

   b. Diagnosis: normochromic-normocytic anemia, sometimes quite severe. Normal retic count. Burr cells may be present.

   c. Therapy: Anemia improves after dialysis, transplantation. Androgens can increase the hematocrit.

2. Marrow infiltration.
3. Hypothyroidism.
4. Cirrhosis.
5. Early Iron deficiency.

III. **Macrocytic Anemias**

A. Etiologies: Vitamin B12 deficiency (malabsorption from pernicious anemia, gastrectomy, Crohn's, sprue), folic acid deficiency (usually due to poor intake--alcoholics,

170 Metabolic, Hematologic, and Electrolyte Disorders

indigent, or increased demand--pregnancy, hemolytic anemias), drugs (including methotrexate, nitrous oxide, phenytoin, phenobarbital).

B. Clinical Presentation.
   1. B12 deficiency:
      a. Symptoms of anemia (weakness, lightheadedness, vertigo, tinnitus, angina, symptoms of CHF). Gastrointestinal symptoms (sore tongue, anorexia, weight loss, diarrhea). Neurological symptoms (numbness, paresthesias, weakness, ataxia, sphincter dysfunction).
      b. Signs include those of anemia (pallor, tachycardia, etc.) and neurological signs of hyper- or hyporeflexia, positive Romberg, impaired positional and vibratory sensation, depressed mentation. Neurologic disease may occur with normal hematocrit.
   2. Folate deficiency. Signs and symptoms are the same as in B12 deficiency, except that the patient is more likely to be malnourished and neurologic abnormalities do not occur.

C. Diagnosis: Elevated MCV, low retic count, thrombocytopenia, leukopenia. Smear shows anisocytosis, poikilocytosis, basophilic stippling, hypersegmentation of neutrophils. Low B12 and folate levels. Once the diagnosis of B12 deficiency is made a Schiller's test can identify the pathophysiology.

D. Therapy.
   1. B12 deficiency. Intramuscular cyanocobalmin 100 micrograms for seven days, then twice weekly for one to two months. In cases of documented B12 deficiency associated with a chronic condition lifelong therapy is usually required with 1000 micrograms of cyanocobalmin IM monthly.
   2. Folate deficiency. One milligram of folic acid p.o. q.d. for two to three weeks.
   3. Blood transfusions are usually not required.
   4. Empiric therapy before a diagnosis is established can be dangerous. A patient deficient in B12 may have a

hematologic response to folic acid, but an exacerbation of neurologic symptoms.

References

Goroll AH, *et al*, eds. <u>Primary Care Medicine: Office Evaluation and Management of the Adult Patient</u>. Philadelphia: J.B. Lippincott Co., 1987.

Petersdorf RG, *et al*, eds. <u>Harrison's Principles of Internal Medicine, 10th edition</u>. New York: McGraw Hill, 1983.

Spivak JL and Barnes HV, eds. <u>Manual of Clinical Problems in Internal Medicine, 3rd edition</u>. Boston/Toronto: Little, Brown & Company, 1983.

172 Hematologic, Electrolyte, and Metabolic Disorders

POTASSIUM

I. **Overview**

Total body potassium is approximately 50 mEq/kg body weight. 98% is intracellular; serum decrease of 1 mEq K^+ corresponds to a 10-20% deficit of total body potassium. Distribution affected by Na-K ATPase activity within cell membranes, H^+ concentration in extracellular fluid, insulin, epinephrine, aldosterone, cell membrane permeability. Serum K^+ concentration is not always a reliable indicator of total body K^+. Total body K^+ is largely controlled by the kidney with 90% of ingested K^+ excreted in the urine. 10% of the daily K^+ load is excreted in the GI tract (in uremic pts this may increase to 33%). Normally there is no significant K^+ loss through the skin; with profuse sweating the K^+ loss through the skin may approach 24% of the daily K^+ load. 5-15 mEq of K^+ are lost daily in the urine even with no K^+ intake.

II. **Hypokalemia**: serum K^+ level below lab's normal limits.

   A. Etiology.

   1. GI losses of K^+ seen in vomiting, NG suction, diarrhea, malabsorption syndrome, laxative or enema abuse. Villous adenomas may excrete K^+, associated with a large amount of mucous in the stools. GI losses distal to the stomach result in a low urine K^+ concentration and metabolic acidosis secondary to high bicarbonate losses. GI losses from the stomach result in a high urine K^+ concentration (usually > 40 mEq/L) and metabolic alkalosis secondary to high HCl loss.

   2. Diuretics. Thiazides, furosemide, ethacrynic acid and bumetanide. Maximal decrease in serum K^+ concentration is usually seen after 7 d of treatment. Degree of K^+ depletion dependent on Na^+ ingestion with severe salt restriction (< 2 g/d) or excessive Na^+ intake (10 g/d) resulting in increased K^+ loss. More likely to be significant K^+ loss if patient has edema (edematous states associated with elevated aldosterone which stimulates K^+ excretion). Serum K^+ concentration should be measured prior to initia-

tion of a diuretic and one week after initiation of or increase in dose of the diuretic. Serum K^+ measurement may be repeated annually in patients without edema on a stable diuretic dose, but more frequently in edematous patients.

3. Other causes of hypokalemia.

   a. Insufficient dietary K^+ is an unusual cause, seen occasionally in alcoholics or cachectic patients.

   b. Excessive renal losses: when hypokalemia occurs with a urine K^+ concentration > 20 mEq/L. Causes: hyperaldosteronism, Fanconi syndrome, glucocorticoid excess, magnesium deficiency, osmotic diuresis, renal tubular acidosis, diuretics and many antibiotics (carbenicillin, aminoglycosides).

   c. Maldistribution of K^+: alkalosis, insulin, and glucose cause a shift of K^+ from the ECF into the cells without depletion of total body K^+.

B. Presentation: weakness (especially of proximal muscles), postural hypotension, decreased GI motility resulting in ileus, muscle cramps, agitation, fatigue, and depression. Hyperpolarization of cardiac cells occurs with hypokalemia and may cause ventricular ectopy, re-entry phenomena, and conduction abnormalities. The EKG frequently shows flatted T waves, U waves and ST segment depression. Hypokalemia also causes increased sensitivity of cardiac cells to digitalis preparations and may result in toxicity at therapeutic plasma levels of digitalis.

C. Treatment.

1. Oral therapy. K^+ supplementation should be given at initiation of diuretic therapy in edematous patients. Recheck K^+ concentration 2-4 weeks after starting supplementation. Recheck every 3 months in edematous patients and every 6-12 months in non-edematous patients after stable. Patient should consume 100 mEq K^+ daily while taking a diuretic. Any K^+ salt may be used if it is to be given prophylactically. However, KCl must be used for correction of hypokalemia secondary to diuretic use since K^+ cor-

rection cannot be achieved without correction of the Cl deficit.

2. IV therapy should be used for servere hypokalemia and in patients unable to tolerate oral supplement. If serum K^+ concentrations >2.4 mEq/L and no EKG changes, K^+ can be given at a rate up to 10 mEq/hr with maximum daily administration of 100-200 mEq. Rapid treatment required if K^+ concentration is <2mEq/L with EKG changes. K^+ may be administered at rates up to 20 mEq/hr in concentrations up to 40 mEq/l via peripheral IV. Serum K^+ concentrations should be measured every 4-6 hours with the patient under continuous EKG monitoring until EKG changes resolve.

III. **Hyperkalemia**

A. Etiology.

1. Inadequate renal excretion: acute or chronic renal failure, potassium-sparing diuretics.

2. Potassium load may result from massive cell death due to crush injuries, major surgery, acute arterial emboli, hemolysis, GI bleeding or rhabdomyolysis. Exogenous sources such as ingestion of potassium supplements and salt substitutes, blood transfusions, IV potassium administration and high dose penicillin therapy must also be considered.

3. Intracellular to extracellular shift: acidosis, digitalis overdose, insulin deficiency, or rapid increase of blood osmolality.

4. Adrenal insufficiency.

5. Pseudohyperkalemia: secondary to hemolysis of blood sample or prolonged tourniquet time.

B. Presentation: weakness, paresthesia, areflexia, confusion and occasionally muscular and respiratory paralysis. Bradycardia, ventricular fibrillation, and asystole usually occur when the serum potassium level exceeds 8 mEq/L. EKG shows sequential changes with a rising serum potassium level. Initially, tall peaked T waves are seen, followed by depressed ST segments, decreased R wave amplitude, prolonged PR intervals, diminished P wave amplitude, widened QRS complexes and prolonged QT intervals which lead to a sine-wave pattern. Ventricular fibrillation or asystole are likely with potassium of > 10 mEq/L.

C. Treatment: Continuous EKG monitoring is warranted for detection of arrhythmias if EKG changes are present or if serum potassium is greater than 7 mEq/L.

1. Calcium gluconate may be administered IV as 5-10 ml of a 10% solution over 2 minutes to stabilize myocardium and cardiac conduction system. Effect is temporary. Administration of calcium may cause digitalis toxicity in patients on digitalis therapy.

2. Sodium bicarbonate alkalinizes the blood causing a shift of potassium from the extracellular fluid to the intracellular space. This is given as one ampule of 7.5% $NaHCO_3$ IV over 5 minutes and may be repeated in 10-15 minutes if needed. The effect is temporary.

3. Insulin causes a shift of potassium from the extracellular fluid into cells. 5-10 units of regular insulin should be administered with 1 ampul of 50% glucose IV over 5 minutes. A response may not be seen for 50-60 minutes and the effect usually lasts for several hours.

4. Cation-exchange resins such as Kayexalate remove potassium from the body by binding potassium in the GI tract in exchange for another cation (sodium in the case of Kayexalate and most other drugs in this class). These drugs may be given orally or rectally. The initial oral dose is 15-30 gr Kayexalate mixed with 50-100 ml of 70% sorbitol to counteract its constipating effect. The dose may be repeated every 3-4 hours to a total of 4-5 doses/day if needed. A retention enema is given as 50 gr Kayexalate mixed with 200 ml of 20% sorbitol or 20% D/W and may be repeated every 1-2 hours initially and then every 6 hours or as necessary. These agents cause a significant sodium load.

5. Dialysis may be required in severe, refractory cases of hyperkalemia.

6. Potassium restriction is indicated in the late stages of renal failure (GFR < 15 ml/min).
7. Adrenal insufficiency is treated with fludrocortisone, 0.05-0.2mg/day.

References

Barker LR, Burton JR, Zieve PD, eds. Principles of Ambulatory Medicine, 2nd edition. Baltimore: Williams and Wilkins, 1986.

Friedman HH, ed. Problem-Oriented Medical Diagnosis, 3rd edition. Boston/Toronto: Little Brown & Company, 1983.

Orland MJ and Saltman RJ, eds. Manual of Medical Therapeutics, 25th edition. Boston/Toronto: Little Brown & Company, 1986.

Rush DR and Hamburger S, eds. Hyponatremia. Southern Medical Journal 77(5):565-575, May 1984.

SODIUM

I. **Hypernatremia**
   A. Etiology.
      1. Occurs if hypotonic fluid losses are not adequately replaced. If fluid losses are extrarenal (GI losses, perspiration, or hyperventilation), the urine osmolality will be greater than that of the serum and urinary Na^+ will be <20 mEq/liter. A urine osmolality less than or equal to that of the serum implies renal fluid losses (diuretic therapy, osmotic diuresis, diabetes insipidus, acute tubular necrosis, postobstructive uropathy, hypokalemic nephropathy or hypercalcemic nephropathy).
      2. Hypernatremia may occur with hyperalimentation or other hypertonic fluid administration.
   B. Signs and symptoms: Muscle irritability, confusion, and seizures secondary to the hypernatremia. Additional manifestations usually occur secondary to the underlying abnormality and volume status (tachycardia and orthostatic hypotension with volume depletion; edema with fluid excess).
   C. Treatment.
      1. Hypernatremia with volume depletion should be treated by administration of isotonic saline until hemodynamic stability is achieved, then correcting the remaining water deficit with 5% D/W or hypotonic saline.
      2. Hypernatremia with volume excess is treated with diuresis or, if necessary, with dialysis. 5% D/W is then administered to replace the water deficit.
      3. Body water deficit is estimated by:
      - Deficit = desired TBW (liters) - Current TBW.
      - Desired TBW = measured serum Na^+ x current TBW/normal serum Na^+.
      - Current TBW = 0.6 x current body weight (kg).

      One half the calculated water deficit should be given in the first 24 hours and the remaining deficit corrected over 1-2 days to avoid cerebral edema secondary to abrupt change in serum sodium concentration.

II. **Hyponatremia**. Serum sodium concentration below the normal range. Not equivalent to sodium depletion.
   A. Etiology.
      1. Pseudohyponatremia: low measured plasma Na concentration secondary to hyperproteinemia, hyperlipidemia or hyperglycemia. Serum osmolality is normal in pseudohyponatremia and low in true hyponatremia (with the exception of true hyponatremia secondary to osmotic diuresis).
      2. Deficit of total body water and larger deficit of total body sodium. Extrarenal losses (protracted vomiting, diarrhea, burns, pancreatitis, traumatized muscle). Urine Na^+ concentration is < 20 mEq/L. Renal losses (diuretic excess, Addison's, renal tubular acidosis, osmotic diuresis) result in urine Na^+ and Cl concentrations of > 20 mEq/L.
      3. Normal or increased extracellular fluid and normal or slightly decreased total body sodium. This may be caused by hypothyroidism, secondary adrenal insufficiency, emotional stress, pain, drugs, SIADH. Urinary Na concentration is > 20 mEq/L in this type of hyponatremia.
      4. Excess total body sodium and larger excess of total body water: chronic sodium retaining disorders (CHF, cirrhosis, nephrotic syndrome) resulting in a urine Na concentration < 10 mEq/L. Acute and chronic renal failure may also cause this form of hyponatremia but with urine Na^+ and Cl concentrations > 20 mEq/L.
   B. Signs and symptoms: depend on severity and rapidity of fall of the plasma Na^+ concentration. A decrease in plasma Na^+ concentration to 10 mEq/L below normal over several hours will produce nausea, vomiting, headache, bloating, and muscle cramps. A more rapid fall may cause severe headache, lethargy, disorientation, increased intracranial pressure, stupor, coma, and seizures. The mortality rate is as high as 50% with a rapid fall in Na^+ concentration to < 113 mEq/L. Other manifestations are

related to fluid status (volume depletion with tachycardia, orthostatic hypotension, decrease skin turgor; sodium and water excess with edema or directly related to more precise etiology.

C. Treatment.

1. Sodium and water deficiency: volume deficit should be corrected with isotonic NaCl solution (see Hypernatremia for calculation of body water deficit). Rate of infusion should be based on CNS symptoms, cardiac and renal function. The underlying disorder must also be corrected.

2. Normal or slightly increased extracellular fluid with normal or slightly decreased total body sodium: fluid restriction to 500-1,000 cc daily with SIADH. Demeclocycline therapy (600 mg-1.2 grams daily in 3-4 divided doses) may be instituted to antagonize the ADH effect on the kidney. Demeclocycline is mainly excreted by the kidney and should be used with caution in patients with renal insufficiency. Acute water intoxication with CNS symptoms should be treated with furosemide and hypertonic saline to increase the plasma Na^+ concentrations halfway to normal within 6-8 hours. Na^+ and K^+ losses in the urine should be replaced hourly.

3. Excess sodium and body water: water restriction and frequently diuretics. Other treatment should be directed at underlying disorder (diuretics, vasodilators, and cardiac glycosides for CHF, steroids for nephrotic syndrome). Hypertonic saline should not be used.

References

Barker LR, Burton JR, Ziebe PD, eds. Principles of Ambulatory Medicine, 2nd edition. Baltimore: Williams and Wilkins, 1986.

Friedman HH, ed. Problem-Oriented Medical Diagnosis, 3rd edition. Boston/Toronto: Little Brown & Company, 1983.

Orland MJ and Saltman RJ, eds. Manual of Medical Therapeutics, 25th edition. Boston/Toronto: LIttle Brown & Company, 1986.

Rush DR and Hamburger S, eds. Hyponatremia. Southern Medical Journal 77(5):565-575, May 1984.

HYPOGLYCEMIA

Chemical hypoglycemia is defined as a plasma glucose less than 50 mg/dl and is frequently asymptomatic.

I. **Symptoms**

   A. Adrenergic symptoms occur when low blood glucose stimulates the release of epinephrine. These include diaphoresis, tremor, anxiety, and sensation of hunger. Irritability and palpitations may also occur. These symptoms usually have sudden onset and resolve spontaneously within 15-30 minutes.

   B. Neuroglycopenic symptoms occur in response to glucose deprivation of the nervous system. Headache, mental dullness, and fatigue are common in mild hypoglycemia. Moderate to severe hypoglycemia results in confusion, visual blurring, loss of consciousness, and seizures.

II. **Diagnosis**

   A. Hypoglycemia is divided into two categories: postprandial and fasting. A careful history is essential to classify the problem into one of these categories. Symptoms of postprandial hypoglycemia tend to be adrenergic, while neuroglycopenic symptoms predominate in fasting hypoglycemia.

   B. Causes of Hypoglycemia.

      1. Postprandial
         a. Idiopathic (reactive).
         b. Early diabetes mellitus.
         c. Alcohol ingestion.
         d. Postgastrectomy state.

      2. Fasting: excess insulin secondary to:
         a. Insulin injection.
         b. Oral hypoglycemic agents.
         c. Other drugs, such as haloperidol, propoxyphene, salicylates, etc.
         d. Insulinoma, alcohol ingestion, hormone deficiencies.

e. Adrenal insufficiency

III. Postprandial Hypoglycemia

Should be evaluated with a 5 hour glucose tolerance test (GTT) measuring fasting plasma glucose prior to ingestion of 75g glucose and repeating plasma glucose measurement every 30 minutes until 5 hours have elapsed. Up to 25% of normal, asymptomatic persons may have 5 hour GTT with plasma glucose values less than 50 mg/dl accompanied by hypoglycemic symptoms. Normal persons may also have plasma glucose values less than 50 mg/dl without symptoms.

A. Hypoglycemic patients with early diabetes mellitus will have a normal fasting glucose, an elevated glucose fulfilling diagnostic criteria for diabetes during first 2 hours, and a low plasma glucose between 3 and 4 hours after a glucose load.

B. Patients with hypoglycemia secondary to the postgastrectomy state will show a rapid rise in plasma glucose peaking by one hour after a glucose load, followed by a rapid decline with a trough at 2-3 hours.

C. Idiopathic hypoglycemia is characterized by normal plasma glucose measurements in the first 2 hours after a glucose load with a low glucose at about 3 hours and a return to baseline by 5 hours.

D. The term "idiopathic postprandial syndrome" denotes a condition with typical postprandial adrenergic symptoms and signs but plasma glucose levels not diagnostic of hypoglycemia during the 5 hour GTT. In these individuals, plasma epinephrine increases abnormally in response to blood glucose levels of 50-70 mg/dl. Measurement of plasma epinephrine levels during the 5 hour GTT has been proposed for diagnosis of this condition.

IV. Fasting Hypoglycemia

Defined as a plasma glucose less than 50 mg/dl greater than 4 hours after a meal. For screening, the plasma glucose is measured after an overnight fast. If this is normal, the duration of fasting may have to be extended to up to 72 hours under close observation. Prolonged fasting may not be useful in all patients, since most premenopausal women have a glucose concentration less than 50 mg/dl after a 72-hour fast. Normal males, however, will have a glucose of greater than 50mg/dl after a 72-hour fast.

- A. Insulinoma. Tumor characterized by large quantities of insulin leading to abnormal hunger, weight gain, and symptoms of hypoglycemia. Several methods are available for determining the presence of excess insulin, including immunoreactive insulin to glucose ratio, proinsulin levels, and provocative tests with tolbutamide, glucagon or leucine. Each may require special laboratory capabilities and the assistance of an endocrinologist. CT and ultrasound are useful in identifying large tumors (2cm or greater), but angiography may be required for smaller tumors.

- B. Surreptitious insulin or sulfonylurea self-administration occasionally accounts for hypoglycemia. The patient is usually a relative of a diabetic or has a medical background. Needle marks on the patient's skin should alert the physician to this possibility. Blood can be analyzed for the presence of sulfonylureas in specialized laboratories. Insulin C-peptide can be measured and will be low if exogenous insulin is being administered. Also, insulin antibodies are formed only with administration of animal insulins.

- C. Alcohol abuse can produce postprandial hypoglycemia in "social drinkers." Chronic alcohol abuse can cause fasting hypoglycemia which frequently occurs when the patient stops eating but continues to drink for 10-20 hours.

- D. Liver disease such as severe hepatitis and chronic congestive heart failure may result in hypoglycemia. Hypoglycemia in a patient with severe cirrhosis should prompt an evaluation for a hepatoma.

- E. Pituitary or adrenal insufficiency may cause hypoglycemia as growth hormone and glucocorticoids are important regulators of glucose metabolism.

V. **Treatment**

- A. Early diabetes is managed with an ADA diet with a high proportion of complex carbohydrates and low simple sugars. The patient should have frequent small meals and restrict alcohol ingestion.

B. Postgastrectomy patients and patients with idiopathic hypoglycemia may be managed with diet similar to the early diabetes. Propantheline 7.5 mg propantheline 30 minutes before meals may also be helpful by delaying gastric emptying. Propranolol may be hazardous as it blocks symptoms without affecting the blood glucose.

Reference

Barker LR, Burton JR, and Zieve PD, eds. Principles of Ambulatory Medicine, 2nd edition. Baltimore: Williams and Wilkins, 1986.

DIABETES MELLITUS

Hyperglycemia secondary to decreased insulin production or peripheral tissue resistance to insulin.

I. **Classification**
   A. Insulin-dependent DM (IDDM or Type I DM).
      1. Onset usually childhood or young adult.
      2. Ketosis and acidosis occur without insulin therapy.
      3. Multifactorial etiology (e.g. genetic predisposition, viral, autoimmune).
   B. Non-insulin-dependent DM (NIDDM or Type II DM).
      1. Accounts for 90% of cases of DM.
      2. Onset usually past age 40; 60-90% of patients are obese.
      3. Not ketosis-prone, but may require insulin therapy to control hyperglycemia. May develop ketosis under conditions of stress, such as infection.
      4. Etiology -- genetic component is stronger than that of IDDM.
   C. Gestational DM.
      1. Onset of diabetes is noted during pregnancy. Hyperglycemia frequently resolves with delivery but patient is at higher risk for developing DM at a later date.
   D. Other (secondary) DM.
      1. Steroid therapy or Cushing's syndrome may cause DM.
      2. Pancreatectomy or pancreatic insufficiency secondary to pancreatitis.
      3. Thyroid disease, acromegaly, other endocrine disorder.

II. **Presentation**
   A. Symptoms may include polyuria, polydypsia, polyphagia associated with weight loss, blurred vision, monilial vaginitis, skin infections, or dehydration.
   B. Many cases will be asymptomatic and picked up on routine screening.

III. Diagnosis

A. Plasma glucose > 200 mg/dl in a symptomatic patient establishes the diagnosis.

B. Normal 2 hour postprandial blood glucose varies depending on age (Figure 5-1).

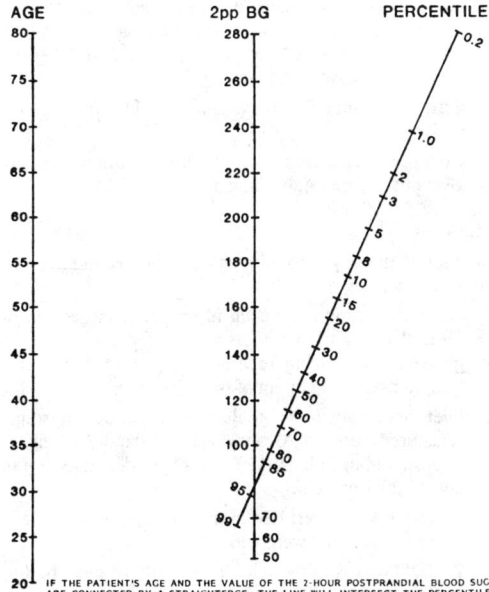

IF THE PATIENT'S AGE AND THE VALUE OF THE 2-HOUR POSTPRANDIAL BLOOD SUGAR ARE CONNECTED BY A STRAIGHTEDGE, THE LINE WILL INTERSECT THE PERCENTILE LINE AT A POINT WHICH INDICATES THE PERCENTAGE OF PATIENTS OF THAT AGE WHO HAVE NORMAL BLOOD VALUES AT THAT LEVEL AND DO NOT HAVE CLINICAL DIABETES.

Fig 5-1.
Adapted from Driscoll CE, et al. Handbook of Family Practice. Chicago: Year Book Medical Publishers, 1986.

186 Hematologic, Electrolyte, and Metabolic Disorders

- C. The diagnosis is made in an asymptomatic patient if the fasting plasma glucose is > 140 mg/dl on more than one occasion, or if an oral glucose tolerance test (OGTT) is abnormal. The GTT must be done when daily carbohydrate intake is > 150 gm, physical activity is unrestricted, and when the patient is not under stress. The patient must fast for 10-16 hours prior to the ingestion of a 75 g glucose load. Plasma glucose is measured initially and at 1/2 hour intervals until 2 hours post glucose administration. The test is normal if the fasting plasma glucose is < 115 mg/dl, the 2 hour plasma glucose is < 140 mg/dl, and no value is > 200 mg/dl. The diagnosis of DM can be made if the 2 hour sample and at least one other sample is > 200 mg/dl. The patient is said to have impaired glucose tolerance if the plasma glucose values are above normal but not diagnostic for DM. Of these patients, 1-5%/year will develop DM.
- C. Criteria are modified for diagnosis of DM in pregnant patients.
- D. Consider reversible factors which promote hyperglycemia before establishing diagnosis of DM.

IV. Treatment

The goal of therapy is to eliminate symptoms and prevent complications.

- A. Patient education is crucial in proper management of DM. Patients must understand diet planning, home glucose monitoring techniques, proper foot care, symptoms and treatment of hypoglycemia.
- B. Diet therapy. Patients should receive instruction from a registered dietician. Alcohol ingestion should be limited. Diet should include 60-65% carbohydrates, 25-35% fat, and 10-20% protein.
  1. NIDDM -- Overt DM in the obese patient is usually reversible with weight loss.
  2. IDDM -- A fairly rigid dietary pattern must be followed to avoid wide fluctuation in plasma glucose. There can be some flexibility if intensive conventional therapy is used. If a meal must be delayed, the patient should ingest 10 g carbohydrate per 1/2 hour. Caloric needs may be estimated at 40 kcal/kg/d for an

adult with average activity. Modest exercise requires 10 g extra carbohydrate per hour while vigorous exercise requires 20-30g/hour.

C. Drug therapy.
1. NIDDM -- If control of hyperglycemia is not achieved with diet alone, then insulin or an oral hypoglycemic agent should be considered. Hgb A1c level may be helpful in deciding need for drug therapy in relatively mild hyperglycemia. Use of insulin or oral agents may impede attempts at weight reduction by stimulating appetite.
2. IDDM -- These patients should be started on insulin therapy at the time of diagnosis.

D. Insulin.
1. Several preparations are available with varying duration of action (See Formulary).
2. Conventional insulin therapy usually involves a single injection once daily. If an intermediate acting agent alone does not provide adequate control of hyperglycemia, then a second agent should be added, using a short-acting insulin if hyperglycemia occurs during the daytime. If fasting hyperglycemia is a problem, a long-acting insulin may be added, or the intermediate acting agent may be given BID.
    a. Initial dose for a NIDDM patient is 20 units of NPH or Lente for a non-obese patient and 30 units for an obese patient given in the AM as a subcutaneous injection.
    b. The insulin dose may be increased by 5 units every 3 to 7 days until adequate control is achieved.
    c. If split dosing is required to control fasting hyperglycemia, start by giving up to 15 units before the evening meal with a concomitant reduction of the AM dose. Usually 2/3 of the total daily dose is given in the morning and 1/3 in the evening.
    d. If addition of a long-acting to an intermediate insulin is desired, add Ultralente or Lente in daily increments of 5-10 units.

- e. Measure preprandial glucose 4 times daily (including bedtime) while adjusting insulin dosage.
- f. Regular and protamine zinc insulins cannot be mixed
- g. Only regular insulin can be given IV

3. Intensive insulin therapy.
   - a. Insulin pumps administer a continuous subcutaneous insulin infusion with small boluses of insulin given at mealtime.
   - b. Intensified conventional insulin therapy requires multiple daily insulin injections as well as frequent self-monitoring of blood glucose.

E. Oral hypoglycemic agents stimulate insulin secretion and reduce insulin resistance of tissues. These drugs are indicated in the management of NIDDM.

1. Contraindications include IDDM, severe renal or hepatic disease, pregnancy, lactation. They should not be used in children.

2. Characteristics of these preparations are described in the Formulary section.

3. Hypoglycemic effects of the sulfonylureas may be potentiated by salicylates, sulfonamides, phenylbutazone, methyldopa, clofibrate, coumadin, monoamine oxidase inhibitors, and chloramphenicol.

4. Complications.
   - a. Hypoglycemia may occur and be severe and prolonged.
   - b. A disulfiram-like effect may be seen when taken in conjunction with alcohol with symptoms of flushing, HA, tachycardia, nausea, and vomiting.
   - c. Severe hyponatremia and fluid retention may result with the use of chlorpropamide in the elderly.

5. Drug Interaction.
   - a. Propranolol and clonidine mask the signs and symptoms of hypoglycemia.

b. Thiazide diuretics, chlorthalidone, furosemide, ethacrynic acid and phenytoin may have antagonistic effects on sulfonylureas.

V. **Complications of DM**

A. Atherosclerotic heart and peripheral vascular disease is increased three-fold in diabetics and is proportionate to the duration of the disease.

1. Peripheral vascular disease causes ischemia thereby predisposing the patient to infections which are resistant to antibiotic therapy.

2. 30% of MI's in diabetic patients are "silent," i.e. painless. The possibility of an MI must be considered whenever a diabetic patient presents with CHF, ketoacidosis, or other secondary events.

B. Diabetic neuropathy.

1. Peripheral sensory nerves are most commonly involved, resulting in hypesthesia first of the distal portion of the lower extremities followed by the distal upper extremities. Hypesthesia may be preceded by hyperesthesia and dysesthesia especially with burning sensations. Sensory loss predisposes to pressure ulcerations which are slow to heal and prone to infection because of peripheral vascular disease.

2. Peripheral motor neuropathy may occur particularly involving the interosseous muscles of the feet and hands.

3. Mononeuropathies can occur in any superficial nerve with sudden onset of intense pain in the distribution of the affected nerve, usually worse at night. Muscle weakness and atrophy may occur, usually with complete recovery within a few months. The cranial nerves may be involved; pupillary function is usually spared with 3rd nerve palsy. Pain management may require potent analgesics.

4. Autonomic neuropathy may be manifested by hyperhydrosis of the upper body with anhydrosis of the lower body, or by generalized anhydrosis. Other symptoms may include resting tachycardia, impotence, neurogenic bladder, diarrhea, and urinary

or fecal incontinence. Postural hypotension may be treated with fludrocortisone, 0.1-0.3 mg/day or with NaCl, 1-4 gm po qid; care must be taken to avoid recumbent hypertension and cardiac failure if these measures are adopted.

C. Diabetic myopathy is a rare complication of DM with proximal muscle weakness and pain, most commonly involving the pelvic girdle. Onset may be rapid and the patient may have a low grade fever and elevated ESR. Prognosis for improvement is good.

D. Neuropathic arthropathy (Charcot's joint). Degenerative changes of the joints of the feet and ankles occasionally occur with progression to complete joint destruction. This is frequently a painless process secondary to recurrent trauma which may have gone unnoticed by the patient.

E. Gastroparesis diabeticorum (gastric atony) may be asymptomatic or manifested by vomiting. Gastric emptying time may be unpredictable making diabetic control difficult in insulin-dependent patients. Metoclopramide may be effective treatment.

F. Care of the diabetic foot is of the utmost importance. Feet should be inspected daily for ulcerations and shoes must be properly fitted. Foot ulcers commonly become infected and osteomyelitis may also develop. Staphylococci and streptococci are the most common pathogens, but gram-negative and anaerobic bacteria may also be involved. Antibiotic therapy should be chosen accordingly. Aggressive therapy with dressing changes and debridement is also essential. Surgical revascularization should be considered if other measures fail to resolve an infected ulcer. Amputation of the foot is occasionally necessary.

G. Diabetic retinopathy is a leading cause of blindness. Typical lesions include microaneurysms, punctate retinal hemorrhages, hard exudates, soft exudates ("cotton wool" spots), microvascular anomalies, and macular edema. With proliferative retinopathy, new vessels and fibrous tissue grow along the posterior surface of the vitreous; this may lead to constriction of the vitreous causing traction on the vessels and on the retina resulting in vitreous hemorrhages and retinal detachment. Diabetics should be periodically evaluated by an ophthalmologist.

References

Barker LR, Burton JR, Zieve PD, eds. <u>Principles of Ambulatory Medicine, 2nd edition</u>. Baltimore: Williams & Wilkins, 1986.

Driscoll CE, *et al*, eds. <u>Handbook of Family Practice</u>. Chicago: Year Book Medical Publishers, 1986.

Orland MJ and Saltman RJ, eds. <u>Manual of Medical Therapeutics, 25th edition</u>. Boston/Toronto: Little, Brown & Company, 1986.

DIABETIC KETOACIDOSIS

I. **Overview:** Occurs primarily in Type I diabetics, but may occur in any diabetic that requires insulin to control sugars. Development of ketosis indicates insulin dependence. Ketoacidosis results from significant insulin deficiency, which causes hyperglycemia, osmotic diuresis and volume depletion, breakdown of free fatty acids to acetoacetate and beta-hydroxybutarate with resulting acidosis, hyperosmolarity, and K+ depletion.

II. **Evaluation:**
   A. Diagnosis suggested by mental status changes (confusion or coma), rapid respirations, acetone ("fruity") odor on breath, nausea/vomiting, evidence of volume depletion (dry membranes, tachycardia, possibly orthostatic changes). History of diabetes is usually present.
   B. Hyperglycemia can be diagnosed at the bedside with portable glucose monitor and ketosis can also be determined with bedside reagents. These determinations with the above symptoms and signs are adequate for the initiation of treatment.
   C. Additional laboratory evaluation should include true glucose, serum ketones, electrolytes, BUN/Cr, serum osmolarity, arterial blood gases. Treatment should not be delayed pending these results.

III. **Treatment**
   A. Initial resuscitation:
      1. Supportive therapy, including airway maintenance, supplemental O_2 as indicated, and treatment of shock.
      2. Fluid: initially 1-2 liters of normal saline without additives should be administered rapidly (at a rate of 1 liter per 30 minutes) if patient has no cardiac compromise. This alone will result in lowering of the blood glucose and restore adequate renal perfusion. If cardiac compromise is present, central venous pressure monitoring is indicated to guide fluid resuscitation.

Diabetic Ketoacidosis

3. Insulin: 10-20 units of regular insulin IV bolus in adults should be given with the initial fluid resuscitation. This should be followed by an insulin infusion of 10 units per hour, adjusted according to subsequent glucose and electrolyte determinations.
4. Bicarbonate: indicated for coma, arterial pH of less than 7.10, severe hyperkalemia. May be administered with one of the initial liters of fluid by placing 2 ampules of bicarb (88 mEq) in a liter of 0.45% saline, which is substituted for one of the liters of normal saline.

B. Continuing treatment:
1. Monitor serum glucoses and potassium, hourly at first. Also urine output. If bicarbonate therapy is administered, arterial blood gases should be followed. Otherwise, monitor ketoacidosis by following plasma bicarbonate levels.
2. Insulin: ideal rate of fall in serum glucose is not greater than 100 mg/dl/hour. If the glucose fails to fall by at least 10%, insulin infusion should be doubled each hour until response occurs. When blood glucose reaches 250-300 mg/dl, glucose should be added to IV fluids, 5-10% solutions, and insulin infusion reduced to 5 u/hr.
3. Potassium: should be added to IV fluids when serum K+ reaches normal range and administered at rate of 10 mEq/ hour, adjusted according to response. If the initial serum K+ is low or low normal, K+ supplementation should be started immediately and serum K+ levels followed closely. Care is required if urine output fails to increase with fluid resuscitation.
4. Phosphate: supplementation may be required if patient not able to initiate oral intake within first few hours. Potassium phosphate (4 mEq K+/93 mg phosphorous), may be added to maintenance fluids if necessary. Should not exceed total dose of 20 mEq K+ and great caution required with renal insufficiency.
5. Maintenance fluids should consist of 0.45% saline with additives as indicated, 150-200 ml/hr adjusted according to urine output.

6. Evaluate for potential precipitating factors, including infection, pregnancy, MI, inappropriate use of insulin.
7. Diet: oral intake may resume when mental status and nausea/vomiting allow. Initial diet should consist of fluids and full diet not resumed until ketoacidosis corrected.

Reference

Orland MJ and Saltman RJ, eds. <u>Manual of Medical Therapeutics, 25th edition</u>. Boston/Toronto: Little, Brown and Company, 1986.

HYPERGLYCEMIC-HYPEROSMOLAR NONKETOTIC SYNDROME

I. **Overview**: Occurs primarily in Type II diabetes, with severe hyperglycemia resulting in dehydration from osmotic diuresis. This may result in impaired renal perfusion. Stresses that can result in DKA can cause this syndrome, as can excess carbohydrate load or stroke. Mortality is high.

II. **Evaluation**
   A. Clinical presentation often includes obtundation or coma, severe hyperglycemia, negative serum ketones, signs of dehydration (including dry mucosa, orthostasis or shock), hypernatremia, and elevated plasma osmolarity. Lactic acidosis may occur and can be severe. The presence of mental status changes, hyperglycemia, and absence of serum ketones is adequate to begin therapy.
   B. Laboratory evaluation includes glucose, serum ketones, serum osmolarity, electrolytes, BUN/Cr, arterial blood gases. EKG should be obtained. Treatment should not be delayed pending the results of these studies.

III. **Treatment:**
   A. Initial resuscitation:
      1. Supportive measures to provide adequate airway and ventilations, and treatment of shock.
      2. Fluid: initial therapy should be with normal saline at 1 liter/hour until intravascular volume is restored. If hypernatremia is present this may be switched to 0.45% saline. Caution must be exercised in the setting of renal impairment, CHF, possible MI.
      3. Insulin: treatment is initiated with 10-20 units of regular IV bolus for serum glucose greater than 600 mg/dl.
   B. Continuing therapy:
      1. Monitor glucose and electrolytes initially every hour. Urine output should be monitored continuously. Arterial blood gases should be followed if bicarbonate is given. Serum osmolarity should be checked every two to 3 hours initially to aid in fluid therapy.

2. Fluid: after intravascular volume is restored, therapy should be guided by electrolyte determinations. Generally 0.45% saline will be appropriate. If significant hypernatremia is present, the initial resuscitation with 0.45% saline should be followed by 0.2% or water. Fluid should be administered at 150 ml/hour, adjusted according to vitals and urine output.

3. Electrolytes: Potassium depletion may occur and supplementation should be provided if levels approach low normal; 10 mEq/hour of KCl initially, adjusted accordingly.

4. Insulin: after initial bolus, constant infusion should be started at 5-10 units of regular insulin per hour. Gradual decline in blood sugar (around 75 mg/dl/hour) is the desired goal. Glucose should be added to the maintenance fluids when blood sugar drops to the 200-300 mg/dl range.

5. Patient should be evaluated for possible precipitating causes, including infection, MI, stroke.

Reference

Holvey DN and Talbott JH, eds. The Merck Manual of Diagnosis and Therapy, 12th edition. New Jersey: Merck & Company, Inc., 1972.

THYROID

I. **Hyperthyroidism:** 12 times more common in women than in men, prevalence of 19 per 1000 women and 1.6 per 1000 men. Remember that the total T4 level is normally elevated when thyroid-binding globulins (TBG) are elevated (estrogen supplementation, pregnant patients). A decrease in TBG may occur with liver disease or in patients on anabolic steroids and normally results in a decreased total T4. Phenytoin, heparin, salicylates, and clofibrate compete with T4 binding to serum proteins.

   A. Signs and symptoms:
   1. Patients may present with nervousness, heat intolerance, palpitations, weight loss, weakness, dyspnea on exertion, emotional lability, poor concentration, itching and burning of the eyes, fullness in the throat, increased number of bowel movements, and decreased menstrual flow. Depression and withdrawal may be seen in older patients.
   2. Exam: usually have an enlarged thyroid, tachycardia, and a tremor. Warm moist palms, lid lag and retraction, thinning of the hair in the temporal regions, Plummers nails (separation of the distal nail from its bed, most commonly found on the fourth digit), skin hyperpigmentation, and vitiligo are also commonly found. A bruit over the thyroid is highly suggestive of hyperthyroidism. Periorbital edema, exophthalmos, conjunctivitis with tearing, and ocular muscle palsies are classic signs of Graves' disease and may occur even in the absence of hyperthyroidism.

   B. Laboratory evaluation:
   1. T4, T3 uptake and free thyroxine index (FTI). If these results are equivocal, a serum T3 level by radioimmunoassay should be performed.
   2. High levels of thyroid antibodies are found in autoimmune thyroiditis, while low levels may occur in many types of thyroid disorders.
   3. Radioactive iodine uptake test helpful in establishing a diagnosis or for determining the dose of I^{131} needed for therapy. It is generally high with Graves' disease

and toxic nodular goiter, while it is low with subacute thyroiditis, autoimmune thyroiditis or factitious hyperthyroidism.

C. Etiology. Common causes of hyperthyroidism include:

1. Graves' disease: most common cause of hyperthyroidism in the 3rd and 4th decades. Causes diffuse symmetrically enlarged thyroid gland with normal to slightly soft consistency. The classic infiltrative ophthalmopathy may occur with or without hyperthyroidism.

2. Toxic multinodular goiter: results in an irregular, asymmetric, nodular thyroid gland. It usually develops insidiously in the sixth or seventh decade in a patient who has had a nontoxic nodular goiter for years. A thyroid scan may be useful in establishing the diagnosis.

3. Solitary hyperfunctioning adenomas: usually occur during the fourth and fifth decades. The thyroid gland contains a smooth, well-defined, soft to firm nodule which shows intense radioactive uptake on scan with absence of uptake in the rest of the gland. Most patients with solitary adenomas do not become thyrotoxic. When they do, they are usually less toxic than those with Graves' disease and they don't develop ophthalmopathy or pretibial myxedema. A bruit is not heard in this form of hyperthyroidism.

4. Autoimmune thyroiditis: normal sized or enlarged non-tender thyroid gland. Thyroid antibodies, when present, are high in titer. I^{131} uptake is suppressed or zero. This disorder improves spontaneously but frequently recurs. Autoimmune thyroiditis, painless thyroiditis, lymphocytic thyroiditis and Hashimoto's thyroiditis are probably all the same disorder.

5. Excess exogenous thyroid may occur due to dosage errors or, occasionally, in individuals taking large doses of thyroid hormones in order to lose weight or increase their energy. The thyroid gland is normal or small in size and I^{131} uptake is suppressed.

6. Subacute thyroiditis: tender, diffusely enlarged thyroid gland with a normal or elevated T4, a

depressed I^{131} uptake, and an elevated sedimentation rate.

7. Rare causes include radiation thyroiditis, thyroid carcinoma, excessive TSH stimulation, excessive iodine intake, struma ovarii, and trophoblastic disease.

D. Treatment

1. Graves' disease:

    a. Drug therapy. Propylthiouracil 100-150 mg every 8 hours, or methimazole 20-30 mg every 12 hours may be used. Clinical improvement may be seen in 1-2 weeks and the patient becomes euthyroid 2-3 months after beginning therapy. After the euthyroid state is reached, the medication dose should be decreased by 1/3 every few months if the patient remains euthyroid. A T4 level should be checked after 1 month of therapy and then every 2-3 months. Low dose thyroxine may be needed during therapy. These drugs are usually continued for 6 months to 1 year. A significant number of patients will experience permanent remission of hyperthyroidism after discontinuing these medications. Side effects include rashes, agranulocytosis, thrombocytopenia, anemia, hepatitis, arthritis, fever. A white count and liver enzymes should be obtained prior to initiating drug therapy and rechecked after 1 month and 3 months of treatment; after that, recheck labs only if new symptoms arise. These drugs cause no permanent thyroid damage.

    b. Inorganic iodine rapidly controls hyperthyroidism by inhibiting hormone synthesis and release from the gland. One drop of saturated potassium iodide solution in juice is taken daily. This should not be used as the sole form of therapy. It may be used alone for 7-10 days prior to surgery to decrease the vascularity of the thyroid gland. It should not be used for at least 3 days after I^{131} therapy but thereafter may be used alone until the I^{131} becomes effective.

c. Propranolol, 80-200 mg/day in divided doses, will reduce symptoms of tachycardia, palpitations, heat intolerance, and nervousness but will not normalize the metabolic rate. It should not be used alone except in the case of transient hyperthyroidism secondary to autoimmune thyroiditis.

d. I^{131}, 5-15 mCi, renders most patients euthyroid within 3-6 months. Therefore, treatment should be preceded and followed by antithyroid therapy. Most will eventually become hypothyroid. Pregnancy is an absolute contraindication to I^{131} therapy.

e. Surgery is usually reserved for those who are unable to take antithyroid drugs.

f. Ophthalmopathy: symptomatic treatment only. Artificial tears or methyl cellulose drops for the discomfort, patching or prisms for diplopia, diuretics and raising the head of the bed for periorbital edema.

2. Toxic multinodular goiter is treated with I^{131} or surgery. Antithyroid drugs will not induce permanent remission and should be used only as interim therapy. Large multinodular goiters do not respond well to I^{131}. Hypothyroidism is rare following I^{131} therapy because normal thyroid tissue is suppressed and so does not take up the I^{131}.

3. Solitary hyperfunctioning adenomas are treated with I^{131} or surgery with antithyroid drugs used only as interim therapy when needed. Hypothyroidism is rare after therapy.

4. Autoimmune thyroiditis is transient and does not require definitive treatment except in those patients with recurrent hyperthyroidism. Propranolol may be used alone if symptoms are mild. Antithyroid drugs may be needed for a short time in some patients.

5. Subacute thyroiditis may be treated with aspirin, 650 mg QID. In more severe cases, prednisone may be used at 40 mg every day, tapering to 10 mg each day over 2 weeks, then continued for 1 month after patient becomes asymptomatic. Resolution of

Thyroid

symptoms usually occurs in 1-6 months and relapse is common. Hypothyroidism may occur but usually is not permanent.

II. **Thyroid Storm**: severe, life threatening hyperthyroidism.
   A. Etiology. Trauma or illness may precipitate thyroid storm in a previously mildly hyperthyroid patient.
   B. Signs and symptoms consist of the usual signs and symptoms of hyperthyroidism with addition of fever. The patient may be markedly agitated or even psychotic.
   C. Treatment:
       a. When suspected, treatment should be instituted immediately. With therapy, defervescence usually occurs within several hours, otherwise infection should be suspected. Other signs of hyperthyroidism may require several days of therapy before improvement is seen.
       b. Treatment consists of propylthiouracil 200 mg every 4 hours and 5 drops supersaturated potassium iodide QID (or 10-20 mg/day IV). Propranolol, 20-40 mg every 4 hours may also be given. Fluid and electrolytes should be replaced and fever controlled with acetaminophen and a cooling blanket. Hydrocortisone, 100 mg IV initially with tapering over a 24 hour period, is frequently administered, but there is little evidence that this is of benefit.

III. **Hypothyroidism**: present in 1-6% of the population. Primary hypothyroidism refers to a thyroid hormone deficiency as a result of thyroid gland disease, secondary hypothyroidism results from TSH deficiency, and tertiary hypothyroidism results from TRH deficiency.
   A. Etiology:
       1. Without thyroid enlargement: Commonly due to I^{131} therapy, thyroidectomy for hyperthyroidism. The second most common cause is idiopathic hypothyroidism. Developmental defects and TSH or TRH deficiency are less common causes.

2. With thyroid enlargement: most commonly due to Hashimoto's thyroiditis. Drugs, iodine deficiency and inherited defects in thyroid hormone synthesis are rare causes.

B. Signs and symptoms include fatigue, weakness, slow movement, cold intolerance, constipation, hair loss, menorrhagia, carpal tunnel syndrome, dry skin, edema of the face and extremities, memory impairment, hearing loss, hoarseness, and occasionally bradycardia and hypothermia. Sparse eyebrows with loss of the lateral half is a non-specific sign. Pericardial effusion and ascites occasionally occur. A delay in the relaxation phase of the deep tendon reflexes, especially at the ankles, is a specific finding. Psychosis may develop with long-standing hypothyroidism and may be precipitated by thyroid hormone replacement. Infants may present with hypotonia, umbilical hernia, and delayed mental and physical development in addition to other signs and symptoms typical of adult patients. Mental retardation may result if hypothyroidism in the first few years of life goes untreated.

C. Laboratory findings include a low T4 and T3U. A low TSH indicates secondary or tertiary hypothyroidism, while a high TSH is diagnostic of primary thyroid failure. The I^{131} uptake is not helpful. Other laboratory abnormalities may include high SGOT, low sodium, low blood sugar, elevated CPK, elevated cholesterol and triglycerides, mild anemia, elevated prolactin levels secondary to high TRH levels, and flat or inverted T waves with minor ST segment depression and low amplitude on EKG.

D. Treatment consists of levothyroxine, 0.15 mg every day. Patients over the age of 40, or those with heart disease, should be started on 1/4 to 1/3 of this dose with increases every 2 weeks until a maintenance dose is reached. The serum TSH usually returns to normal within a few weeks after maintenance dose is reached. Elective surgery should be avoided in hypothyroid patients as respiratory depression commonly occurs. Increased sensitivity to narcotics and hypnotics is common in the hypothyroid patient.

IV. **Myxedema Coma:** may occur with severe, chronic hypothyroidism and is life-threatening. May be precipitated by exposure to cold, infection, hypoglycemia, narcotics, or allergic reactions. Treatment consists of 0.2-0.4 mg thyroxine IV followed by an oral dose of 0.1 mg daily. Hyponatremia and hypoglycemia frequently occur and should be treated appropriately. Care should be taken to avoid heat loss by wrapping the patient in blankets.

Reference

Orland MJ and Saltman RJ, eds. <u>Manual of Medical Therapeutics, 25th edition</u>. Boston/Toronto: Little, Brown & Company, 1986.

THYROID ENLARGEMENT

I. **Goiter**: simple enlargement of the thyroid gland. More common in females with the highest incidence in the second through sixth decades of life in endemic areas.

   A. Diffuse goiters: caused by iodine deficiency or excess, congenital defects in thyroid hormone synthesis, and drugs (e.g. lithium).

   B. Most are asymptomatic. Unusual to have pain and rare to have hoarseness and tracheal obstruction. Thyroid function tests should be performed on all patients with goiter, as it can be associated with hypothyroidism, euthyroidism or hyperthyroidism.

II. **Multinodular Goiter**: multinodular enlargement of the thyroid gland.

   A. Etiology: unknown.

   B. Clinical presentation:

      1. Symptoms: thyromegaly, occasionally with rapid enlargement and tenderness secondary to hemorrhage into a cyst. Rarely, tracheal compression may occur, causing coughing or choking. Some patients may complain of a lump in the throat.

      2. On physical exam, many nodules of varying sizes are usually palpable. Occasionally, it may be difficult to distinguish from the typically lobulated, irregular Hashimoto's gland.

      3. Thyroid function tests should be performed to rule out toxicity. A thyroid scan is useful only if the diagnosis of multinodular goiter is in doubt based on physical exam. A scan will show a patchy radioisotope distribution. Malignancy is rare, but should be considered if the gland is enlarging rapidly or hoarseness develops.

   C. Treatment: exogenous thyroid hormone suppression of TSH to prevent further growth of the gland. The gland usually will not shrink significantly with therapy. Synthroid is begun at 0.15-0.20 mg daily and thyroid function tests, including TSH, should be monitored. Occasionally hyperthyroidism may develop in a patient with multinodular goiter. Synthroid suppression should not be given to patients with angina or other known heart disease. If thyroid enlargement persists despite adequate TSH suppression, a needle biopsy and/or subtotal thyroidectomy should be considered.

III. **Solitary Nodules**: usually benign. Suspect malignancy in a patient with a history of radiation exposure, rapid enlargement, hoarseness on obstruction, and a solid nodule that is cold on scan.

   A. A thyroid scan should be done on every patient with a solitary nodule. High risk lesions should be surgically removed. Low risk lesions may be aspirated for cytology if pathologist is experienced in cytology.

IV. **Subacute Thyroiditis**: Presents with diffuse enlargement of the thyroid gland and may be associated with hyper-, hypo-, or euthyroidism. See section on hyperthyroidism for discussion.

V. **Thyroid Carcinoma**: Rare. Incidence in women is 3 times higher than in men and occurs at all ages with its peak incidence in the sixth decade. Up to one-third of patients who have received radiation to the head and neck as children will develop thyroid carcinoma.

   A. Most carcinomas are papillary or follicular and grow slowly. Undifferentiated tumors spread rapidly and are often metastatic at time of diagnosis. Medullary carcinoma may be familial and is occasionally associated with pheochromocytoma or other endocrine abnormality.

   B. Clinical presentation:
   1. Symptoms may include hoarseness, tracheal obstruction, rapidly enlarging gland, and rarely, pain. A history of radiation exposure or family history of thyroid malignancy should be sought.
   2. An enlarged, indurated, fixed thyroid gland on physical exam is suspicious for malignancy. The neck should be carefully palpated for lymphadenopathy.

   C. Laboratory evaluation should include a thyroid scan on every patient suspected of having a thyroid carcinoma. A single cold nodule on scan and a solid nodule on ultrasound suggest carcinoma.

D. Treatment:
  1. Resection of the thyroid gland.
  2. Thyroid hormone suppressive therapy given prior to surgery prevents continued growth; given after surgery, it improves prognosis as many tumors are TSH dependent.
  3. When lymph nodes are involved, one or more doses of ^{131}I should be given after surgery to ablate residual thyroid tissue.
  4. Monitor: Total body scans should be performed periodically and additional ^{131}I given if metastases are demonstrated. Euthyroid patients should receive stimulating doses of TSH prior to scan. Serum calcitonin levels should be followed in patients with medullary carcinoma as this rises with recurrence or metastasis of the tumor. Likewise, serum thyroglobulin levels should be followed in patients with differentiated thyroid carcinoma.

References

Driscoll CE, *et al*, eds. Handbook of Family Practice. Chicago: Year Book Medical Publishers, 1986.

Rakel RE and Conn HF, eds. Textbook of Family Practice, Third edition. Philadelphia: W.B. Saunders Company, 1984.

6/RHEUMATOLOGY/ORTHOPEDICS

Charles A. Bolick, M.D.

RHEUMATOID ARTHRITIS

I. **Overview:** Chronic systemic inflammatory disorder principally involving joints but also with extra-articular manifestations. Prevalence is 0.3 - 1.5 %, with females 2-3 times more affected than males.

II. **Clinical Features**
   A. Initial Presentation and Course.
      1. Malaise, fatigue, joint pain and tenderness, may have diffuse musculoskeletal pain. Low grade fever, weight loss, depression. Stiffness in morning or after periods of inactivity with symmetrical joint involvement, particularly hands, wrists, elbows and shoulders, but can affect almost any joint.
      2. Course ranges from limited period of disease to gradual progressive course to rapid joint destruction and incapacitation. 10-20% have acute onset over a period of days, but usually intermittent at first with more problems as disease progresses.
   B. Articular involvement.
      1. Synovium is the site of onset of inflammation, with proliferation of synovium ("pannus") and inflammatory destruction of soft tissue resulting in laxity of ligaments and tendons.
      2. Joint destruction occurs with erosion of juxta-articular bone around the margins of pannus and invasion of subchondral tissue by pannus. Can see cysts, loss of cartilage and bony erosion.
      3. Hands.
         a. Fusiform swelling of fingers and MCP joints, ulnar deviation of fingers, palmar subluxation of proximal phalanges.
         b. Swan neck deformity (severe cases): hyperextension of PIP with flexion of DIP.

c. Boutonniere deformity: flexion of PIP with extension of DIP.
4. Wrists.
    a. Dorsiflexion is limited early in course.
    b. Common early sign of disease is erosion of pisiform and triquetrium.
    c. Carpal tunnel syndrome results secondary to synovial proliferation.
5. Elbows: flexion contractures and swelling are common.
6. Shoulder: tenderness, particularly below and lateral to coracoid process along with limitation of motion.
7. Neck.
    a. Significant spinal involvement is usually limited to upper cervical spine.
    b. Neck pain and stiffness are common.
    c. Progressive erosion can produce atlantoaxial subluxation leading to cord compression with neurological deficits.
    d Impingement on vertebral arteries may result in vertebrobasilar insufficiency.
    e. Usually see decreased rotatory movement of head, with less effect on flexion/extension.
8. Hips.
    a. Abnormal gait and limitation of motion.
    b. Discomfort often localized to groin.
9. Knee.
    a. Synovial hypertrophy and effusion, with quadriceps atrophy.
    b. Destruction of bone and soft tissue leads to joint instability
10. Feet and Ankles.
    a. X-ray signs may appear here before in hands.
    b. Cock-up toes and fibular deviation of first through fourth toes.
C. Extra-articular.

1. Skin.
   a. Rheumatoid nodules: subcutaneous nodules found in 24% of patients (almost all seropostive). Often associated with more severe and destructive disease. Common to periarticular regions and areas subject to pressure (elbows, occiput and sacrum). Usually asymptomatic.
   b. Vasculitic processes: manifested by easy bruising and ecchymosis.
2. Cardiac: Symptomatic cardiac disease is not common. Most common type is acute pericarditis, usually in seropositive individuals (unrelated to duration of arthritis). Rheumatoid nodules can involve valves and myocardium.
3. Pulmonary: Diffuse interstitial fibrosis with pneumonitis is very common in mild form. Several forms of COPD are more common than in general public. Pleural disease is usually asymptomatic; can see subpleural nodules, exudative pleural effusions.
4. Neurological.
   a. Mononeuritis multiplex, associated with vasculitis.
   b. Nerve compression from proliferating synovium.
   c. CNS involvement is uncommon.
5. Ophthalmologic: Sjogren's syndrome: dryness of eyes with corneal and conjunctival lesions.
6. Felty's syndrome: chronic RA with splenomegaly, lymphadenopathy, anemia, thrombocytopenia, and neutropenia with systemic symptoms (fever, anorexia, fatigue, and weight loss).

D. Laboratory.
   1. CBC, ESR.
      a. May have mild anemia (normochromic) usually resistant to iron therapy even if serum iron is low.
      b. ESR elevated in most, can be a rough index of disease activity.

2. Serology.
    a. Rheumatoid factor: useful but not diagnostic. High titers usually associated with more generalized disease and more destructive arthritis. Extremely high titers are associated with the presence of rheumatoid nodules.
    b. Other serologic tests, such as antibody to DNA occur in a small percentage of patients.
3. Synovial fluid white count range is 5 - 20,000/mm^3 with 50-70% neutrophils.

III. **Treatment**
   A. First line drugs are NSAID's.
      1. Aspirin: long history of effective use. May try buffered or enteric coated forms to reduce GI side effects.
      2. Non-acetylated salicylates: fewer side effects plus bid dosing.
      3. Special considerations.
         a. Sulindac (Clinoril): considered to have least effect on kidneys. This effect appears to be lost at higher doses.
         b. Piroxicam (Feldene): once daily dosing.
         c. Aspirin, tolmetin (Tolectin), and naproxen (Naprosyn) are the only NSAID's approved in the U.S. for juvenile rheumatoid arthritis.
   B. Corticosteroids: Intraarticular for acute inflammatory synovitis. Systemic for severe vasculitis, unremitting disease with systemic symptoms, and to control symptoms until slower-acting agents take effect.
   C. Antimalarials: primarily hydroxychloroquine, dosed 200 mg once or twice a day. May cause retinal lesions with loss of vision so patients need an ophthalmologic exam q 6 months.
   D. Gold.
      1. Felt to work best in seropositive patients, especially males, and those early in the course of the disease.
      2. Administered I.M. or orally.

a. Parenteral is 10 mg IM week 1, 25 mg week 2, then 50 mg q week until response. Then reduce to every other week and eventually monthly.

b. Oral: average dose is 6 mg/day. Overall not as effective as parenteral.

3. Side effects.

   a. Common: Pruritic skin rash, mouth ulcers, transient leukopenia, eosinophilia, diarrhea (oral). Treatment can sometimes be temporarily halted then restarted at lower doses and side effects may not recur -but need to let the rash clear because it can lead to an exfoliative dermatitis.

   b. Transient proteinuria: 3-10% of patients. Usually only require cessation of treatment until the urine clears.

   c. Less common: thrombocytopenia, pancytopenia, agranulocytosis, and aplastic anemia. Usually responds to stopping drug. Gold chelating agent (dimercaprol) can be used if response is not fast enough.

E. Penicillamine.

1. Dose: 250 - 750 mg/day.

2. Side effects: Thrombocytopenia, leukopenia, taste alterations, nephrotic syndrome, skin reactions, GI symptoms, immune mediated syndromes, obliterative bronchiolitis.

F. Methotrexate (now FDA approved)

1. Weekly pulse therapy used to reduce bone marrow suppression and hepatotoxicity.

2. Most patients get mildly elevated LFT's but usually not significant.

3. May get mild rashes or GI side effects but may not have to stop the drug.

G. Physical Therapy to maintain mobility.

H. Orthopedic surgery: preventive measures and to repair damage.

OSTEOARTHRITIS

I. **Overview**

   A. Progressive loss of articular cartilage with reactive changes at joint margins and subchondral bone.

   B. Clinical manifestations include joint pain, stiffness, and swelling with limitation of motion, and occasionally secondary synovitis.

   C. Prevalence increases with age, approaching 100% in patients 65 and over.

   D. Two types

      1. Primary or idiopathic most common.

      2. Secondary to an identifiable cause or predisposing factor. Examples include inherited metabolic diseases (such as Wilson's disease or hemachromatosis), slipped capital femoral epiphysis, congenital dislocation of hips, neuropathic arthropathy, Paget's disease, hemophiliac arthropathy, rheumatoid arthritis, gout, pseudogout, and septic arthritis.

II. **Clinical Features**

   A. Signs and symptoms.

      1. Early: pain after use of joint.

      2. Late: pain with minimal movement, at rest, and night pain become common.

      3. Joint stiffness is usually localized and of short duration.

      4. Patients often demonstrate pain on passive movement, crepitus, and joint enlargement.

      5. Local tenderness seen if synovitis is present.

   B. Commonly involved joints.

      1. Hands -- DIP joints (Heberden's nodes are spurs formed on the dorsolateral and medial aspects of the DIP joints), 1st MCP joint, trapezioscaphoid joint.

      2. Knees -- patients have pain, tenderness, crepitus, and often secondary muscle atrophy.

a. May develop genu valgus or varus deformity if there is a disproportionate loss of cartilage on one side.
  b. Pseudolaxity of collateral ligaments develops with degeneration of cartilage.
 3. Hips -- pain and limp.
  a. Pain may be described in groin or inner thigh, and can be referred to buttocks, sciatic region, or knee.
  b. Limitation of motion, especially internal and external rotation.
 4. Foot -- especially the 1st metatarsophalangeal joint.
 5. Spine -- pain and stiffness, with radicular pain if a nerve root is compressed.
  a. Lumbar spine is most commonly involved, especially L3-4.
  b. Cervical spine can be involved.
C. Diagnostic tests.
 1. Laboratory tests are mainly used to rule out other diseases.
  a. Synovial fluid shows minimal abnormalities, possibly a mildly elevated cell count.
  b. Crystal exam may reveal calcium pyrophosphate dihydrate or apatite crystals.
 2. X-rays.
  a. Early in course of disease may be normal.
  b. Later can see joint space narrowing, subchondral bony sclerosis (eburnation), marginal osteophyte formation, cyst formation.

III. Treatment

A. Analgesics -- Tylenol and others, but should limit narcotics.
B. Nonsteroidals -- aspirin is prototype but all are effective at providing analgesia and anti-inflammatory effect.
C. Physical therapy.
 1. Heat, range-of-motion exercises.

    2. Protect from overuse by proper use of appliances such as canes, walkers, and cervical collars.
- D. Weight reduction if indicated.
- E. Oral corticosteroids are contraindicated.
- F. Intraarticular steroids.
    1. Can be quite helpful in acute flares.
    2. Should limit frequency, especially in weight-bearing joints, as overuse can lead to accelerated joint destruction.
- G. Surgical options include arthroplasty, osteotomy, fusion, and partial or total joint replacement.

CHONDROCALCINOSIS

Chondrocalcinosis: degenerative joint disease characterized by accumulation of calcium pyrophosphate crystals in articular cartilage and periarticular tissues. May be idiopathic or associated with a variety of metabolic diseases.

I. **Clinical Features**
   A. Pseudogout: acute inflammatory attacks involving one or more joints and lasting for several days.
      1. Can be very similar to gout although usually not as severe.
      2. Patients often have smaller, less painful attacks between flares.
      3. Knees involved in about half of patients but any joint can be affected.
      4. Surgery or illnesses can predispose to attacks.
      5. Crystal deposition can occur in tendons, ligaments and synovium as well as in cartilage.
   B. Pseudo-osteoarthritis.
      1. Progressive degeneration of multiple joints similar in many ways to osteoarthritis.
      2. Knees most commonly affected, followed by wrists, MCP joints, hips, shoulders, elbows, and ankles.
      3. Involvement tends to be symmetric.
   C. Pseudorheumatoid arthritis.
      1. 5% of patients present with an illness similar to rheumatoid arthritis, characterized by morning stiffness, fatigue, synovial thickening, elevated ESR.
      2. About 10% of patients with CPPD have a (+) rheumatoid factor, but it is not more common in patients with pseudorheumatoid arthritis.
   D. Many patients with CPPD crystal deposits actually have no joint symptoms.
   E. Laboratory.
      1. Crystals composed of calcium pyrophosphate dihydrate (CPPD).

2. Crystals are rod-shaped, often intracellular and are positively birefringent, or blue when parallel to the axis of a polarizing microscope compensator.
3. Evaluation should include serum calcium, magnesium, phosphorus, alkaline phosphatase, ferritin, serum iron and iron binding capacity, glucose, T4, TSH, and uric acid.

II. Radiologic Findings

A. Typical findings are punctate and linear densities in articular hyaline or fibrocartilaginous tissues.

B. Characteristic sites include articular cartilage of knee, acetabular labum, symphysis pubis, articular disc of wrist, and anulus fibrosis of intervertebral discs.

C. Radiological screen for CPPD disease should include AP of both knees, AP of pelvis including hips and symphisis pubis, and a PA of both hands.

III. Treatment

A. Nonsteroidals.
   1. Effective. No one is superior. May be used in similar fashion to use in acute episodes of gouty arthritis.

B. Colchicine.
   1. Particularly effective when given I.V.
   2. Oral form is less predictable than with gout, but has been proven to reduce the number and duration of attacks (with 1.2 mg daily).

C. Corticosteroid injections--often combined with aspiration in large joints.

GOUT

I. Clinical Features

A. Commonly affects middle-aged men and post menopausal women.

B. Acute attack.
   1. Acute onset of monoarticular arthritis, usually involving first MTP joint but others including ankle, tarsal and knee can be affected.
   2. Joint is erythematous, hot, swollen, and exquisitely tender.
   3. Attacks last 3-10 days without treatment, and the skin overlying the joint may desquamate.
   4. Often triggered by an identifiable event (illness, trauma, drugs, or alcohol).

C. Course.
   1. Asymptomatic intervals between attacks.
   2. Attacks tend to come more frequently with time.
   3. Well-recognized associations with obesity, hypertriglyceridemia, and alcohol.

D. Chronic tophaceous gout.
   1. Seen in more advanced cases (those with more frequent and severe attacks), appearing 10 or more years after onset of disease, more commonly in inadequately treated cases.
   2. Tophi are commonly found in synovium, olecranon bursa, prepatellar and Achilles tendons, subchondral bone, and subchondral tissue of extensor surface of forearms.

E. Chronic gouty arthritis.
   1. Involves any joint.
   2. May mimic rheumatoid arthritis although it is less symmetrical.

II. Diagnostic Features

A. Diagnosis usually made from the clinical presentation.

- B. Recommendation is to demonstrate crystals on joint aspirate at least once to document the diagnosis.
    1. Synovial fluid white count ranges for 2000 to 100,000 cells/mm^3, commonly majority are neutrophils.
    2. Crystals may be recovered from joints during asymptomatic periods.
    3. Crystals are rod or needle shaped, intra or extracellular, and negatively birefringent.
    4. Fluid should be cultured because presence of crystals does not exclude infection.
- C. Serum uric acid levels are not helpful in acute attack (can be normal).
- D. Urinary uric acid excretion of over 750 mg in 24 hours suggests overproduction of uric acid.
- E. X-Ray Findings.
    1. Acute phase: usually only see soft tissue swelling.
    2. Chronic arthritis.
        a. Oval or round periarticular or intra-articular bony erosions with a sclerotic margin, often called "rat-bite lesions."
        b. Joint spaces are generally preserved until late in the course of disease.

III. Treatment of Acute Attacks

- A. Colchicine: very effective.
    1. Oral dose: 0.6 mg po every hour until improvement, GI side effects (usually diarrhea), or maximum dose of 6-8 mg in 24 hour period.
    2. IV: 1 mg, repeated in one hour. (Avoids GI side effects, but very irritating and potentially damaging to tissues if extravasates). Maximum IV dose is 4 mg in 24 hours
    3. Side effects.
        a. GI, particularly diarrhea, quite common.
        b. With high doses can get marrow suppression, D.I.C., renal failure, and shock.
    4. Adjust dose for renal or hepatic impairment.

- B. NSAID's: considered by many to be the treatment of choice. Almost all effective. Start at high dose and taper.
    1. Indocin: (very effective) start at 50 mg po t.i.d. or q.i.d until the patient responds and taper to 25 mg t.i.d. until the attack resolves.
    2. Clinoril: (sulindac) is considered to have less effect on renal function and thus may be safer with decreased renal function.
    3. Ibuprofen: nonsteroidal of choice in patients on warfarin.
- C. Corticosteroids: effective. Indicated if nonsteroidals and colchicine are contraindicated or have failed.
    1. Prednisone 30 mg or equivalent p.o. or parenterally will usually control attacks.
    2. ACTH 20 units IV or 40-80 units IM q 6-12 hours for 1-3 days.
    3. Rebound attacks after discontinuation of steroids are not uncommon. Begin prophylactic colchicine 0.6 mg po bid before stopping steroids.
- D. Uric acid lowering agents should not be initiated during an acute attack as they can exacerbate or prolong inflammation.

IV. Prevention of Attacks

- A. Colchicine.
    1. Effective in preventing attacks at lower doses (caution is still required in patients with hepatic or renal impairment).
    2. Dose is 0.6 mg once or twice a day. Some patients are managed on lower doses.
- B. Nonsteroidals have also been used.
- C. Drugs to lower uric acid levels; indicated if visible tophi, severe overproduction of uric acid, frequent intractable attacks, renal calculi from hyperuricemia.
    1. Probenecid.
        a. Acts by blocking the tubular reabsorption of filtered urate. Best suited for patients who are not overexcretors of uric acid.

- b. Dosing range 0.5 to 1.5 + grams per day orally. Start at lower dose and increase as needed.
- c. Encourage patients to increase their fluid intake during the first months of therapy.
- d. Recommend concurrent administration of low dose colchicine for the first 6-12 months because of an increased risk of flares.
- e. Patients with renal impairment or on aspirin therapy usually should not be treated with probenecid.
- f. Probenecid interferes with renal excretion of many drugs (penicillin, indomethacin, acetazolamide and others).

2. Allopurinol.
   - a. Xanthine oxidase inhibitor, blocks conversion of hypoxanthine to xanthine, and xanthine to uric acid.
   - b. Dosing range is 100-800 mg orally, given once a day. Average dose is 300 mg. Recommendation is to start low and increase if necessary.
   - c. Drug of choice for patients with renal impairment, renal stores, hyperexcretors.
   - d. Frequency of side effects is about the same as with probenecid but more serious side effects are usually associated with allopurinol.
   - e. Side effects include rashes, allopurinol hypersensitivity syndrome, and bone marrow suppression.

4. Low purine diet.
5. Increase fluid intake to approximately 3 liter/day to try to reduce the uric acid concentration in the urine.

ANKYLOSING SPONDYLITIS

I. **Overview**
   A. Disease primarily affecting the sacroiliac joints with varying involvement of the spine and less so the appendicular skeleton.
   B. May have extrartricular involvement.
   C. Males more commonly involved, females tend to have milder disease with more peripheral involvement.
   D. Offspring have a 10-20% risk of disease.

II. **Clinical Features**
   A. Historical.
      1. Insidious onset, lasting over 3 months.
      2. Age less than 40.
      3. Morning stiffness, improvement with exercise.
      4. May have fatigue, weight loss, low grade fever.
      5. 25% develop uveitis at some time.
      6. Up to 10% have cardiac involvement (aortic insufficiency, cardiomegaly, conduction defects).
   B. Physical Exam.
      1. Muscle spasm.
      2. Loss of lumbar lordosis.
      3. Mobility of lumbar spine decreased in both anterior and lateral planes.
      4. Peripheral joint involvement in 20-30%, with hips, shoulders and knees typically involved.
      5. Characteristic posture -- patient with lumbar, hip, and knee flexion.
   C. X-ray findings.
      1. Early--squaring of superior and inferior margins of vertebral bodies.
      2. Later--bamboo spine.
      3. X-ray evidence of sacroiliitis.

4. Findings tend to by symmetrical (as opposed to Reiter's syndrome and psoriatic arthritis which are asymmetrical).

D. Laboratory tests.
 1. HLA-B27 present in 95% of caucasians with ankylosing spondylitis, but also 6-8% of normal population.
 2. HLA-B27 should not be obtained as a screening measure, diagnosis is made on clinical and x-ray findings.

III. **Treatment**
  A. Nonsteroidals. Indocin is very effective, but others can be used.
  B. Physical therapy for exercises, local modalities, and bracing as needed.
  C. Patient education and genetic counseling.
  D. Smoking cessation -- because of decreased pulmonary ventilation with disease involving chest wall.

METABOLIC BONE DISEASE

I. **Clinical Features**

   A. Presents as musculoskeletal pain, weakness, and fractures as a result of osteopenia.

   B. Osteopenia is defined as the loss of bone mass greater than expected for age, race, and sex.

   C. Laboratory evaluation.

      1. X-rays. 30-50% loss of bone mass is required before plain x-rays can detect osteopenia. (Newer and more sensitive techniques include dual photon densitometry and computerized tomography.)

      2. Fasting serum calcium, phosphorus, alkaline phosphatase, and parathyroid hormone.

      3. 24 hour urine calcium excretion.

II. **Osteoporosis** (the most common cause of osteopenia)

   A. Osteoporosis is defined as osteopenia with loss of both bony matrix and mineral.

   B. Average bone mass is greater in males and in blacks. White and Asian women are at greatest risk of osteoporosis.

   C. Accelerated bone loss occurs in women at menopause, especially from appendicular skeleton.

   D. Predisposing factors include family history, small body build, decreased physical activity, decreased dietary calcium intake, decreased exposure to sunlight, smoking, alcohol, and chronic glucocorticoid use.

   E. Treatment--limited success.

      1. Calcitonin--inhibits bone resorption and may also have an effect on increasing bone formation, thus slowing bone mass decline.

         a. Has been shown to be therapeutically effective in some patients.

         b. Dose of 100 units per day is effective, although doses as low as 50 units 3 times a week have shown some effect.

- c. Problems include cost, route of administration (currently requires subcutaneous administration), and development of resistance (overcome by changing species of calcitonin used).
- d. Human and salmon calcitonin are most commonly used.
2. Fluoride--stimulates osteoid formation and increases density of bone when it is incorporated into the hydroxyapatite crystal, in axial skeleton more than appendicular.
    - a. Studies have shown decreased incidence of fractures in treated patients.
    - b. Dose is 25 mg of sodium fluoride po b.i.d.
    - c. Requires concurrent administration of calcium and vitamin D to avoid a mineralization defect.
    - d. Common side effects include gastrointestinal (nausea and vomiting, epigastric pain), lower limb pain syndrome, osteomalacia, fasciitis, and arthropathy.

F. Prevention--the best treatment option, ideally began prior to menopause.
1. Regular exercise (against gravity).
2. Adequate intake of calcium and vitamin D.
    - a. Calcium 1000 mg/day in premenopausal women, 1500 mg/day in postmenopausal women.
    - b. Vitamin D 400-800 I.U. p.o. daily.
3. Estrogen replacement.
    - a. Women treated with estrogen within 3 years of menopause have a significantly lower rate of bone loss and incidence of fractures.
    - b. Recommendation is to treat until age 65 and then reevaluate, although can continue longer.
    - c. Minimum effective dose is 0.625 mg of conjugated estrogen or equivalent per day (alternate would be 2 mg 17 B estradiol per day).
    - d. Adverse effects of long-term estrogen therapy are minimized by giving in cyclical fashion with progestins.

- Medroxyprogesterone acetate 5-10 mg daily for 10-14 days per month.
- Use to prevent endometrial hyperplasia but may lower HDL cholesterol.
- Usually causes withdrawal bleeding which may be unacceptable to some patients.
  e. Studies show 0.3 mg estrogen plus 1500 mg calcium per day is as effective as 0.625 mg estrogen. This regimens does not cause endometrial hyperplasia so progestins are not needed, eliminating the nuisance of withdrawal bleeding.

III. **Other Causes Of Osteopenia**
  A. Osteomalacia--inadequate mineralization of bone matrix
     1. Vitamin D deficiencies.
     2. Phosphate wasting syndromes.
  B. Osteitis fibrosa--increase in mineral and matrix resorption due to parathyroid hormone excess.
  C. Corticosteroid induced osteopenia.
     1. Overproduction of adrenal corticosteroids.
     2. Chronic glucocorticoid therapy.
        a. Treatment to reduce steroid osteopenia is suggested, using calcium 500 mg per day plus vitamin D 50,000 units once or twice weekly.
        b. Monitoring of serum and urinary calcium levels are necessary because hypercalcemia and hypercalciuria can occur.

SYSTEMIC LUPUS ERYTHEMATOSUS

I. **General Considerations**: Systemic autoimmune disorder producing a chronic inflammatory disease affecting all organ systems. Genetic, environmental, and hormonal factors play a role in its etiology. Prevalence 2.9-4/100,000, more common in blacks and some Asian populations. Certain drugs can cause a systemic reaction similar to lupus.

II. **Clinical Features**: Course is one of exacerbations and remissions. If onset after age 50, usually milder course. Onset during childhood is associated with more severe course with higher incidence of nephritis and pericarditis. Survival with lupus nephritis is 85% at 5 years, 65% at 10 years.

   A. Joints.
   1. Symmetric arthritis and arthralgias are among most common features (can be confused with rheumatoid arthritis early in course). No articular destruction on x-ray but joint deformities may occur due to contractures.
   2. Tenosynovitis occurs in up to 10%, sometimes in absence of arthropathy.

   B. Skin.
   1. Acute cutaneous lupus: characteristic butterfly malar rash, often accompanied by a more widespread morbiliform eruption. Will flare with exacerbation of systemic disease or from sun exposure.
   2. Discoid Lupus: erythematous plaques with scale, mostly on scalp, face, or neck and occasionally on chest and arms. May be pigmented early with later central depigmentation and atrophy. Alopecia and scarring are common. Many with discoid lupus have no other systemic involvement.
   3. Subacute Cutaneous Lupus: Skin lesions are symmetric, superficial, non-scarring, often annular, occurring on shoulders, upper arms, chest, back, and neck. Over half will have diffuse non-scarring alopecia and 20% will have discoid lesions. Photosensitivity is prominent, but low incidence of nephritis.

   C. Cardiac involvement.

1. Pericarditis: may occur in up to 30% and may be asymptomatic. Often accompanied by pleural effusions. Rarely complicated by tamponade or restrictive pericarditis.
2. Myocarditis: may occur in up to 25%, often associated with pericarditis. Suggested by tachycardia, ST-T wave changes, and cardiomegaly. CPK-MB elevation may occur and can result in CHF or arrhythmias.
3. Endocarditis: first described by Libman and Sachs. Typically asymptomatic without murmur or hemodynamic dysfunction. Mitral and aortic are the most commonly involved valves and can be severe. Emboli are relatively rare.
4. Myocardial infarction: usually considered secondary to accelerated atherosclerosis from long term steroid use.

D. Renal involvement: affects 50% of patients, with the glomerulus the most commonly affected site. Any pathological form of glomerulonephritis can occur, with variable level of dysfunction and prognosis. Clinical presentations include hematuria, proteinuria, hypertension, and uremia.

E. Pulmonary: lung or pleura involved in 40-50%, with pleuritis or pleural effusion most common. Myopathy may affect diaphragm.

F. Central nervous system: frequently involved with highly varied presentation, depression is common. Strokes, TIA's, epilepsy, chorea, and frank psychosis also occur.

G. Gastrointestinal: less commonly involved. Serositis, oral ulcerations, and esophageal dysmotility may occur. Liver involvement not uncommon but jaundice is rare.

H. Other systems.
    1. Vascular: terminal arterioles may be involved in vasculitis.
    2. Reticuloendothelial: lymphadenopathy is common.

III. ANA Negative and Drug Induced Lupus, Lupus Anticoagulant

A. ANA negative lupus.
   1. High incidence of photosensitive cutaneous involvement (subacute cutaneous lupus).
   2. Arthritis and Raynaud's phenomena common.
   3. Decreased frequency of renal and CNS involvement.
   4. Many have positive latex rheumatoid factor.
   5. Overall increased survival.

B. Drug induced lupus.
   1. Clinical features: arthralgias, myalgias, fever, pleuritic pain. CNS and renal disease is rare.
   2. ANA and LE prep are often positive.
   3. Drugs involved are numerous. Procainamide has a high incidence (50%) of +ANA, and half of these patients will have symptoms. Hydralazine also commonly involved, females more than males.

C. Lupus Anticoagulant: characterized by antibody against the phospholipid cardiolipin. Associated with thrombosis. Atypical lupus; frequently ANA negative, not fitting SLE criteria, with high incidence of CNS involvement (especially stroke) and other thrombotic complications.

IV. Diagnosis

A. Clinical Diagnosis: based on presence of at least 4 of 11 criteria.

B. Laboratory test.
   1. Antinuclear antibodies: present in almost all lupus patients but not specific for SLE. High titers helpful. Most common pattern is homogeneous and diffuse (pattern resulting in "LE cell"). Antibody to double-stranded DNA almost unique to SLE while antibody to single-stranded DNA can be seen with other rheumatic diseases. Anti-smooth muscle antibodies are also almost exclusive to SLE.
   2. Hematologic abnormalities: anemia (up to 40% of patients), usually normochromic and normocytic, often autoimmune hemolytic. Leukopenia also may

be seen. Thrombocytopenia in up to 25% of patients. ESR usually elevated, does not always correlate with disease activity.

V. Treatment

A. Preventive care.

1. Regular monitoring: patients should be seen every 3-6 months even if they are doing well.

2. Energy conservation: fatigue is a common complaint.

3. Photoprotection: sunscreen and avoidance of excess sun.

4. Infection control: pneumococcal vaccine and yearly influenza vaccine. Consider antibiotic prophylaxis for procedures.

5. Contraception: avoid pregnancy at time of increased disease activity or while on immunosuppressive therapy.

B. Medications.

1. Nonsteroidal anti-inflammatory drugs: used to treat minor manifestations, all equally effective. Often used in combination with steroids to minimize steroid dose. Must watch for adverse renal effects, especially in patients that already have lupus nephritis. Aseptic meningitis due to NSAID may also occur.

2. Anti-malarials: hydroxychloroquine is most commonly used. Effective for cutaneous, musculoskeletal, and mild systemic symptoms. Mechanism of action is unknown. Begin 400 mg po daily for four weeks then taper to maintenance dose. Relapse is frequent with discontinuation of drug but control can be maintained on low dose. Ocular toxicity may occur, including corneal deposits (which are not necessarily a contraindication to continued use) and retinopathy.

3. Corticosteroids: topical for cutaneous manifestations. Low oral dose for minor disease activity, higher dose for more significant disease activity. Dose should be once daily in a.m. to reduce effect on pituitary-adrenal axis and high dose limited to 4-6 weeks if possible. Maintenance should be lowest possible dose, using alternate day therapy if possible. NSAID's used to try

to lower steroid dose or for symptomatic treatment on the off day of alternate day therapy.
4. Immunosuppresive agents: experimental, reserved for patients who fail conventional therapy. Associated with significant toxicities. Agents include cyclophosphamide, chlorambucil, and azothioprine.

LOW BACK PAIN

I. **Etiology:** Often never specifically identified.
   A. Disc injury.
      1. Herniation of nucleus pulposus, usually posteriorly since posterior longitudinal ligament is weaker than anterior. Posterior portion of anulus fibrosis is also the weakest portion. May impinge upon nerve roots. Chance of herniation increases after age 40 as discs lose elasticity.
      2. Typically pain increases with coughing, sneezing, or trunk flexion and includes radicular symptoms and signs.
   B. Degenerative changes of facet joints.
      1. Results in nerve root impingement at foramina.
      2. Sudden attacks lasting for a few days with symptom-free intervals. Typically pain worse with trunk extension.
   C. Spondylosis: degenerative changes of vertebral bodies.
      1. May result in nerve root impingement.
   D. Spondylolisthesis.
      1. Slippage of anterior portion of superior vertebral body on inferior vertebra of unknown significance.
      2. 80% occurs at L5-S1, then L4-5.
   E. Fractures, traumatic or pathologic.
   F. Spinal canal stenosis.
      1. Thought to result from narrowing of canal with impingement of the cauda equina.
      2. Irritation during activity results in pain in one or both extremities while walking. Relieved with rest. Can be confused with claudication.
   G. Soft tissue injury.
      1. History of trauma, heavy work or unusual activity.
   H. Functional: more of a concern with chronic low back pain.
      1. Usually duration over 3 months, may have symptoms of an affective disorder.
   I. Post-Surgical: possibly related to scarring.

J. Inflammatory Back Pain: ankylosing spondylitis.
   1. Insidious onset, morning stiffness, improves with exercise.
K. Malignancy.
   1. Primary tumors: multiple myeloma most common.
   2. Metastatic disease: majority are carcinomas.
      a. Enter via bloodstream.
      b. 85% (in order of frequency) are from breast, prostate, lung, kidney, and thyroid and cause lytic lesions (except for prostate and treated thyroid carcinomas, which are sclerotic).
   3. 24-30% bone loss required before changes are seen radiographically.
L. Vascular: dissecting abdominal aortic aneurysm.
M. Abdominal pathology: pancreatitis, perforated duodenal ulcer.
N. Genitourinary: urolithiasis, pyelonephritis, pelvic inflammatory disease.
O. Infection: bone or disc.
P. Children
   1. Under 10 years old: infection, tumor, A-V malformations, osteomyelitis.
   2. Over 10 years old: spondylolisthesis, herniated discs, Scheuermann's disease, overuse syndrome, tumor.

II. Physical Exam

A. With patient standing.
   1. Examine for obvious defects. Palpate for tenderness or muscle spasm. Test mobility of lumbar spine with flexion, extension, and lateral flexion.
   2. Observe patient's normal gait and have patient walk on toes (plantar flexion tests S1) and up on heel (dorsiflexion tests L5).
B. With patient sitting.
   1. Sitting straight leg raise: passive extension of knee. Positive test is radicular pain at less than 60 degrees.

2. Reflexes: Patellar reflex tests L4 root, Achilles reflex tests S1 root.
3. Babinski: if present indicates pathology above the lumbar region, such as cord tumor.
4. Sensation:
   - L4: medial border of feet.
   - L5: triangular area at base of middle toes on dorsum of feet.
   - S1: lateral margin of feet and distal calf.

C. With patient supine.
   1. Straight leg raise: flex one leg at hip and knee, passive flexion of the other hip with knee in full extension. Positive test is pain radiating down the back of the leg at less than 60 degrees of hip flexion. In addition, can compress midline of popliteal fossa (Bowstring test) or dorsiflex foot, when leg is raised to just short of pain threshold. These maneuvers should also cause the pain. Pain in non-lifted leg may indicate central disc herniation.

D. With patient on side.
   1. Check hip abduction (L5 motor).

E. With patient prone.
   1. Perianal sensation (S3,4,5; also controls anal and urethral sphincter tone).
   2. Hip extension.

F. Saddle anesthesia, decreased anal sphincter tone, and cross-over leg pain are signs of a central disc herniation which is considered a surgical emergency. Must be suspected if there is a history of new bowel or bladder incontinence.

G. Considerations regarding the question of malingering.
   1. Suggested by migratory tenderness and dramatic pain reactions.
   2. Axial loading: vertical loading on a standing person's head should not reproduce low back pain.
   3. True muscle weakness is a slow giving way with constant resistance. Factitious is suggested by sudden giving way or cog-wheeling. If a patient is apparently straining against an examiner and the examiner sud-

denly gives way, active movement should occur immediately.

4. Straight leg raise: if both legs are elevated simultaneously one can go higher before reproducing pain because the spine is flexed and the nerve roots are not tethered. Sitting straight-leg raise should produce pain at about the same degree flexion as lying.

III. Laboratory Evaluation

A. Lumbar spine films: Not necessary in most routine patients because they are usually not helpful in acute low back pain without a history of trauma. Should be obtained if there is a history of trauma or symptoms lasting over 8 weeks.

B. Computerized tomography: Preferred over myelogram for disc lesions, spinal stenosis, and bony abnormalities. Less radiation than standard lumbosacral spine series and more cost effective than myelogram. Not as good for intradural lesions or postoperatively.

C. Magnetic resonance imaging: becoming more popular but not routine yet.

D. Radionuclide imaging (bone scan): Useful for localizing infections and metastatic lesions.

E. EMG/NCV: can be used for suspected nerve root involvement.

F. Blood tests: Primarily used in older patients or those with systemic complaints. Consider CBC with differential, ESR, calcium, phosphorous, alkaline phosphatase, acid phosphatase, and urinalysis.

IV. Treatment

A. Hospitalization indicated for:
1. Cauda equina syndrome.
2. Severe neurological deficit.
3. Progressive neurological deficit.
4. Multiple nerve root involvement.

B. Outpatient treatment:
1. Bedrest in position of comfort: many prefer semi-Fowler's (hips and knees flexed, low back slightly

flexed) or on side in fetal position. Opinion varies as to length of time, but early mobilization (by 3 - 5 days) is being encouraged. Need not be strict (patients can be up to meals and bathroom) but emphasize getting weight off back. Avoid activities that aggravate the back.

2. Analgesia.

   a. NSAID's: most commonly used. Provide pain relief and decrease inflammation.

   b. Acetaminophen: analgesia but no anti-inflammatory properties. May be used with NSAID's.

   c. Narcotics: used short term only for severe pain.

   d. Muscle relaxants: commonly used with the intent to relieve muscle spasm, but most feel these have no real benefit. All sedating to some degree, which may be useful in helping patients with bedrest. None superior to others.

3. Physical therapy: Traction requires use of significant (50-100 lbs) weight and provides only transient (if any) benefit so not usually recommended. Local modalities (heat, cold, ultrasound) may provide short term relief. Corsets provide abdominal support which assists lumbar support and may provide short term relief, but long term use leads to muscle atrophy. Transcutaneous Nerve Stimulation (TENS) units provide short term symptomatic relief but have no proven long term benefits.

4. Epidural and facet injections: steroids have proven useful in some. May use lidocaine first to localize facet joint pain.

5. Rehabilitation exercise: Trunk extensors, abdominal muscles, aerobic conditioning. Most useful in preventing and shortening duration of back pain.

6. Surgery: Majority of patients with acute disc injuries will respond to conservative treatment, but surgery can be helpful in many who do not.

7. Chymopapain: very controversial, most feel this is not useful.

C. Regardless of method of treatment, 40% better within 1 week, 60-85% in 3 weeks, and 90% in 2 months. Negative prognostic factors include more than 3 episodes of back pain, gradual onset of symptoms, and prolonged absence from work.

V. Chronic Low Back Pain

A. Bedrest.

B. Mild analgesia, avoid narcotics.

C. Tricyclics (such as amitriptyline) are useful for chronic pain syndromes.

D. Surgery has had poor results and may even worsen problem.

E. Consider psychological referral for MMPI.

OVERUSE SYNDROMES

I. **Tendonitis**
   A. Clinical features.
      1. Most cases represent an overuse syndrome where the body responds to acute or chronic injury with inflammation.
      2. Patients typically complain of pain, increased with activity and decreased with rest.
      3. Physical examination reveals tenderness over involved tendon, erythema, warmth, and crepitus.
      4. Commonly involved tendons include the long head of the biceps, patellar tendon (also known as jumper's knee) and Achilles tendon.
      5. X-rays are not helpful.
   B. Treatment.
      1. Initial treatment is rest - usually for 7-10 days.
         a. Important factor is discontinuation of repetitive stresses.
         b. Immobilization is usually not necessary except in severe cases or in noncompliant patients.
      2. Local modalities.
         a. Ice is initial treatment of choice.
         b. After several days may switch to heat or use heat before warming up and ice after activity.
      3. Medications.
         a. Nonsteroidals are quite useful for analgesia and anti-inflammatory effect.
         b. Cortisone injections have very limited usefulness in tendonitis and have been implicated in tendon ruptures.
      4. Physical therapy.
         a. Flexibility and strengthening exercises are important.
         b. Cardiovascular fitness is maintained utilizing activities which do not stress the involved tendon (biking or swimming).

c. Phonophoresis and iontophoresis - modalities using ultrasound and direct galvanic current respectively, to introduce a topical steroid into inflamed tissue.

C. Prevention.
1. Recognition of repetitive stresses that lead to tendonitis.
    a. Strengthening and flexibility exercises.
    b. Proper training methods - avoiding abrupt increases in intensity or duration.
    c. Emphasis on proper fitting equipment and athletic techniques.
2. Equipment modification may be useful at times, example - heel lift for Achilles tendonitis.

II. **Stress Fractures**
A. Clinical Features.
1. Loss of bony integrity as a result of abnormal repetitive stresses.
2. Onset of pain usually gradual, often over a period of weeks.
3. A change in type or level of physical activity can usually be demonstrated.
4. Physical Examination.
    a. Tenderness over the fracture site or the overlying soft tissue.
    b. There may be swelling of the involved bone or soft tissue.
    c. Percussion of the involved bone at a site distant from the fracture may elicit pain over the fracture site.
B. Radiologic Test.
1. Plain films: Radiographic signs depend on the age of the fracture.
    a. Early periosteal changes may be seen at three weeks.
    b. Maximum periosteal new bone formation seen at 6 weeks.

c. Trabecular changes, such as those seen in compression fractures, may be seen earlier.
 2. Technetium 99 Bone Scan.
    a. May show changes as early as 3 days after injury.
    b. False positives are uncommon unless complicating factors such as osteomyelitis, bone cysts, or sprains are present.
    c. False negatives are rare.
 3. Tomography and C.T. scans have been helpful with particularly difficult fractures (tarsal navicular, femoral neck).
C. Treatment.
 1. Rest is treatment of choice, followed by rehabilitation.
    a. Casting or non-weight bearing is usually not recommended except for tarsal navicular fractures.
    b. Average time for return to activity is 3 to 8 weeks depending on location and severity of fracture.
    c. Patient should be pain free with a full range of motion.
 2. Drug Therapy.
    a. Analgesics: Tylenol or NSAID's.
    b. Specific therapy for patients with a metabolic abnormality such as osteomalacia.
 3. Adjunctive Therapies.
    a. Ice and massage are useful.
    b. Ultrasound is contraindicated (increases pain at fracture site).
    c. Emphasis is on regaining flexibility and conditioning before return to full activity.
    d. Conditioning can usually be maintained by utilizing activities which do not stress the involved bone.
    e. Bracing is useful on occasion to limit motion, but care must be taken to avoid creating stress in a previously asymptomatic region.

4. Surgical repair should be considered in areas which would have serious consequences if they progressed to a complete fracture (femoral neck fractures).

D. Prevention.
   1. Introduction of periods of rest within strenuous activity to allow stressed areas an opportunity to heal before a fracture develops.
   2. Proper fitting equipment.

III. **Bursitis**
   A. Clinical Features.
      1. Inflammatory condition of joint bursa resulting from two types of injury: acute trauma (direct blow resulting in acute hemorrhagic bursitis), and chronic repetitive stresses.
      2. Need to consider possibility of infection, especially if overlying skin is not intact or if history of therapeutic/diagnostic aspirations. If infection is considered obtain a CBC, ESR, aspirate bursa and send for culture and sensitivities and gram stain, and obtain plain x-rays of the joint.
      3. Physical exam will reveal pain, tenderness, swelling, and decreased range of motion of the joint. X-rays are usually negative.
   B. Specific clinical syndromes.
      1. Subacromial bursa: injured by repetitive motions of the shoulder (often throwing). Often accompanied by rotator cuff tendonitis. Characterized by point tenderness beneath the tip of the acromion, often with swelling and redness.
      2. Olecranon bursa: usually injured by direct trauma, either acute or chronic. Swelling at the tip of the elbow may be nontender in chronic cases.
      3. Greater trochanteric bursa: results from trauma to the bursa. Patients limp with antalgic gait and have well-localized tenderness. May be associated with leg length discrepancies.
      4. Knee: Prepatellar bursitis most common. Pes anserine bursa--lying between medial collateral liga-

ment and pes anserine tendon (common insertion of gracilis sartorius, and semitendonosus tendons)--commonly inflamed in running sports.
    5. Heel: bursa around Achilles tendon frequently becomes inflamed, especially with overuse, with pain and tenderness in the retro-calcaneal area. Often patients can identify a change in their running routine.
C. Treatment.
    1. Reduction in the level of activity that precipitated the injury, with immobilization considered at times.
    2. Ice to affected areas acutely; may use heat in chronic cases.
    3. Nonsteroidals.
    4. R.O.M. exercises early, with strengthening as inflammation resolves.
    5. Bursal aspiration; only as adjunct to other therapy.
    6. Steroid injections: can be helpful in greater trochanteric and olecranon bursitis, or in those cases resistant to other measures. Avoid injecting into adjacent tendons.
    7. Adequate padding for cases of repetitive trauma.
    8. Consider heel lift for Achilles bursitis.
    9. Correct leg length discrepancies of > 1/2 inch.

ORTHOPEDIC INJURIES

I. **Acromioclavicular Joint Injuries**: usually result from a direct blow or fall on the tip of the shoulder.
   A. Grade I (sprain): partial tear of joint capsule.
      1. Joint is tender to palpation; there may be swelling. Abduction past 60 degrees causes pain.
      2. A-C joint films (with and without weights) are normal.
      3. Treatment consists of ice, immobilization with a sling, and rest until pain free range of motion restored. Rehabilitation with strengthening and R.O.M. exercises.
   B. Grade II (subluxation): tear of the joint capsule usually involving the superior acromioclavicular ligament.
      1. Joint is tender and swollen. The distal clavicle may protrude slightly upward at the A-C joint. Abduction past 60 degrees is painful.
      2. X-rays without weights usually normal, but with weights may show widening of the joint.
      3. Treatment: ice, sling, rest for 3-4 weeks, rehabilitation with strength and R.O.M. exercises.
   C. Grade III (dislocation): complete disruption of joint with tearing of acromioclavicular and coracoclavicular ligaments.
      1. Joint is markedly tender and swollen. Distal clavicle usually clearly projects superiorly. Usually pain with any attempt at abduction although some patients may abduct to 60 degrees.
      2. X-rays show superior displacement of clavicle even without weights, and complete dislocation of joint with weights.
      3. Treatment options:
         a. External brace (such as Kenny Howard splint) which depresses clavicle into a more normal position while supporting arm in a sling or simple immobilization in a sling. Immobilize approximately 6 weeks then begin rehabilitation.

Orthopedic Injuries 243

      b. Surgical repair: usually not necessary although may result in quicker return to full function.

II. Glenohumeral Dislocations

A. Clinical features.
1. Vast majority (98%) are anterior, most commonly subcoracoid, then subglenoid.
2. Patients complain of severe pain and usually hold the arm tightly against their body.
3. Shoulder appears shortened and lowered. Acromion process is prominent so shoulder appears squared off. Often can palpate humeral head in subcoracoid region. Examiner must check neurovascular status of involved extremity since the brachial plexus, axillary nerve and artery, and rotator cuff may all be injured.
4. X-rays: standard views include an A.P. of the shoulder and a lateral of the scapula. Axillary view can be useful if standard views cannot identify the dislocation.

B. Reduction:
1. Modified Stimson reduction:
    a. Analgesia or relaxation obtained using Demerol, diazepam, or Versed (self administration of 50% mixture of nitrous oxide and oxygen works well).
    b. Patient placed prone on a table with the injured shoulder hanging free.
    c. Weight (up to 10 pounds) is suspended from the wrist and the patient is left for 5-15 minutes.
    d. Further manipulation often required--consisting of gentle internal and external rotation with downward traction.
2. Traction-Countertraction reduction:
    a. Patient placed supine on a table with a folded sheet placed around the patient in the axillary region.
    b. The sheet is pulled in the opposite direction while the examiner places gentle traction on the arm. Internal and external rotation may be applied.

c. Usually a noticeable click occurs when humeral head relocates.

3. External rotation method:
   a. Patient placed supine, with arm adducted against chest wall, elbow flexed to 90%.
   b. Examiner holds elbow in position against patient's side, and guides the forearm of the patient outward, externally rotating the shoulder. No pressure is applied to the forearm to force external rotation; arm is allowed to fall outward to full external rotation "under its own weight."
   c. Reduction usually occurs silently, unnoticed by patient.

C. Post-reduction care:
   a. Post reduction x-rays are obtained to assure good relocation.
   b. Arm immobilized using shoulder immobilizer or sling and swathe technique.
   c. Early orthopedic follow-up recommended.
   d. Recurrent dislocation or subluxation is common.
   e. Recurrent dislocations may require surgical repair.

III. Elbow Dislocation

A. Clinical features
   1. Posterior is most common, followed by medial or lateral, then anterior (rare). Usual mechanism is a fall on an outstretched hand.
   2. Exam reveals a painful deformed elbow, markedly swollen. Needs to be reduced quickly to avoid vascular compromise. Absence of distal pulses mandates attempted reduction or at least traction along the axial line of the arm. There can be distal pulses even in spite of an injured artery so arteriography is indicated if vascular injury is suspected. A careful neurovascular exam should be performed both before

Orthopedic Injuries 245

and after reduction. Anterior dislocations are associated with a higher incidence of vascular injury.

B. Reduction: may be attempted without anesthesia, but some form usually needed.
   1. Posterior.
      a. Assistant immobilizes the humerus.
      b. Traction is applied distally at the wrist.
      c. Elbow is flexed and then posterior pressure applied to the distal humerus.
      d. There is a distinctive sound when the capitellum slides over the coronoid process.
   2. Medial and lateral dislocations utilize the same technique except for varying the direction of pressure on the distal humerus.
   3. Anterior dislocation usually results from direct blow to olecranon process with the elbow flexed.
      a. Reduction obtained by traction on the wrist with posterior pressure on the forearm.

C. Post-reduction.
   1. Post reduction x-ray to check placement.
   2. Immobilize elbow in approximately 120 degrees of flexion.
   3. Repeat the neurovascular exam.
   4. Recurrence is rare.
   5. Full range of motion may take some time to return.

D. Radial Head subluxation (Nursemaid's elbow).
   1. Mechanism is sudden longitudinal pull on forearm while arm is pronated, occurring almost exclusively in 1 to 4 year olds.
   2. Child holds arm in pronation and usually refuses to move it. Pain on supination and palpation of radial head.
   3. X-rays usually normal, many feel not indicated in classic case.
   4. Reduction obtained by supinating forearm while palpating the radial head and extending the elbow. Examiner may feel a click over the radial head as it

reduces. (Reduction often occurs in process of x-ray evaluation).

5. Successful reduction indicated by prompt relief of discomfort and use of arm. Return of full function may take several hours.

IV. **Metacarpophalangeal Joint Dislocation**

A. Clinical features.

1. Most commonly occurs at 1st MCP joint. Usually results from a hyperextension injury.
2. The articular surface of the proximal phalanx is displaced dorsally and proximally.

B. Reduction.

1. If anesthesia is necessary, use a metacarpal block approximately 2 cm proximal to the joint.
2. Grasp the hand with a flexed thumb on the dorsum of the metacarpal against the base of the phalanx.
3. Push distally with gradually increasing force against the phalangeal base.
4. As the phalanx engages the articular surface of the metacarpal redirect pressure in an arc to push the base into articulation, leaving the phalanx in slight flexion.
5. Immobilization usually not necessary except perhaps to prevent hyperextension.
6. Treat with active flexion exercises.

V. **Interphalangeal Joint Dislocations**

A. Proximal interphalangeal joint.

1. Mechanism is usually a hyperextension injury with the base of the middle phalanx displaced dorsally and proximally.
2. Can attempt reduction before x-ray unless there is difficulty distinguishing from an angulated fracture of the phalangeal shaft.
3. Reduction may be done without anesthesia or with a metacarpal block.
4. Reduction:

    a. Push with thumb straight distally on the base of the dorsally displaced phalanx.
    b. As base of middle phalanx engages the joint surface the direction of force changes to an arc to follow the phalanx into slight flexion.
    c. Examiner usually feels a sense of giving way as the joint reduces.
   5. Post reduction.
    a. X-ray to rule out avulsion fractures.
    b. Check active extension.
    c. Splint in full extension for 3 weeks then begin exercises to restore range of motion.
  B. Mallet finger.
   1. Injury resulting from forced flexion of distal tip of a finger. Result is a stretching or rupture of extensor digitorum profundus tendon or avulsion of part of the distal phalanx with tendon attached.
   2. Exam reveals swelling, tenderness, DIP joint held in flexion with patient unable to extend it.
   3. Treatment
    a. Splint finger in extension across DIP joint leaving PIP joint free to allow continued function. Splint for several weeks (6-12), longer times for injuries with delayed diagnosis.
    b. Operative repair is necessary for the minority of cases which don't respond to splinting.

VI. **Patellar Dislocations**
  A. Clinical features
   1. Patients complain of knee giving way or popping out.
   2. Patella may remain dislocated on presentation, but many have already spontaneously reduced (often patients reduce it themselves). Effusion (hemarthrosis) is usually present. Medial retinaculum tender. Apprehension test: displace patella laterally, patients feel as if patella is going to dislocate and will be very apprehensive and tender.

3. Examination between occurrences: Patella noted to have marked lateral mobility, particularly during active extension. Patellar ligament may be noted to angulate laterally from axis of quadriceps muscle.

B. Reduction.
   1. Encourage patient to relax quadriceps.
   2. Push patella medially back into place.
   3. If unable to get patella over lateral femoral condyle, push patella anteriorly while passively flexing the knee (patella usually reduces by 30 degrees flexion.)
   4. If effusion is tense, aspiration is helpful.

C. Post-reduction care:
   1. Many feel that adequate immobilization is obtained with use of knee immobilizer for 6 weeks. Some feel that full leg cylinder cast is required.
   2. Have patient on full weight bearing as well as quadriceps isometric exercises while immobilized.
   3. After immobilization, patients are on partial weight bearing while quadriceps strengthening is initiated. Rehabilitation needs to include vastus medialis which only operates in the last 15 degrees of extension. Resume full weight bearing when flexion to 30 degrees is painless. Elastic knee support may add some patellar stability during strenuous activity.
   4. Dislocation more than 3 times may require surgical treatment (lateral retinuclar release).

FRACTURES

I. **Terminology**
   A. Open fracture -- fracture associated with an open wound extending from skin surface to bony injury.
   B. Incomplete -- involving only 1 cortex.
   C. Complete -- involving both cortices.
   D. Comminuted -- fracture consisting of 3 or more fragments.
   E. Compression -- type of impacted fracture characterized by crushed bone.
   G. Avulsion -- fragment of bone pulled from its normal position by a muscular contraction or resistance of a ligament.
   H. Greenstick fracture -- incomplete angulated fracture of long bones, particularly in children.
   I. Angulation -- fragments are out of a linear relationship.
   J. Rotation -- one or both fragments rotate on its axis in relation to the other.

II. **Epiphyseal Plate Fractures**
   Described using the Salter & Harris classification.
   A. Salter I (approximately 6%).
      1. Separation of the epiphysis from the metaphysis without evidence of a metaphyseal fragment.
      2. Usually the result of a shearing force, can be associated with birth injury.
      3. Most common in infants and young children.
      4. High index of suspicion is necessary because spontaneous reduction can occur.
      5. Prognosis is excellent because epiphyseal blood supply is usually intact and growing cells of epiphyseal plate are undisturbed.
   B. Salter II (approximately 75%).
      1. Fracture extends transversely through the epiphyseal plate then out through the metaphysis on the side opposite the fracture intitiation resulting in a triangular metaphyseal fragment.

2. Most frequent in children over age 10
3. Usually treated with closed reduction.
4. Prognosis is excellent because the blood supply is almost always intact.

C. Salter III (8%).
   1. Intraarticular fracture which extends from the joint surface across the epiphysis to the epiphyseal plate and out to the periphery.
   2. Commonly involves the lower tibial epiphysis.
   3. Caused by an intraarticular shearing force.
   4. Often requires open reduction.
   5. Prognosis is good if the blood supply is intact and reduction is maintained.

D. Salter IV (10%).
   1. Intraarticular fracture consisting of a vertical fracture through the epiphysis which crosses the epiphyseal plate and exits through a portion of the metaphysis.
   2. Frequently involves lateral condyle of humerus.
   3. Treated with anatomic reduction and internal fixation.
   4. Prognosis is poor unless reduction is maintained.

E. Salter V (1%).
   1. Results from a crush injury through the epiphysis to a portion of the epiphyseal plate.
   2. Usually occurs in a joint which has only one plane of movement.
   3. Most commonly seen in the knee and ankle.
   4. Initial x-rays tend to be normal so must suspect this fracture from the mechanism of injury.
   5. Results are poor with premature cessation of growth.
   6. Nontraumatic events causing a Salter V type injury are metaphyseal osteomyelitis and epiphyseal aseptic necrosis.
   7. Salter V can occur in conjunction with Salter I, II, and III fractures and not be recognized until growth arrest occurs.
   8. Treat with 3 weeks of non-weight bearing.

SEPTIC ARTHRITIS

I. **Bacterial Arthritis**
   A. Any infectious agent can cause arthritis but bacterial arthritis is the most rapidly destructive form.
   B. Two major classes.
      1. Arthritis due to Neisseria gonorrheae or other Neisseria species.
      2. Nongonococcal bacterial arthritis.
   C. Source of infection.
      1. Hematogenous spread.
      2. Puncture wound or skin infection.
      3. Adjacent osteomyelitis.
      4. Rarely from intra-articular injection or joint aspiration (incidence ranges from 1 in 500 to 1 in 5000).
      5. Patient with systemic connective tissue disorders are more prone to bacterial arthritis.
      6. IV drug use.
         a. Often involves unusual joints, i.e. sternoclavicular or sacroiliac.
         b. Frequently involves unusual organisms such as Pseudomonas, Serratia, and methicillin-resistant Staph.

II. **Clinical Appearance and Diagnosis**
   A. Clinical Features.
      1. Acute onset of a warm swollen joint.
         a. Usually 1 or 2 joints involved, perhaps more with gonococcal arthritis.
         b. Knee most commonly affected in adults.
         c. Hip and knee most commonly involved joints in children.
      2. Fever is common but can be low-grade, chills are less common.
   B. Diagnosis.
      1. Definitive test is joint aspiration with fluid sent for:

- a. Gram-stain [+ in 75% of gram (+) cocci, 50% of gram (-) rods].
- b. Synovial fluid culture [(+) in less than 50% of patients with Neisseria].
- c. Synovial fluid leukocyte count and differential [greater than 50,000 cells/ml in 70% of patients, with over 80% neutrophils].
- d. Synovial fluid glucose should be much lower than serum glucose.
- e. Synovial fluid for latex agglutination. Useful for N. meningitidis, H. influenzae, and S. pneumoniae but not other gram (+) cocci or N. gonorrheae.

2. Blood cultures -- (+) in 50% of nongonococcal arthritis but rarely in gonococcal arthritis.
3. Elevated white count with a left shift and an elevated ESR are often present but nonspecific.
4. Radiological exams.
    - a. Plain films obtained for baseline and to look for osteomyelitis. Usually no initial changes except effusions and perhaps juxta-articular osteopenia. Changes of osteomyelitis take 10-20 days to appear on plain films.
    - b. Radionuclide imaging, gallium scanning, and computed tomography can be helpful, particularly with suspected hip or axial joint infections.
5. Surgical exploration may be necessary to obtain fluid from joints such as sternoclavicular or sacroiliac.

III. Gonococcal Arthritis

A. Incidence.
   1. Disseminated gonoccal infection (DGI) occurs in 0.1-0.5% of patients with gonorrhea.
   2. Most common cause of bacterial arthritis in urban areas.
   3. 5% of patients with meningococcal infections will have arthritis -- much less common than gonococcal but with a similar clinical picture.

- B. Clinical features.
    1. Most patients have migratory polyarthralgias.
    2. Some will have purulent arthritis involving 1-2 joints, usually knees, ankles, and wrists.
    3. Fever.
    4. 25% have genitourinary symptoms.
    5. Physical exam.
        a. Synovitis and/or tenosynovitis.
        b. Two-thirds of patients have a dermatitis, with multiple, usually asymptomatic, lesions which can be macular, papular, vesicular or pustular.
- C. Laboratory features.
    1. Synovial fluid white count averages over 60,000 per ml, but low numbers have been reported.
    2. Only 25% of synovial fluid cultures are (+).
    3. Blood cultures and synovial fluid cultures are usually not (+) at the same time.
    4. In 75% of patients, organism can be isolated from a genitourinary source.

IV. Nongonococcal Bacterial Arthritis

- A. Causative organisms.
    1. Staph aureus most common, followed by various strep species, with pneumococcal infections becoming much less common.
        a. Most Staph are resistant to penicillin, many are methicillin resistant.
    2. Anaerobic infections with Fusobacterium Necrophorium, Peptococcus anaerobius, and Bacteroides fragilis. More often seen after joint replacements, with postoperative sepsis, or in patients with chronic debilitating illnesses.
    3. Polymicrobial infections often with both aerobic and anaerobic organisms are being described more frequently.
    4. Gram negative infections now being implicated in 1/4 to 1/3 of nongonococcal arthritis, most commonly in elderly patients and I.V. drug abusers.

5. Special clinical situations.
   a. Neonates (under 6 months) E. Coli and other gram (-).
   b. Infants (6 months to 2 years) H. flu is most common organism.
   c. Patients with sickle cell anemia and other hemoglobinopathies frequently have Salmonella or other gram (-) organism.

B. Prosthetic joint infections.
   1. Types.
      a. Acute (within 3 months of surgery).
      b. Subacute.
      c. Chronic (over 1 year since surgery).
   2. Usually more insidious onset and harder to diagnose.
      a. Pain, fever, elevated ESR, synovial fluid analysis with evidence of infection.
      b. X-rays and radionuclide scans may be required to make the diagnosis.
   3. Acute infections are due to Staph epidermides, Staph aureus, and anaerobes.
   4. Late infections are due to Staph aureus.
   5. Removal of the prosthesis is usually required, although salvage procedures may succeed.
   6. Prophylactic antibiotics before and for a few days after prosthetic joint surgery are recommended.

V. **Treatment**

A. Antibiotic Therapy.
   1. D.G.I.
      a. Penicillin usually yields response within 48 hours. Example: Penicillin G 10 million units IV/day for 7-10 days followed by one week of oral therapy.
      b. For areas with known or suspected penicillin-resistant gonorrhea: Ceftriaxone 1 gram IV qD x 7 days followed by oral therapy according to sensitivities.

Septic Arthritis

      c. For penicillin-allergic patients: erythromycin or spectinomycin.

  2. Nongonococcal arthritis.

      a. Make initial choice based on gram stain and clinical likelihood.

      b. Essentially all antibiotics reach high levels of activity within an inflamed joint following oral or parenteral administration.

      c. Consider penicillinase-resistant penicillin (such as methicillin or nafcillin) or vancomycin plus an aminoglycoside or aztreonam.

      d. Imipenim has been proposed for single-agent therapy.

      e. Neonates -- methicillin, nafcillin, or vancomycin plus 3rd generation cephalosporin.

      f. Infants and young children -- methicillin, nafcillin or vancomycin plus cefuroxime.

      g. Prosthetic joint infections: vancomycin plus aztreonam.

  3. Duration of therapy.

      a. D.G.I.: 7-10 days IV followed by one week p.o. -- longer for purulent arthritis than arthralgias with tenosynovitis alone.

      b. Nongonococcal -- at least 2 weeks parenteral therapy followed by one or more weeks p.o.

      c. Reassess therapy if:

- Synovial fluid cultures are not negative within 72 hours.
- Synovial fluid white count is not markedly lower after 7 days.

B. Drainage.

  1. Needle drainage.

      a. As good as open drainage in most situations.

      b. Not adequate for hip infections, especially in children.

      c. Aspirate with large bone needle, daily while effusions accumulate rapidly, can facilitate with sterile saline.

2. Open drainage. Method of choice for hip infections.

3. Arthroscopy. Early arthroscopy has been reported to be helpful with bacterial arthritis of the knee.

C. Immobilize joint in functional position during acute phase of infection, with early mobilizaton and muscle strengthening exercises.

D. Prognosis.

1. Mortality up to 10%.

2. Only 60% recover completely, with many left with a joint problem.

3. Results depend on organism, duration of symptoms, and health of individual.

   a. Patients symptomatic more than 7 days before treatment do poorly.

   b. Staph aureus and gram negatives tend to be more destructive.

   c. Gonorrhea and pneumococcus are rarely destructive.

   d. Healthy individuals do better than IV drug users, and all do better than the elderly, patients with multiple problems, and those with a preexisting severe arthritis.

4. Sterile synovitis may develop after treatment. Usually self-limited and responds to nonsteroidals.

References

Chapman C, ed. Emergency Department Orthopedics. London: Aspen Systems Corporations, 1982.

Gartland JJ, ed. Fundamentals of Orthopedics, 3rd Edition. Philadelphia: W.B. Saunders Company, 1979.

Gentry LO. Osteomyelitis: Options for diagnosis and management. Journal of Antimicrobial Chemotherapy Supplement C 21:115, 1988.

Green NE and Edwards K. Bone and joint infections in children. Orthopedic Clinics of North America 18(4):555, October 1987.

Hunter SC and Poole RM. The chronically inflamed tendon. Clinics in Sports Medicine 6(2):371, April 1987.

Karlin JM. Osteomyelitis in children. Clinics in Podiatric Medicine and Surgery 4(1):37, January 1987.

Markey KL. Stress fractures. Clinics in Sports Medicine 6(2):405, April 1987.

Ramamurti CP and Tinker RV, eds. Orthopedics in Primary Care. Baltimore: Williams and Wilkins, 1979.

Reilly JP and Nicholas JA. The chronically inflamed bursa. Clinics in Sports Medicine 6(2):345, April 1987.

Rockwood CA, *et al*, eds. Fractures in Children, 3rd edition. Philadelphia: J.B. Lippincott Company, 1984.

Rodnam GP and Schumacher HR, eds. Primer on Rheumatic Diseases, Ninth edition. Arthritis Foundation, 1988.

Rosen P, ed. Emergency Medicine: Concepts and Clinical Practice, 2nd edition. St. Louis: C.V. Mosby Company, 1988.

Wallach S. Calcitonin therapy in osteoporosis. Current Concepts Report of Seventh Ross Conference on Medical Research, Ross Laboratories, 1987.

7/ GYNECOLOGY

Timothy Momany, M.D. and Candace F. Shanks, M.D.

CONTRACEPTION

Table 7-1. Methods of Contraception

Method	Mechanism of Action	Failure Rate Optimal/Typical	Contraindications	Comments
Diaphragm and spermicide	Barrier, Inactivation of sperm	3%/2-18%	Allergy to rubber or spermicide, recurrent UTI's	↑ risk of UTI
Condom	Barrier	2%/12%	Allergy to rubber	↓ enjoyment, ↓ risk of STD's
Oral contraceptives				
combined	Inhibition of ovulation "hostile" cervical mucus	0.1%/3%	See next page	See next page
Progestin only	Same	0.5%/2%	See next page	Irregular menses, acne, hirsuitism, wt. gain, amenorrhea
IUD	Inhibition of sperm migration, fertilization or ovum transport	-/6	Active pelvic infection or strong h/o PID, h/o ectopic, impaired response to infection, valvular heart disease, impaired coagulation, multiple sexual partners	PID, loss of fertility, uterine perforation; ectopic pregnancy; menstrual blood loss.
Progesterone T		-/2.0		
Copper T380A		-/0.8		
Cervical cap with spermicide	Barrier, inactivation of sperm	5%/18%	Allergy to rubber or spermicide	↑ risk of vaginal infections, ↑ incidence of abnormal pap smears
Sponge with spermicide	Barrier, inactivation of sperm	5-8%/18-28%	None known	↑ risk of candidiasis
Spermicide	Inactivation of sperm	3%/21%		Irritation can occur

Method	Mechanism of Action	Failure Rate Optimal/Typical	Contraindications	Side Effects
Rhythm	Avoidance of coitus during presumed fertile days	2-10%/20%	Irregular menstrual cycles. Irregular BBT charts	↓ number of days to safely have intercourse
Medroxyprogesterone acetate injections	Changes in cervical mucous & endometrium, suppression of ovulation	0.3/0.3%	? breast tumors	Irregular, unpredictable bleeding, question of ↑ breast tumors

Gynecology

I. Contraindications to Oral Contraceptives

A. Absolute.

- Thromboembolic disorder.
- Cerebrovascular disease.
- Coronary artery disease.
- Malignancy of the breast or reproductive system.
- Pregnancy.
- Impaired liver function-hepatic adenoma.
- Undiagnosed abnormal genital bleeding.
- Obstructive jaundice in pregnancy.
- Congenital hyperlipidemia.
- Wilson's disease.

B. Relative.

- Migraine headache.
- Diabetes.
- Hypertension.
- Gallbladder disease.
- Women over 35 years old who smoke.
- Women over 40 years old.
- Heavy cigarette smoking.
- Long leg cast, lower extremity injury, immobilization.
- Cardiac or renal dysfunction.
- Lactation.
- Uterine leiomyomas.
- Varicose veins.
- Sickle cell disease.
- Undiagnosed abnormal vaginal bleeding.
- Undiagnosed breast lumps.

C. Possible Side Effects.

1. Very Serious.

- Thromboembolism.
- Myocardial infarction.
- Hepatocellular adenoma.
- Cerebral vascular accident.

2. Serious.

- Hypertension.
- Elevated serum lipids.
- Gallbladder disease.
- Abnormal glucose tolerance.
- Ocular lesions.

3. Minor (may be eliminated by changing pills).
   - Breakthrough bleeding.
   - Weight gain.
   - Depression, fatigue, anxiety.
   - Headaches.
   - Acne.
   - Hair loss.
   - Cystic breast changes.
   - Amenorrhea.
   - Monilial vaginitis.
   - Nausea, vomiting.
   - Growth of uterine myomas.
   - Chloasma.
   - Hirsutism.
   - Decreased libido.
4. Beneficial
   a. Decreased:
   - menstrual blood loss.
   - dysfunctional uterine bleeding.
   - dysmenorrhea.
   - fibrocystic disease.
   - premenstrual syndrome.
   - functional ovarian cysts.
   - acne and/or hirsutism.

   b. Increased:
   - libido.
   - breast size.

Reference

Abramowiczs M, ed. The Medical Letter on Drugs & Therapeutics: Choices of Contraceptives. 30:779, November 18, 1988.

PELVIC PAIN

I. Diagnostic Approach to Pelvic Pain
   A. History.
      1. Pain -- onset, location, duration, description, intensity, relationship to menses.
      2. Menstrual history -- changes, LMP, spotting, birth control, sexual activity, signs of pregnancy (nausea, breast tenderness, urinary frequency).
      3. Systems -- specific questions with above differential diagnosis in mind (GU, GI, GYN systems). Evidence of hypovolemia.
   B. Physical Exam.
      1. Abdomen -- peritoneal signs, masses, tenderness, bowel sounds, rectal exam with guaiac, flank tenderness.
      2. Pelvic -- complete vulvar and vaginal exam, cervix (dilation, tissue at os, lesions, tenderness to movement), uterine tenderness and size, adnexae (masses, tenderness, unilateral or bilateral).
   C. Diagnostic aids.
      1. Bloods -- CBC with differential, ESR. Elevated with infections or inflammations, H/H may be decreased with hemorrhage. Useful with repeat testing over time.
      2. Cultures -- blood, cervical, urine, as indicated.
      3. Urinalysis -- helpful to differentiate GU pathology. May still be negative if complete obstruction is present.
      4. Stool guaiac -- points toward GI tract if positive.
      5. Pregnancy test -- must know sensitivity of the test you are using. Urine pregnancy test may miss up to half of all ectopics. Serum RIA is very sensitive and picks up virtually all pregnancies.
      6. Culdocentesis -- positive with any intraperitoneal bleeding (eg., ectopic pregnancy, bleeding corpus luteum cyst, ruptured liver adenoma, ruptured spleen, peptic ulcer).

Pelvic Pain

7. Ultrasound -- useful to distinguish intrauterine from extrauterine pregnancy, may also be abnormal in appendicitis, luteal cysts, PID, spontaneous abortion.
8. Abdominal films -- may show ureteral stone, bowel obstruction.
9. Radiologic studies -- e.g., barium enema, IVP, CT scan.
10. Laparoscopy -- sometimes performed prior to laparotomy.

II. Management (Table 7-2)

Table 7-2. Differential Diagnosis.

GI	GU	GYN
appendicitis	pyelonephritis	ectopic pregnancy
diverticulitis	ureteral stone	spontaneous abortion
inflammatory bowel	cystitis	pelvic inflammatory disease
irritable bowel		bleeding corpus luteum cyst
bowel obstruction		adnexal torsion
inguinal hernia		mittleschmerz
		endometriosis

A. Assess vital signs, stabilize if necessary.
B. Order CBC with diff, UA, urine or serum pregnancy test.
C. Consider culdocentesis if patient has unstable vital signs or peritoneal signs.
D. If evidence of peritoneal irritation (surgical abdomen), intraperitoneal bleeding with signs or symptoms of pregnancy, positive pregnancy test--consult with OB/GYN. If suspect hemorrhage (unstable vital signs), do not order more time consuming tests (eg., ultrasound) prior to surgical consultation.
E. If findings are as in D, but without signs or tests suggesting pregnancy, consult OB/GYN or general surgery.
F. If patient is stable and without signs of a surgical abdomen, consider further workup to determine cause of pain as indicated by the history (eg., cultures, ESR, ultrasound, barium enema, sigmoidoscopy, colonoscopy, IVP, abdominal flatplate).

References

Hospital Medicine. Hospital Publications, Inc. Oct. 1988, pg. 134-135.

Mills J, *et al*, eds. <u>Current Emergency Diagnosis and Treatment, 2nd edition</u>. Los Altos: Lange Medical Publications, 1985.

ADNEXAL MASSES

I. Overview

A. Adnexae are the potential spaces between the uterus and the lateral pelvic walls.

B. Normal Structures.

1. Ovaries, usually 3-5 cm. in length but influenced by hormones.
2. Fallopian tubes, normally cannot be felt.
3. Ninety percent of adnexal masses involve the fallopian tube and/or ovary.

II. Differential Diagnosis by Organ System

A. Ovary.

1. Functional cysts.
   a. Hemorrhagic cysts.
   b. Delayed resolution of corpus luteum cyst.
   c. Follicle cyst.
2. Neoplasm.
   a. Benign.
   b. Malignant.
3. Endometriosis.

B. Fallopian tube.

1. Tubo-ovarian abscess.
2. Ectopic pregnancy.
3. Hydrosalpinx.
4. Parovarian cyst.
5. Neoplasm.

C. Uterus.

1. Pregnancy in horn of bicornate uterus.
2. Pedunculated or interligamentous myoma.

D. Bowel.

1. Cecal or sigmoid gas and/or feces.
2. Diverticulitis with cellulitis or abscess.
3. Ileitis.

       4. Appendicitis with cellulitis or abscess.
       5. Colonic cancer (especially with perforation and abscess).
    E. Miscellaneous.
       1. Distended bladder.
       2. Mesenteric cyst.
       3. Pelvic kidney.
       4. Abdominal wall hematoma or abscess.
       5. Retroperitoneal neoplasm.
       6. Lymphocyst.
       7. Urachal cyst.

III. Evaluation

   A. History.
      1. Ovarian neoplasms are often clinically silent except for nonspecific "pressure" symptoms. These include urinary frequency, constipation, and pelvic heaviness.
      2. Very large tumors may cause abdominal swelling and may be confused with pregnancy.
      3. Pain may result from stretching of the ovarian capsule, torsion, rupture, or intracystic hemorrhage.
      4. Functional cysts may cause menstrual abnormalities.
   B. Physical exam.
      1. Benign tumors are characteristically unilateral, cystic, mobile, and do not cause ascites.
      2. Malignancies are usually solid, fixed, nodular, and may cause ascites.
   C. Diagnostic evaluation may include ultrasound. Other tests such as chest x-ray, abdominal films, IVP, bowel x-rays, and laparoscopy may be indicated.

IV. Treatment of Ovarian Masses

   A. Women of childbearing age with clinically benign ovarian cysts under 6 cm. in diameter may be observed monthly. If a cyst persists or increases in size during a period of observation, proceed with evaluation and probably surgical excision. If the cyst persists but decreases in size, it may be observed through another cycle.

B. Premenstrual and postmenopausal females are at high risk for malignancy. One should proceed to full evaluation without a period of observation. Early diagnosis is essential and usually necessitates surgical excision.

C. Cysts greater than 10 cm. in diameter are more likely to be malignant and require immediate evaluation and probable excision.

D. Solid ovarian tumors (by ultrasound) are almost always malignant and demand immediate and aggressive evaluation and treatment. An exception to this is the rare luteoma of pregnancy.

References

Obstetrics and Gynecology: A pocket Reference. Main and Main, Year Book Medical Publishers, 1984.

Rivlin ME, *et al*, eds. Manual of Clinical Problems in Obstetrics and Gynecology with annotated references. Second edition. Boston/Toronto: Little, Brown, and Co., 1986.

DYSPAREUNIA

Dyspareunia is defined as painful intercourse. It may have a psychologic or organic origin. Even if the basic cause is organic, psychologic factors may secondarily emerge resulting in patterns of behavior that must be addressed as well as the organic cause of pain.

I. **Types of Dyspareunia**
   A. Superficial dyspareunia--pain is perceived at or near the introitus.
   B. Deep dyspareunia--pain is perceived deep in the vagina or lower abdomen.
   C. Non-organic dyspareunia.

II. **Differential Diagnosis**
   A. Superficial dyspareunia.
      1. Inflammatory disease of the vulva, vagina, bladder; e.g., vulvovaginitis, trigonitis, urethritis, bartholinitis; vestibulitis; causes are fungal, bacterial, viral (herpes, condylomata), irritant (tight fitting clothes).
      2. Tender, contracted scars; e.g., following episiotomy, vaginal repair.
      3. Atrophic vaginitis or vulvar dystrophy in the older patient. Atrophic vaginitis also occurs with anorexia, breast-feeding, pelvic irradiation.
      4. Rigid hymen or developmental anomaly in the younger patient.
      5. Errors in sexual technique; e.g., too little foreplay leading to poor lubrication, overzealous clitoral stimulation.
      6. Medications that decrease lubrication; e.g., anticholinergics, antihistamines, diet pills.
      7. Foreign bodies; .eg., coital aids.
      8. Anal intercourse without sufficient lubrication.
      9. Vaginitis medicamentosa from contraceptive chemicals, feminine deodorant sprays, douches.
      10. Vaginismus.

B. Deep dyspareunia.
   1. Endometriosis.
   2. Pelvic inflammatory disease
   3. Ovarian cysts, pelvic surgery causing adhesions, scarring, ovary sutured to vaginal cuff.
   4. Radiation therapy effects.
   5. Pelvic neoplasm.
   6. Retrodisplaced uterus causing an ovary displaced to the cul-de-sac.
   7. Uterine prolapse.
   8. Cervical lacerations or scars.
   9. Rectal pathology.
   10. Orthopedic problems.
C. Psychologic dyspareunia.
   1. Sexual, e.g., fear, disinterest, ignorance, anxiety involving the relationship, (partner with sexual dysfunction, feelings of hostility).
   2. Negative experience, e.g., rape, homosexual encounter

III. Evaluation

A. History.
   1. Onset -- first attempt at intercourse vs. recent onset suggesting recent change or situational problem.
   2. Occurrence of pain -- before penetration, on penetration, with deep penetration. Failure to localize pain suggests psychologic cause.
   3. Duration of pain. Pain existing for several years may not resolve even after a medical condition is identified and corrected.
   4. Establish whether a tampon can be inserted; if so, mechanical obstruction is unlikely.
   5. History of surgery, PID, radiation.
   6. History regarding sexual fears, time spent on foreplay, feelings toward the partner.
   7. Interview the partner.
B. Physical examination.

1. Pelvic exam -- look for signs of vulvovaginitis, atrophic vaginitis, narrowed introitus, cervicitis, congenital abnormalities. Observe for involuntary spasm on attempted examination. Palpate for uterine mass; retroverted uterus; tenderness of uterus, adnexae or with movement of cervix. Examine for loss of support, cystocoele, rectocoele.

C. Laboratory exam.
   1. Pap smear.
   2. Wet prep.
   3. CBC, ESR, cervical cultures if evidence of PID.
   4. Pelvic ultrasound if mass suspected.
   5. Referral for laparoscopy if endometriosis, adhesions, or adnexal mass is suspected.

IV. Treatment

A. Organic diseases should be appropriately treated, eg., infectious diseases (vaginitis, Bartholin's gland duct cyst, PID); atrophic vaginitis; endometriosis.

B. Inadequate lubrication without organic pathology should be treated with reassurance and advice regarding prolonging foreplay and use of a water-soluble lubricant. Changing coital positions, guiding the penis for insertion and oral-genital foreplay are other possible suggestions.

C. Specific surgical procedures may be required (introital dyspareunia), e.g., excision of painful scars or nerve endings damaged by herpetic infection; hymenotomy; plastic surgery for congenital or surgically-acquired disorders not amenable to progressive self-dilatation.

D. Specific surgical procedures (deep dyspareunia), e.g., ventral suspension of uterus or ovaries, hysterectomy, lysis of adhesions.

E. Marital-sexual therapy if indicated, e.g., emphasis on communication skills, sensate focus exercises, relaxation, masturbatory techniques.

F. Behavioral techniques, e.g., changes in coital position (avoidance of deep pain), Kegel's pelvic floor exercises, vaginal self-dilatation.

G.

Blocking or deconditioning spastic vaginal response of vaginismus.

H. Patient education in all cases.

References

Gorol A, *et al*, eds. <u>Primary Care Medicine, 2nd edition</u>. Philadelphia: J.B. Lippincott Co., 1987.

Rivlin ME, *et al*, eds. <u>Manual of Clinical Problems in Obstetrics and Gynecology With Annotated Key References, Second edition</u>. Boston/Toronto: Little, Brown and Company Publishers, 1986.

PEDIATRIC GYNECOLOGY

Gynecology of infancy and childhood is an often neglected area, primarily because gynecologic problems are uncommon prior to onset of puberty; however, when such problems arise, they must be appropriately evaluated.

I. **Pediatric Gynecologic Exam** (performed as needed, not routinely)
   A. Newborn/young infant.
      1. Inspection of external genitalia and palpation of abdominal and inguinal regions.
      2. Assess vaginal patency with soft neonate feeding catheter or "butterfly" catheter tubing after removal of needle.
      3. Rectal exam combined with palpation of abdomen to assess uterus, masses (adnexal/vaginal, etc.).
      4. Vaginoscope or veterinary otoscope for direct visualization of vagina/cervix.
   B. Child.
      1. Inspection as per newborn/young infant.
      2. Pelvic exam performed in either modified frog-leg, Sims, or knee chest positions. Relaxation, comfort, minimal anxiety, good eye contact all important.
      3. Instrumentation as per young infant or use of Huffman-Graves virginal bivalved speculum.

II. **Common Disorders of Infancy and Childhood**
   A. Vulvovaginitis -- most common complaint (85%).
      1. Symptoms include pruritus, soreness, vaginal discharge/bleeding, abdominal/pelvic pain.
      2. Requires exam, microscopic evaluation of vaginal secretions (wet prep), UA, possible cultures.
      3. Etiologies include infections (Candida, Gardnerella, Trichomonas, gonorrhea, beta-strep), foreign bodies, neoplasms-rare.
      4. Treatment.
         a. Removal of foreign body if identified.

- b. Educate concerning perineal hygiene, wiping.
- c. Sitz baths.
- d. Candida -- miconazole nitrate vaginal cream q HS for 7-14 days.
- e. Gardnerella/Trichomonas -- metronidazole 35-50 mg/kg/d up to 750mg divided TID for 7 days.
- f. Gonorrhea -- probenecid 25 mg/kg PO plus amoxicillin 50 mg/kg or procaine PCN G 100,000 Units/kg IM or spectinomycin 40 mg/kg IM.
- g. B-strep -- PCN G 200,000 Units PO QID x 10 days
- h. UTI -- Amoxicillin 20-40 mg/kg/d divided TID x 7-10 days or dependent on sensitivities.
- i. Scabies -- wash clothing and bedding, gamma benzene hexachloride 1% lotion/shampoo once.

B. Pinworms (Enterobias vermicularis).
  1. May cause vulvovaginitis, rectal itching common.
  2. May visualize perianal worms or ova using scotch-tape test (apply adhesive side of tape to perianal skin in early morning hours when worms migrate to area to deposit eggs).

C. Diaper dermatitis (primary contact irritant dermatitis).
  1. Caused by irritants in excreta, mainly urine, producing red, papulo-vesicular, shiny rash sparing skin folds; may fissure.
  2. Secondary infection with Strep, Staph, Candida may occur.
  3. Treat with frequent changing allowing skin to dry completely, good hygiene, mechanical protection with zinc oxide or white petroleum.
  4. Treat secondary infection if present.

D. Labial adhesions.
  1. May have congenital origin or form secondary to inflammatory process, also seen with sexual abuse.
  2. Form visual adhesions of labia preventing complete visualization of introitus.
  3. Treat with topical estrogen cream BID for 7-14 days.

Gynecology

- E. Neonatal vaginal bleeding.
    1. May occur at 3-5 days age representing withdrawal of placental estrogens; normal physiologic process.
    2. No treatment necessary, reassure parents.
- F. Urethral prolapse.
    1. Inadequate support tissue in distal urethra because it is estrogen dependent, further stress placed on tissue with straining, increased intraabdominal pressure.
    2. Findings of a painful, friable mass at vaginal orifice; catheter passed through center of mass enters bladder.
    3. Treat initially with topical estrogens and antibiotic creams; may require surgical excision if medical therapy fails.
- G. Vaginal foreign body.
    1. May present with putrid, purulent, blood-tinged discharge.
    2. Confirmed by direct visualization, cultures taken to evaluate for concurrent infection.
    3. Remove foreign body and treat infectious process if identified.

III. Rare But Serious Disorders of Infancy/Childhood

- A. Sarcoma botryoides.
    1. Presents with bloody vaginal discharge and originates in upper vagina/cervix.
    2. Cluster of grapes appearance, may appear as a single polyp.
    3. Survival is rare and early radical surgery is imperative.
- B. Ovarian tumors.
    1. Usually germ or mesenchymal cell origin.
    2. Symptoms include pain, mass, pressure; may cause vaginal bleeding if hormonally active.
    3. Require complete evaluation by experienced gynecologist.

References

Behrman RE and Vaughan VC, eds. <u>Nelson Textbook of Pediatrics, 12th edition</u>. Philadelphia: W.B. Saunders Co., 1983.

Driscoll CE, *et al*, eds. <u>Handbook of Family Practice</u>. Chicago: Year Book Medical Publishers, 1986.

ABNORMAL VAGINAL BLEEDING

Abnormal vaginal bleeding is a symptom representative of a variety of different possible conditions, most of which are benign yet troublesome.

I. **Introduction**
   A. Normal menstrual bleeding occurs every 3-5 weeks lasting 5-7 days, is less regular and with greater variance in flow at the extremes of reproductive functioning, ie menarche and menopause.
   B. Terminology for abnormal bleeding:
      1. Menorrhagia -- bleeding at expected time but heavier than normal. Bleeding requiring > 1 pad/hr. or with excessive amount of clotting.
      2. Metrorrhagia -- bleeding which occurs between menstrual periods, commonly referred to as spotting or break-through-bleeding.
      3. Polymenorrhea -- cyclical bleeding at intervals less than 21 days.
      4. Oligomenorrhea -- cyclical bleeding at intervals greater than 35 days.
      5. Amenorrhea -- absence of menstrual bleeding.
   C. 5-20% women experience menorrhagia at some point in time, symptom most commonly evaluated.

II. **Etiology** (Five Major Categories)
   A. Pregnancy -- normal and complicated pregnancies including spontaneous abortions, threatened abortions, ectopics, molar pregnancies, etc.
   B. Dysfunctional uterine bleeding- most often associated with anovulatory cycles and irregular sloughing of estrogen stimulated endometrium. Represents abnormal hormonal regulation with tonic hormone levels rather than cyclical fluctuating gonadotropins and sex hormones. Common causes include: puberty, climacteric, anorexia nervosa, PCOD and obesity.
   C. Benign organic lesions -- include chronic cervicitis, cervical polyps, endometrial polyps, leiomyomata, chronic en-

dometritis including low grade form associated with IUD use.

D. Malignant lesions -- including vaginal, uterine, cervical carcinomas; estrogen producing ovarian neoplasms with most common being granulosa-thecal cell tumor.

E. Coagulopathies -- most common is Von Willebrand's disease. Also consider leukemias.

F. Miscellaneous causes -- viral illnesses, hypothyroidism, liver disease, oral contraceptive break-through bleeding, ovulatory bleeding, etc.

III. **Evaluation** (Somewhat Age-Dependent)

A. History including prior menstrual history, drug history, symptoms of mononucleosis, hepatitis, pregnancy, bleeding tendencies, contraceptive use (oral contraceptives or IUD).

B. Physical exam (including pelvic) noting hirsutism, virilization, vaginal/cervical lesions, uterine size and shape, adnexal masses.

C. Initial lab evaluation to include: CBC, PT, PTT, platelet count, T4, TSH. Consider BHCG, androgens, FSH/LH as indicated.

IV. **Treatment of Irregular Bleeding**

A. Differs between adolescent, woman in mature reproductive years, and postmenopausal bleeding.

B. Adolescent usually represents dysfunctional (anovulatory) bleeding.

1. After history and PE have excluded organic disease, treat with norethindrone 5 mg PO BID x 21 days and expect withdrawal bleeding. Repeat a second cycle from day 5-25.

2. Alternative therapy includes medroxyprogesterone acetate 10 mg PO BID x 5 days.

3. Consider oral contraceptive therapy for regulation until maturation of hypothalamic-pituitary-ovarian axis.

4. Profuse bleeding (Hb < 10, orthostatic) may require high dose estrogens (conjugated estrogens 25 mg IV

q 4 hours) followed by combined estrogen-progestin therapy or currettage.

    5. If repeated episodes of excessive, irregular bleeding occur, consider polycystic ovarian disease, obtain appropriate studies to confirm and treat with oral contraceptives or cyclical medroxyprogesterone acetate 10 mg PO q day x 10 days starting 20 days after beginning withdrawal period.

C. Reproductive mature female--first rule out pregnancy and evaluate for organic causes. Also consider oral contraceptive related bleeding.

    1. Medical currettage using norethindrone 5 mg PO TID x 21 days. If bleeding continues beyond day 7 of progestin, perform D&C.

    2. After initial progestin therapy, cycle with medroxyprogesterone acetate 10 mg PO q day or norethindrone 5 mg PO BID x 10 days each cycle beginning 20 days after onset bleeding for 3-4 months.

    3. Repeated episodes of irregular bleeding should be treated with D&C and hysteroscopy to evaluate for organic lesions, ie polyps, submucosal fibroids.

    4. Hysterectomy may be considered for recurrent bleeding if reproductive potential not desired.

D. Postmenopausal bleeding

    1. Always requires complete evaluation for carcinoma including endometrial biopsy, possibly full surgical D&C under anesthesia.

    2. Treat benign lesions if identified.

    3. Surgical therapy with adjunctive radiation therapy for carcinoma.

Reference

Goldfarb. Evaluating menstrual dysfunction. <u>Patient Care</u>, Sept. 15, 1982, pp 12-48.

DYSMENORRHEA

I. **Dysmenorrhea is:** (Painful Menses)
   A. Types of dysmenorrhea.
      1. Primary --pelvic organs are normal.
      2. Secondary -- pathologic lesions are found on pelvic exam or at laparoscopy.
   B. Importance.
      1. Painful menstruation may be the most common gynecologic disorder. Over half of menstruating women experience some discomfort. 10% of these women are incapacitated for 1-3 days each month.
      2. Dysmenorrhea is a significant cause of lost time from work and school and is responsible for over 140 million wasted hours annually.
   C. Diagnosis.
      1. Primary dysmenorrhea must be differentiated from premenstrual syndrome.
      2. Differentiation of primary and secondary dysmenorrhea depends on history, physical examination and, possibly, laboratory findings.

II. **Primary Dysmenorrhea**
   A. Definition. Primary dysmenorrhea is menstrual pain in women whose pelvic organs are normal.
   B. Etiology. The cramping is accepted as being secondary to exaggerated uterine contractility. Stimulation of the contractility is through increased prostaglandin activity from hormonal and psychologic factors.
   C. Clinical features.
      1. Pain characteristically begins a few hours before to 12 hours after the onset of flow, lasting 24-36 hours.
      2. Typical history is of pain-free menses for the first few months to years following menarche with gradual onset of pain with menstruation which may become increasingly severe.
      3. Absence of pain with menarche is thought to be related to early cycles being anovulatory. With ovula-

tion, hormonal stimulation of prostaglandin activity increases pain.

4. Most women with primary dysmenorrhea are younger than 20 years.

D. Evaluation.

1. After obtaining a history compatible with primary dysmenorrhea (see II. C.):

    a. Obtain a general medical history. Certain debilitating medical conditions can increase symptoms.

    b. Investigate possibility of pregnancy, colitis, UTI.

    c. Gently probe into psychologic areas. Asking "What do you remember of your first period?" may allow information regarding knowledge about periods, ability to talk with friends or mother about periods, source of information about periods or sexual matters, as well as information regarding pain and other characteristics of menarche to be presented.

    d. Assess how much the pain interferes with her life. Reassurance may be all that is sought and necessary.

2. General physical exam and pelvic exam are mandatory.

3. Laboratory tests are usually not necessary unless history or physical exam suggest other abnormalities (eg., pregnancy, colitis, UTI).

E. Treatment.

1. Reassurance may be all that is needed, with or without over-the-counter drugs.

2. Prostaglandin inhibitors (e.g., ibuprofen 400 mg PO TID), three days before the onset of flow through the second day of flow. If dysmenorrhea is relieved, continue and reassess need for meds in one year; if not, try another NSAID or go on to ovulation suppression.

3. Oral contraception for ovulation suppression, unless contraindicated. Try for one or two months. If pain is relieved, continue for one year and reevaluate.

4. If above treatments are unsuccessful, consider an organic disease or psychosomatic problem.
    a. Consider laparoscopy.
    b. If laparoscopy is negative, suspect psychosomatic origin and offer to refer for counseling.

III. Secondary Dysmenorrhea

A. Definition. Secondary dysmenorrhea is pain with menstruation noted in the presence of other pelvic disease.

B. Etiology. This "acquired dysmenorrhea" is due to a demonstrable factor. Possibilities include endometriosis, intrauterine or submucous myomata, endometrial cancer and IUD use (all of which can also cause increased prostaglandin synthesis and so increased cramping as in primary dysmenorrhea). Other possiblities are endometrial polyps, pelvic inflammatory disease, mechanical obstruction from cervical stenosis or sharply anteverted or retroflexed uterus. The etiology may also be congenital as in a congenital blind pouch of the uterus or congenitally imperforate hymen.

C. Clinical features.
    1. Pain usually begins after the age of 20 years and is a change from the woman's normal pattern.
    2. Pain is less characteristically related to the beginning of the cycle and may be present before or after the actual menses; tends to be progressive with age rather than decreasing with age as with primary dysmenorrhea.
    3. Review of systems can differentiate the possible etiologies.

D. Evaluation.
    1. History is most important in the diagnosis of secondary dysmenorrhea. See details in section III. C.
    2. Physical Exam. Careful general physical and pelvic exams are mandatory to help distinguish between causes of secondary dysmenorrhea.
    3. Laboratory tests. Appropriate tests as indicated (e.g., cultures, ESR). Radiologic tests may be indicated.

E. Treatment
   1. Laparoscopy is often indicated.
   2. Other treatments appropriate to the underlying cause of the pain (e.g., dilation of the os for cervical stenosis).

References

Friederich MA, ed. Lifting the Curse of Menstruation. Haworth Press, Inc., 1983.

Goldfarb. Evaluation menstrual dysfunction. Patient Care, Sept. 15, 1982, pp. 17-23.

Jones HW and Jones GS, eds. Novak's Textbook of Gynecology, 10th edition. Baltimore/London: Williams & Wilkins, 1981.

Patient Care Flow Chart Manual, 4th edition. Medical Economics Co., 1988.

INFERTILITY

Involuntary infertility, defined as the inability to conceive during one or more years of regular, unprotected intercourse, is increasing in incidence with a larger number of involved couples seeking medical evaluation.

I. General Information
A. Primary infertility -- conception never has occurred.
B. Secondary infertility -- at least one prior pregnancy has occurred.
C. Affects 10-15% of all couples.
D. Average time to conception is three months.
E. Increase in infertility rate possibly secondary to delay in childbearing age, increased incidence of PID and subsequent tubal damage, and apparent increase secondary to unavailability of babies for adoption.
F. May present as family dysfunction problem rather than medical problem.
G. 10-15% couples without identifiable cause after evaluation.

II. Overview of Evaluation
A. Important to define infertility as a couple, avoid pointing guilt.
B. Acknowledge emotional nature of problem and carry out evaluation in a sensitive manner.
C. Four Major Factors (each which require evaluation).
   1. Male factor -- accounts for 40-50%.
   2. Cervical factor -- accounts for approximately 5%.
   3. Tubal factor -- accounts for approximately 40%.
   4. Ovulation factor -- accounts for 5-15%.
D. Screening of male factor prior to expensive, prolonged, female evaluation may be warranted.
E. Each individual should have a thorough general history and physical.

III. Male Factor

A. Semen analysis is most important evaluation.
   1. Optimally performed after 2-4 days abstinence for accurate count, and collected in a glass receptacle, not condom which contains spermacide.
   2. Normal analysis includes 20-40 million sperm/cc, volume of 1.5-4.0 cc, sperm mobility of >60% at 2 hours with good forward motion, and normal liquification.
   3. If analysis normal, no further work-up may be needed. If abnormal, repeat in two weeks to rule out transient abnormalities.

B. If female work-up negative, perform sperm penetration assay.
   1. 20% male infertility secondary to inability to penetrate egg.
   2. Test sperm's ability to penetrate hamster egg.

C. Causes of male infertility.
   1. Genetic disorders, ie Klinefelter's syndrome.
   2. Primary testicular disorders -- cryptorchidism, mumps orchitis, etc.
   3. Endocrine disorders -- panhypopituitarism, prolactinoma, etc.
   4. Ductal obstruction -- epididymal, usually secondary to infection, congenital absence of vas, previous surgical ligation.
   5. Retrograde ejaculation.
   6. Varicocele -- present in 30% all males with infertility.
   7. Hypospadias -- or other conditions leading to lack of deposition of sperm in the vaginal vault.

D. Treatment is etiology specific.
   1. Surgical therapy for vas reversal, spermatic vein ligation of varicocele, hypospadias repair.
   2. Gonadotropin therapy if pituitary failure.
   3. Homologous split ejaculate insemination if low counts or mobility.

4. Artificial insemination with donor semen for untreatable infertility.

IV. Cervical Factor

A. Ovulatory cervical mucus normally allows for prolonged sperm survival. Mucus is clear, acellular, with increased elasticity (spinnbarkeit) and decreased viscosity.

B. Huhner test -- evaluates hostility of cervical mucus.
1. Cervical mucus aspirated 8-12 hours post-intercourse about the time of ovulation to assess sperm number, survivability, motility.
2. Normal exam is >5 sperm with good, linear motility.
3. Immobile sperm of normal number suggests sperm antibodies.
4. Many WBC's suggest infection or chronic cervicitis.

C. Treatment.
1. Antibiotics for cervicitis guided by cervical culture results.
2. Corticosteroids if immunologic cause.
3. Cryotherapy or electrocautery for chronic cervicitis.
4. Estrogen therapy for poor quality mucus.

V. Tubal Factor

A. Tubal obstruction increased in patient with history of PID, abdominal surgery, prior IUD use, previous ectopic pregnancy.

B. Tubal patency does not necessarily equal tubal function.

C. Patency assessed by hysterosalpingogram.
1. May identify uterine anomalies, fibroids, synechiae.
2. May provide therapeutic effect by mechanically lysing adhesions.
3. May not identify pelvic adhesions or endometriosis.

D. Laparoscopy offers advantage of direct visualization.

E. Treatment -- salpingostomy, usually with poor results.

VI. Ovulation Factor

A. Documentation of ovulation should be first step in female evaluation.
   1. Symptoms of ovulation helpful, i.e., Mittleschmerz, PMS symptoms.
   2. Perform basal body temperature (BBT) charting.
      a. Should see 0.5-1.0 F increase with ovulation.
      b. Elevation < 10 days suggests luteal phase defect.
   3. Obtain progesterone measurement on day #21 (>3-5 ng/ml).
   4. Consider endometrial biopsy.

B. May require endocrine work-up if amenorrhea or dysfunctional bleeding (See appropriate sections).

C. Correctable endocrinopathies must be treated before attempting pregnancy.

D. Treatment -- should be performed by those with expertise in the field.
   1. Clomiphene citrate 50 mg/day days 5-9 of menstrual cycle. If not successful after the first cycle, may increase dose to 100 mg/day for 2nd and 3rd cycles. Expect ovulation between days 10-16.
      a. Side effects include ovarian enlargement, vasomotor flushes, multiple gestation in 5-10%.
      b. 80% will ovulate.
   2. Clomiphene as above followed by 10,000 IU HCG 5-7 days after clomiphene.
   3. Human menopausal gonadotropin (Pergonal) to stimulate ovaries.
      a. Treatment of choice if hypothalamic-pituitary insufficiency.
      b. Hyperstimulation syndrome may occur.
      c. Multiple gestation occurs in 20-35%.

E. Luteal phase defect may occur in 3% of infertile women.
   1. Abnormal ovarian function with inadequate progesterone production or duration by corpus luteum.

2. Diagnose by endometrial biopsy 1-2 days prior to expected menses.
    a. Biopsy should be in phase with onset period and date of ovulation estimated by BBT.
    b. Diagnosis confirmed by biopsy out of phase >2 days in 2 cycles.
3. Treatment is supplemental progesterone.
    a. Progesterone in oil 12.5 mg IM daily or vaginal suppositories 25 mg BID starting 3 days after ovulation as determined by BBT.
    b. Continue treatment until menses which should not be delayed.
    c. If pregnancy occurs, continue until week 10 at which time placental progesterone is sufficient to support pregnancy.

References

Branch, ed. Office Practice of Medicine. Philadelphia: W.B. Saunders Co., 1982.

Rivlin ME, et al, eds. Manual of Clinical Problems in Obstetrics and Gynecology. Boston: Little, Brown and Co., 1982.

ENDOMETRIOSIS

I. **Overview**

   A. Definition -- Endometriosis is the presence of functioning endometrial tissue outside its normal location, most frequently confined to the ovaries, uterosacral ligaments, cul-de-sac and occasionally uterovesical peritoneum.

   B. Pathogenesis: Three major theories.

   1. Retrograde transport and implantation.

   2. Retrograde transport with metaplastic transformation of adjacent peritoneum.

   3. Lymphatic or hematogenous dissemination.

II. **Evaluation**

   A. History.

   1. The most common symptoms associated with pelvic endometriosis are dysmenorrhea (66%), dyspareunia (33%), infertility (70%), and pelvic pain.

   2. Less common symptoms include dyschezia (painful defecation), premenstrual spotting, dysfunctional uterine bleeding and dysuria.

   3. One-third of women have no symptoms.

   B. Physical examination.

   1. Fifty percent of women have a normal clinical examination.

   2. Findings may include a fixed, tender, retroverted uterus; tender nodules of the uterosacral ligaments (with obliteration of the cul-de-sac) ; nodules on the back of the uterus and cervix; bilateral fixed adnexal masses.

   C. Diagnostic aids.

   1. Laparoscopy. As the clinical diagnosis may be wrong 30-40% of the time, it is necessary to confirm the diagnosis of endometriosis by laparoscopy prior to beginning an intensive treatment. Laparoscopy will assess the extent and stage of the disease as well as tubal patency.

Endometriosis

III. **Management**
  A. Key points.
    1. Because ectopic endometrial tissue is unable to regenerate after it is removed hormonally or surgically, it is responsive to treatment.
    2. Normal endometrial tissue, if removed from its underlying regenerative layer, will regenerate with appropriate hormonal stimulation.
    3. Diagnosis should be confirmed by laparoscopy before undertaking these intensive treatments.
    4. Minimal disease is not associated with infertility.
  B. Mild disease.
    1. Endometriosis with peritoneal cul-de-sac involvement is often not progressive, particularly when the ovaries are not involved.
    2. Treatment options include:
      a. Observation.
      b. Mild analgesics.
      c. Cyclic birth control pills (estrogen and progesterone) to create anovulatory cycles.
  C. Moderate disease in women not desiring pregnancy.
    1. Treatment options include:
      a. "Pseudo-menopause" -- Danazol treatment for six months. This treatment suppresses gonadotropins and causes endometrial tissue to slough. 10% of women get side effects comparable to menopause.
      b. "Pseudo-pregnancy" -- estrogen and progesterone in 2-10 x the dose in birth control pills. Treat for six months to a year. This treatment has antigonadotrophic effects as well as a direct effect on endometrial tissue. 100% of patients have severe side effects.
      c. Conservative surgery-may use hormones 6 weeks prior to and 3-6 months after surgery.
  D. Moderate disease in women desiring pregnancy.
    1. Treatment options are as above in III. C.

2. Pseudo-menopause and conservative surgery have a better success rate for subsequent pregnancy than pseudo-pregnancy.

E. Severe disease.
  1. Treatment options are as above in III. C.
  2. Radical surgery--hysterectomy with removal of ovaries if they are involved.

References

Obstetrics and Gynecology:A Pocket Reference. Main and Main, Year Book Medical Publishers, Inc., 1984.

Rivlin ME, *et al*, eds. Manual of Clinical Problems in Obstetrics & Gynecology, 2nd edition. Boston/Toronto: Little, Brown & Company, 1982.

PELVIC INFLAMMATORY DISEASE

Includes wide variety of clinical infections, i.e., puerperal and post-op infections, septic abortions, and salpingitis. Term often used interchangeably with acute salpingitis--sexually transmitted, ascending infection of the upper genital tract.

I. **Pathogenesis**
   A. Microbiology -- polymicrobial, N. gonorrhoeae, C. trachomatis, mycoplasma hominis, Ureaplasma urealyticum, facultative enteric gram-negative bacilli, and various anaerobes have been cultured; however, N. gonorrhoae and C. trachomatis are considered causative agents.
   B. Ascending infection from cervix to fallopian tubes. Initial mucosal damage to tubes by N. gonorrhoeae with secondary infection by other organisms.

II. **Predisposing Factors**

   Multiple sexual partners, nonbarrier contraceptive use especially IUD, transvaginal instrumentation of cervix/uterus, recent menstrual period, history of PID.

III. **Diagnosis**
   A. Differential diagnosis includes appendicitis, ectopic pregnancy, septic abortion, pyelonephritis, inflammatory bowel disease, endometriosis, corpus luteum hemorrhage, ovarian cyst.
   B. Important to obtain appropriate cultures--endocervix, rectum, urethral, consider blood and peritoneal fluid as well.
   C. Laparoscopy most reliable method of diagnosis. Culdocentesis may also aid in diagnosis (see procedure section).
   D. Specific criteria for diagnosis. All three of the following:
      1. Lower abdominal pain and tenderness with or without rebound.
      2. Cervical motion tenderness.
      3. Adnexal tenderness.

E. Plus one or more of the following:
 1. Temperature >38 C.
 2. WBC > 10,500.
 3. Culdocentesis positive for WBC's and bacteria.
 4. Inflammatory mass on pelvic or ultrasound exams.
 5. Elevated ESR.
 6. Endocervical gram stain with gram-negative intracellular, diplococci or endocervical smear positive for C. trachomatis by monoclonal antibodies.

IV. Treatment

Precise bacteriological diagnosis often unknown at time therapy initiated, therefore must provide antibiotic coverage for all likely pathogens.

A. Outpatient Therapy.
 1. Ceftriaxone 250 mg IM or cefoxitin 2 grams IM plus probenecid 1 gram PO.
 2. Either of above followed by doxycycline 100 mg PO BID x 10 days.

B. Inpatient therapy.
 1. Cefoxitin 2 grams IV q 6 hrs plus doxycycline 100 mg IV q 12 hrs until improvement, then doxycycline 100 mg PO BID to complete 10 days.
 2. Alternative therapy: clindamycin 600 mg IV q 6 hrs plus gentamicin 2 mg/kg IV x one dose followed by gentamicin 1.5 mg/kg IV q 8 hrs until improvement. Then clindamycin 450 mg PO QID to complete 10-14 days.

C. Criteria for Hospital Admission
 - Uncertain diagnosis.
 - Suspected pelvic abscess.
 - Concurrent pregnancy.
 - Severity of illness precludes outpatient therapy.
 - Patient unable to follow outpatient regimen.
 - Failure of outpatient therapy.
 - Follow-up after 48-72 hrs of therapy not possible.

V. **Complications**

Infection rarely remains confined to fallopian tubes, i.e., peritonitis is common and occasionally becomes generalized. Increased risk of ectopic pregnancy, infertility, rupture of a tubo-ovarian abcess, adnexal torsion, bowel obstruction secondary to adhesions, and septicemia.

References

Abramowiczs M, ed. The Medical Letter on Drugs & Therapeutics: Pelvic Inflammatory Disease. 30:757, Jan. 15, 1988.

Hager WD, *et al*, Criteria for diagnosis and grading of salpingitis. Obstet Gynecol 61:113-114, 1983.

SPONTANEOUS ABORTIONS

I. **Definitions**

A. Threatened abortion -- mild vaginal cramps with bleeding, usually minimal and transient. Cervix is long and closed. Uterus is appropriate size for pregnancy. Fetus remains viable.

B. Inevitable abortion -- persistent uterine cramps and moderate vaginal bleeding. Cervical os is open (finger or 0.5 cm sponge stick passes). Fetal or placental tissue is found in the vagina or protrudes through the cervical os, or the patient gives a history of passing tissue.

C. Incomplete abortion -- as per inevitable abortion but uterine cramps and vaginal bleeding are persistent and excessive.

D. Complete abortion -- entire conceptus is expelled. Uterine cramps markedly diminish or stop. Vaginal bleeding stops.

E. Missed abortion -- products of conception are retained two months or more after fetal death. Symptoms and signs of pregnancy abate and pregnancy test becomes negative. Brownish vaginal discharge (rarely frank bleeding) occurs. Uterine cramps are rare. Uterus is soft and irregular. Abdominal x-ray may reveal fetal parts or uterine gas. Ultrasound rules out live fetus.

II. **Possible Causes of Abortion** (Table 7-3)

Table 7-3. Possible Causes of Abortion

Chromosomal abnormality of ovum	Age of gametes
Radiation exposure	Viral infection
Chemical exposure	Diabetes
Hyperthyroidism/ hypothyroidism	Chronic renal vascular disease
Chronic infection (mycoplasma, toxoplasmosis)	Endometrial polyp
	Incompetent cervix
Chronic glomerulo nephritis	Acute illness
Uterine myomas	Abdominal trauma/surgery
Cervical laceration	Malnutrition
Severe mental shock	Immunologic disease

III. Evaluation

A. History suggests pregnancy, e.g., intercourse without adequate contraception, missed period(s), nausea, vomiting, breast tenderness. Patient then experiences uterine cramps and vaginal bleeding often with passage of tissue.

B. Physical exam includes evaluation of vital signs, rule out orthostasis. Perform pelvic exam to determine if cervix is open or closed, if tissue is visible, if uterus is appropriate size. Evaluate for other causes of vaginal bleeding (e.g., cervical eversion, polyp, vaginal lesion, infection, ectopic pregnancy). Check for fetal heart tones by ultrasound (if gestation > 10-12 weeks).

C. Laboratory exam.
   1. Pregnancy test positive in 75% of cases.
   2. Blood typing and antibody testing required in all patients for Rh status.
   3. Obtain hemoglobin/hematocrit.
   4. Ultrasound and/or pathologic exam of tissue passed if indicated.

IV. Treatment

A. Examine all patients with bleeding that soaks one or more pads per hour or with symptoms of orthostasis (e.g., faintness or dizziness upon standing, diaphoresis, pale skin). Other patients may be followed closely by phone. Remember patients must be seen within 48 hours for Rho-gam if indicated.

B. Rule out orthostasis, and treat with intravenous normal saline or lactated ringers if present. Consider transfusion if indicated (hemoglobin < 8 gm/dl).

C. Threatened abortion.
   1. Bed rest.
   2. Because of possible teratogenicity, use analgesics and sedatives only if absolutely necessary.
   3. Do not use hormones, douches, tampons. Avoid coitus.
   4. Consider ultrasound to check for gestational sac, fetal cardiac activity, or to rule out ectopic pregnancy.

5. A realistic prognosis may be made by monitoring quantitative BHCG levels or with serial ultrasonography after 8 weeks gestational age.

D. Incomplete or inevitable abortion.

1. Hospitalize if hypovolemia or anemia present or if gestation is > 12 weeks. Treat hypovolemia or anemia as above.

2. Patients with inevitable abortion may be observed if stable or treated as with incomplete abortion.

3. Patients with incomplete abortion (tissue passed with continued bleeding) usually require suction curettage or dilation and curretage. Consider an oxytocin drip as an alternative (20 IU of oxytocin in 1000 ml of crystalloid solution infused at a rate of 50-100 ml/hr). If unsuccessful, proceed with D&C.

E. Complete abortion.

1. Discharge home after vital signs and hemoglobin are documented to be stable and vaginal bleeding has decreased.

2. Consider methergine 0.2 mg po tid for three days if diagnosis is certain or after uterine evacuation.

F. Missed abortion.

1. Hospitalize if there are signs of infection, DIC, or if fetus has been retained longer than 4 weeks.

2. Obtain CBC with differential, platelet count, PT, PTT and DIC panel if indicated.

3. Prepare to perform D&C.

4. Outpatient management may be considered if fetus has been retained less than 4 weeks, if weekly fibrinogen levels are obtained, and if the patient is monitored closely for DIC. Fibrinogen levels less than 150 mg/dl call for evacuation of the uterus.

References

Driscoll CE, *et al*, eds. Handbook of Family Practice. Chicago: Year Book Medical Publishers, 1986.

Jones HW and Jones GS, eds. Novak's Textbook of Gynecology, 10th edition. Baltimore/London: Williams & Wilkins, 1981.

Spontaneous Abortions

Mills J, *et al*, eds. <u>Current Emergency Diagnosis & Treatment, 2nd edition</u>. Los Altos: Lange Medical Publications, 1985.

ECTOPIC PREGNANCY

Ectopic pregnancy is potentially life-threatening and though common, may be difficult to diagnose. It must be suspected in any woman with vaginal bleeding and lower abdominal pain.

I. **Etiology**
   A. 98% of ectopic pregnancies are tubal.
   B. Incidence of ectopics is increased in women with the following entities: infections (eg., salpingitis, PID), tubal surgery, previous tubal pregnancies, IUD use, history of surgery (appendectomy to major pelvic surgery).
   C. Ectopics are theoretically increased in incidence in women with altered fallopian tube physiology such as abnormal ovum (multiple gestation) and endometriosis causing abnormal contractions.

II. **Evaluation Overview**
   A. History.
      1. Funny pain, funny period, funny bleeding.
      2. 98% of women have pain as a major symptom ranging from mild cramping to severe searing pain. The key is that it is an unusual pain for the patient in her cycle.
      3. 80% of women experience abnormal bleeding which may be any amount, type and duration, with or without tissue.
      4. 65% of women have missed their usual period.
      5. Other symptoms seen less often include low grade fever (often confused with chronic PID), syncope, lightheadedness, or shock. Symptoms of early pregnancy (eg, breast tenderness, nausea) may be present.
   B. Physical Exam.
      1. Check vital signs. Check for orthostatic changes. Young healthy women may tolerate a 1000-1500 cc blood loss with few symptoms.
      2. Pelvic exam may be normal early on. In more advanced cases, a tender adnexal mass (70% of all cases), enlarged uterus, or blood in the cul-de-sac (doughy cul-de-sac) may be found.

C. Laboratory Exam.
   1. Pregnancy test.
      a. Common urine pregnancy test is positive in only 50-75% of ectopics, newer urine tests are more sensitive (from 50-200 m IU HCG/ml).
      b. The optimal test is the serum quantitative radioimmunoassay (RIA) for the Beta subunit of HCG (sensitive from 5 to 25 m IU HCG/ml).
D. Ultrasound.
   1. Can identify an intrauterine pregnancy at five weeks from the last menstrual period. If seen, an ectopic is virtually ruled out.
   2. With an ectopic pregnancy, ultrasonic evaluation is characterized by the presence of a complex unilateral adnexal mass adjacent to a slightly enlarged uterus, absence of an intrauterine sac, and usually an abnormal intrauterine echo pattern. Fluid (blood) in the cul-de-sac may be present.
   3. If the serum quantitative RIA for Beta HCG reveals a value less than 6500 m IU HCG/ml (correlating with five weeks gestation), an intrauterine sac, if present, will not yet be detectable by ultrasonography.
E. Culdocentesis will demonstrate the presence of free blood in the peritoneum. Unclotting blood or pieces of old clot designate a positive test.

III. Work-up of the Unstable Patient

A. When an acute abdominal emergency and/or hemorrhagic shock is suspected, immediate culdocentesis will confirm hemoperitoneum. When combined with a positive quick urine pregnancy test, a positive culdocentesis indicates an ectopic in over 99% of cases.
B. Time should not be wasted obtaining an RIA for HCG or an ultrasound.

IV. Work-up of the Stable Patient

A. Serum quantitative RIA for Beta HCG should be obtained.
B. If negative, the diagnosis is ruled out.

C. If positive, obtain ultrasound.
   1. If the RIA is >6500 m IU HCG/ml, the ultrasonic absence of an intrauterine sac is highly suggestive of an ectopic pregnancy, and the presence of an intrauterine sac by ultrasound virtually rules out the diagnosis of ectopic.
   2. If the RIA is <6500 m IU HCG/ml, remember that the ultrasound cannot yet detect a sac. The RIA can detect a pregnancy two weeks earlier than either the ultrasound or the surgeon's eye.
   3. Consider obtaining serial HCG values to differentiate ectopic from intrauterine pregnancy. If HCG does not rise by 66% in 48 hours, suspect ectopic pregnancy.

V. **Treatment of Ectopic Pregnancy is Surgical**

References

Mills J, *et al*, eds. <u>Current Emergency Diagnosis & Treatment, 2nd edition</u>. Los Altos: Lange Medical Publications, 1985.

Pelosi MA and Apuzzio J. Ectopic pregnancy: Latest diagnostic tests, <u>Emergency Decisions</u>, Nov/Dec 1987, pp 38-44.

PREMENSTRUAL TENSION SYNDROME

Constellation of physical, emotional, and/or behavioral symptoms occurring during the luteal phase of the menstrual cycle (7-14 days prior to onset menses), with resolution of symptoms soon after menstrual flow begins. There must be a symptom-free interval during the follicular phase of the menstrual cycle.

I. **Epidemiology**
   A. 90% women with a least minimal symptoms, approximately 10% with severe symptoms.
   B. Affects primarily women in 30-40's, sometimes worse after pregnancy. No association with race, socioeconomic status, other demographics.

II. **Etiology** -- Unclear, but multiple theories proposed.
   A. Hormonal imbalance. Estrogen excess or relative progesterone deficiency.
   B. Prostaglandin effect. Similar to affect in dysmenorrhea.
   C. Endorphins pathologically low.
   D. Vitamin B6 deficiency. May play a role in dopamine and seratonin metabolism.
   E. Prolactin excess. Possible osmoregulatory function.
   F. Aldosterone excess/fluid retention.
   G. Reactive hypoglycemia. Secondary to post-ovulatory increase in insulin release/sensitivity.
   H. Biopsychosocial. Patient's expectations, beliefs, personality, coping style, level of control, adoption of sick role, sexual experiences/relationships, social support network, etc., all play a role.

III. **Diagnosis**
   A. By history. Other pathology excluded by physical exam and lab.
   B. No blood test or radiographic procedure confirms diagnosis.
   C. Prospective charting of symptoms helpful in making diagnosis.

- D. Physical symptoms -- fatigue, breast tenderness, bloating, fluid retention, weight gain, acne, headache, constipation, appetite changes.
- E. Emotional symptoms -- anxiety, anger, depression, irritability, decreased concentration, change in libido, oversensitivity to rejection.

IV. Treatment

- A. Validation. Acknowledgement that PMS is real, suffering from an illness with an unknown biologic basis.
- B. Education. Also educate spouse/family. Make aware of support groups, relaxation techniques, theories of etiology, treatment regimens.
- C. Diet
    1. Limit salt, refined sugar, red meat, fats, caffeine, alcohol.
    2. Increase complex carbohydrates and fiber.
    3. Vitamin supplementation of questionable benefit. Vitamin B6 may be helpful. Dose: 50mg TID. Risk of peripheral neuropathy.
- D. Exercise. May decrease depressive symptoms. Aerobic activity 30-45 minutes 3-4 times weekly.
- E. Medications. Very strong placebo effect. Most studies to date not placebo-controlled.
    1. Diuretics -- spironolactone 25 mg QID during luteal phase. Best results for symptoms of weight gain, edema, bloating, breast tenderness.
    2. Prostaglandin inhibitors -- naproxen 500 mg BID or mefenamic acid 500 mg TID 10 days before period through day #2 of menses.
    3. Progestrone -- 200-400 mg/day natural progesterone as vaginal or rectal suppository during luteal phase (12 days prior to menses).
    4. Oral Contraceptives -- reasonable option if patient <35 and requires birth control.
    5. Danazol -- 200 mg/day. Side effects include weight gain, nausea, androgenic changes.

6. Bromocriptine --2.5 mg BID during luteal phase. Best for mastalgia. Expensive. Side effects include nausea, vomiting, dizziness.

References

Benson, ed. Handbook of Obstetrics and Gynecology. Los Altos: Lange Medical Publishers, 1983.

Wickes SL. Clinics in office practice. Primary Care, 15(3): 473, Sept 1988.

MENOPAUSE

Menopause is the physiological cessation of menstrual function. By definition, cessation of periods for six months must occur before diagnosis is made. The time period about menopause, the climacteric, is full of various bothersome symptoms. Hormonal replacement may abolish many of the symptoms associated with the natural failing of ovarian function and may prevent further health risks.

I. **General Information**
   A. Average age is 51.5 years.
   B. FSH > 40 is pathognomic.
   C. 15% women have disabling symptoms; symptoms secondary to rapidly declining estrogen.

II. **Clinical Features**
   A. Vasomotor symptoms (hot flush).
      1. Occur in 80% women.
      2. Warmth in upper body followed by flush; lasts approximately two minutes.
   B. Atrophic symptoms.
      1. Vaginal atrophy (atrophic vaginitis, dyspareunia, pruritis vulvae).
      2. Breast atrophy.
      3. Atrophic distal urethral syndrome (frequency, dysuria, nocturia with sterile urine, later develop urgency and urge incontinence, eventually develop stricture or narrowing).
   C. Psychological symptoms (irritability, depression, and insomnia).
   D. Cardiovascular (increased risk CAD with increased LDL, decreased HDL).
   E. Osteoporosis.
      1. 50% bone loss in first 7 years of estrogen deficiency.
      2. Accounts for large percentage of hip fractures, forearm fractures, vertebral compression fractures in elderly females.

III. Management

A. Osteoporosis prevention -- must be started early.
   1. Calcium 1000 mg pre/perimenopausal; 1500 mg postmenopausal.
   2. Exercise 30 minutes walking/bicycle riding 3 times weekly.
   3. Consider hormone replacement (see below).
   4. Vitamin D 400 Units/day.

B. Treat vasomotor/atrophic symptoms with hormone replacement.

IV. Hormone Replacement Therapy

A. Benefits (cardioprotective, controls vasomotor/atrophic symptoms, osteoporosis prevention).

B. Risks.
   1. Endometrial hyperplasia/neoplasia 2 x normal if estrogen therapy alone; however, if progestin added less than nonhormonally treated.
   2. Breast cancer: no study confirms increased risk, but risk decreased if combined estrogen/progestin therapy used.
   3. Hypertension: small but significant risk, usually reversible, incidence less than that with oral contraceptives.
   4. Thromboembolic disease: rare, more common with oral contraceptives.

C. Initial assessment.
   1. History. Evaluate for contraindications, i.e., liver disease, thromboembolic disease known/suspected endometrial, breast, or other estrogen dependent neoplasms.
   2. Physical exam highlighting breast and pelvic exams.
   3. Baseline mammography.
   4. Evaluate for the need of endometrial biopsy.
      a. Not necessary when no history of postmenopausal bleeding.
      b. Mandatory if any postmenopausal or abnormal perimenopausal bleeding.

c. Not necessary if withdrawal bleeding occurs at expected time.

d. Necessary if bleeding/spotting occur other than at time of expected withdrawal.

e. Consider sampling every 2 years despite no abnormal bleeding.

D. Standard replacement therapy includes conjugated estrogens e.g., (Premarin) 0.625 mg po days 1-25 and medroxyprogesterone acetate 10 mg po days 16-25.

1. Current trend toward longer course of progestin (12-14 days) with smaller dose of 5 mg.

2. Transdermal estrogen therapy becoming popular; data on effectiveness not yet available.

    a. Patches changed twice weekly on days 1-25, progestin added as per oral estrogen regimen.

    b. 0.05 mg patch equals 0.625 mg orally administered estrogen.

3. May also be given Monday through Friday, conjugated estrogens 0.625 mg, medroxyprogesterone acetate 5 mg.

References

DeFazio and Speroff. Estrogen replacement therapy: Current thinking and practice. <u>Geriatrics</u> 40(11):32, Nov. 1985.

Wickes SL. Clinics in office practice. <u>Primary Care</u> 15(3):473, Sept, 1988.

8/ OBSTETRICS

Pamela L. Brown, M.D.

PRENATAL CARE

I. **History at Initial Evaluation:**
   A. Menstrual history: cycle, duration, LMP, contraception
   B. Medical history: Underlying problems or illnesses, history or sexually transmitted diseases, medications, family history, and genetic history.
   C. Habits: Tobacco, alcohol, other drugs, diet, activity.
   D. Obstetric history: Dates of all pregnancies including terminations and miscarriages. Outcome and gestational length. Duration of labor, complications. Type: NSVD, forceps, C-section, weight, sex, and apgars of liveborn infants. Neonatal complications. Number of living children.
   E. Social history: Support network, father of child involved?, wanted pregnancy?, expectations, potential stresses, need for social/financial services.

II. **Physical Examination**
   A. General physical exam. Particular attention to Ht, Wt, BP, thyroid, dentition, heart, breasts, deep tendon reflexes, signs of underlying heart disease.
   B. Pelvic Examination.
      1. External: Look for evidence of condylomata accuminata (These lesions may progress during pregnancy and a small percentage of infants born through involved vaginal tissue will develop laryngeal papillomas. Podophyllin is contraindicated during pregnancy, but cryotheraphy and laser may be used). Also look for and culture lesions suspicious for herpes.
      2. Vaginal/Cervical: Look for evidence of condylomata and herpes. Examine vaginal discharge, culture cervical discharge for GC and chlamydia. Rule out cervical anomalies. PAP smear should be obtained if patient has not had one in past 6 months.

3. Bimanual: Rule out adnexal abnormalities. Determine uterine size: 8 weeks = 2 x normal, 10 weeks = 3 x normal, 12 weeks = 4 x normal, 16 weeks = halfway to umbilicus, 20 weeks = at umbilicus. Thereafter, rely on fundal height.
4. Clinical pelvimetry. (See same heading under labor.)

III. Laboratory Evaluation

A. First visit.
1. Routine: Cervical cytology, complete blood count (CBC), urinalysis (UA) and screen for bacteriuria, blood group, Rh factor, and antibody screen, serology for syphilis, and Rubella antibody titer.
2. When indicated: Cervical culture for Neisseria gonorrhea and chlamydia, Toxoplasmosis antibody test, Hepatitis B surface antigen (HBsAg) titer, sickle cell preparation or hemoglobin electrophoresis in all previously unscreened black women, tuberculin skin testing, HIV antibody testing.

B. During pregnancy:
- serum alpha-fetoprotein (AFP) 16-18 wks.
- Amniocentesis, when indicated, 16-20 wks.
- Blood glucose screen 24-28wks.
- Urine culture 24-28wks.
- Hematocrit 28-32 wks, 36 wks optional.
- Rh antibody screening along with Coombs testing, when indicated at 28-32 weeks. Consider GC, chlamydia, and herpes rescreening at 36 weeks.

IV. Expected Weight Gain

- First trimester: Should gain 2-5 lbs total.
- After first trimester, 3/4 to 1 lb per week.
- Average total wt gain 25 +/- 5 lbs.

V. Risk Factor Analysis

Obstetric risk factors are obtained by history and physical examination. This form is utilized at the University of Iowa Family Practice Clinic.

OBSTETRIC RISK FACTORS

(enter those checked in blanks below)

FIRST VISIT

DEMOGRAPHIC
- [ ] Disruptive social/economic environment
- [x] Marital Status: Single
- [ ] Age: <18; >35
- [ ] Low educational level

PAST OBSTETRIC HISTORY
- [ ] Para 5 or more
- [ ] Previous cesarean section
- [ ] Previous perinatal death
- [ ] Previous baby with congenital anomaly
- [ ] Previous child with mental retardation or epilepsy
- [ ] Previous abnormal presentation at delivery
- [ ] Previous toxemia
- [ ] Habitual aborter (3 or more, spontaneous)
- [ ] Previous third trimester or postpartum bleeding
- [ ] Previous low birth weight infant (<2500g)
- [ ] Previous excessive size infant (>4000g)
- [ ] Blood group isoimmunization
- [ ] History of uterine anomaly or mid-trimester abortion
- [ ] Previous delivery at <37 or >42 weeks

MEDICAL FACTORS
- [ ] Chronic Viral Infections
- [ ] Hypertension
- [ ] Cardiac Disease
- [ ] Diabetes Mellitus
- [ ] Other endocrine disorder, or history thereof
- [ ] History of phlebitis
- [ ] History of coagulation disorder
- [ ] Chronic pulmonary or gastrointestinal disease
- [ ] Epilepsy
- [ ] Anemia
- [ ] Renal disease, including previous urinary tract infection
- [ ] Other significant chronic illnesses or conditions

OTHER
- [ ] Small pelvis on examination
- [ ] Glucosuria
- [ ] Proteinuria
- [ ] Drug or alcohol abuse
- [ ] Weight <100 or >200 lbs.
- [ ] Late registration for antenatal care
- [ ] Religion - Jehovah's Witness
- [ ] History of DES exposure
- [ ] Genital Herpes or history thereof
- [ ] Unwanted pregnancy
- [ ] Pregnancy without family support
- [ ] Cigarette smoker (> 1 ppd)

---

30 weeks - IN ADDITION TO ABOVE:

- [ ] Low weight gain (<12 lbs)
- [ ] Proteinuria; Bacteriuria; Glucosuria
- [ ] Anemia (Hematocrit <30)
- [ ] Isoimmunization
- [ ] Abnormal uterine size (twins, hydramnios, intrauterine growth retardation)
- [ ] Significant bleeding after 12 wks
- [ ] Incipient or early pre-eclampsia
- [ ] Few prenatal visits
- [ ] Cervical dilatation
- [ ] Venereal disease

ADMISSION TO LABOR + DELIVERY - IN ADDITION TO ABOVE:

- [ ] Premature rupture of membrane (12 hours without labor)
- [ ] <37 or >42 weeks gestation
- [ ] Estimated fetal weight <2500g or >4000g
- [ ] Abnormal presentation
- [ ] Twins
- [ ] Pre-eclampsia
- [ ] Fever
- [ ] Significant uterine bleeding
- [ ] Meconium stained amniotic fluid
- [ ] Abnormal fetal heart rate

References

Hacker N and Moore JG, eds. *Essentials of Obstetrics & Gynecology*. Philadelphia: W.B. Saunders & Company, 1986.

Johnson CA. Prenatal screening. *American Family Physician* 37(5):175, May 1988.

Pritchard JA, *et al*, eds. *Williams Obstetrics, 17th edition*. Connecticut: Appleton-Century-Crofts, 1985.

PRENATAL PATIENT EDUCATION

I. **Nutrition in Pregnancy**
   A. Caloric Requirements.
      1. Requirements: 30-35 kcal/kg/24 hr plus 300 kcal.
      2. Additional requirements: adolescence, multiple gestation.
   B. Calcium.
      1. Requirements: 1200-1500 mg elemental calcium/day.
      2. Calcium supplement:
      - Milk, 8oz glass: 300 mg.
      - Generic calcium carbonate 600 mg tablet.
      - Oscal oyster shell 500 mg tablet.
      - Calcium gluconate chewable 45 mg tablet.
      - Tums regular strength 200 mg tablet.
   C. Iron.
      1. Requirements: 30 mg elemental iron/day.
      2. Additional requirements: If the pregnant woman is iron deficient or has a multiple gestation pregnancy, she should take 60-100 mg elemental iron/day. If her Hgb is < 10, then she requires 200 mg day.
      3. Iron supplements.
      - Ferrous sulfate 65 mg Fe (elemental)/325 mg tablet.
      - Ferrous fumarate 100 mg Fe/325mg.
      - Ferrous gluconate 38mg Fe/325mg.
   D. Folic acid.
      1. Requirements: 1 mg/day.
      2. Sources: Green leafy vegetables, broccoli, mushrooms, liver. Prenatal vitamins.

II. **Exercise in Pregnancy**
   A. ACOG guidelines for pregnancy and postpartum.
      1. Regular (3 or more times/week) exercise is preferable to intermittent.
      2. Avoid vigorous activity in heat and humidity.
      3. Avoid ballistic movements.
      4. Avoid deep flexion or extension of joints.

5. Vigorous activity should be preceded by 5 minute warm-up.
6. Vigorous activity should be followed by a period of cool-down.
7. Heart rate should be measured at peak activity.
8. Caution regarding orthostatic hypotension.
9. Liberal liquids.
10. Sedentary lifestyle before pregnancy indicates low intensity activity with very gradual increase in level.
11. Stop activity if any unusual symptoms. (During pregnancy: heart rate should not exceed 140, strenuous activity should not exceed 15 minutes, no exercise in the supine position after 4 months gestation, no Valsalva maneuvers, caloric intake must be adjusted for level of exercise, and maternal core temp should not exceed 38° C.).

B. Contraindications:
1. General: heart disease, cervical incompetence, uterine bleeding, IUGR, fetal distress, previous miscarriages, previous premature labors, uncontrolled HTN, uncontrolled diabetes, uncontrolled renal disease, hemodynamically significant anemia.
2. Relative: essential HTN, controlled diabetes, excessive obesity, malnutrition, multiple gestation, thyroid disease, anemia.

III. **Activity**

Occupation:

A. Abstinence from physical work may be recommended if the woman has a history of two previous premature deliveries, an incompetent cervix, or fetal loss secondary to uterine anomalies. Women with multiple gestations beyond 28 wks, premature rupture of membranes, CHF, hemoglobinopathies, Marfan's syndrome, or diabetes with multiple end organ involvement are also at risk for complications and may benefit from reduced activity. Furthermore bedrest is indicated if there is a suspicion of IUGR or preeclampsia.

B. Other: There are no routine restrictions on sexual relations, other than comfort and position. Caution should be used if any of the conditions apply that are listed in A.

IV. Habits/Miscellaneous

A. Alcohol. Increased risk of mid-trimester abortion, mental retardation, behavior and learning disorders. Ten to thirty percent risk of fetal alcohol syndrome in offspring of women who drink three to five drinks a day. Risks with lesser consumption unknown.

B. Tobacco. Increased risk of low birth weight infants, premature labor, miscarriages, stillbirth, and birth defects. Three times greater incidence of upper respiratory infections and otitis media in young children of smoking parents.

C. Seatbelts: Seatbelt should be worn such that the belts do not directly cross the gravid uterus.

D. Medications: In general, no medications with the exception of acetaminophen should be used without checking with the physician.

E. Infections: Avoid children with viral illnesses, especially if not rubella immune. Avoid direct contact with cat litter and eating raw meat to minimize contact with toxoplasmosis.

V. Potential Problems

A. Contact physician: The patient should be instructed to consult her physician if any of the following problems arise.
1. Vaginal bleeding.
2. Leakage of fluid.
3. Fever.
4. Persistent nausea or vomiting.
5. Burning on urination.
6. Severe abdominal pain.
7. Severe headache or unusual disturbance.
8. Marked decrease in fetal movement.

B. Measuring fetal movement. Generally after quickening, one should expect 4 or more fetal movements per hour.

References

Kruse J. Alcohol use during pregnancy. <u>American Family Physician</u> 29(4):199, April 1984.

Niswander KR, ed. <u>Manual of Obstetrics, 3rd edition</u>. Boston/Toronto: Little, Brown & Company, 1987.

Paisley JE and Mellion MB. Exercise during pregnancy. <u>American Family Physician</u> 38(5):143, Nov. 1988.

Walbroehl GS. Sexuality during pregnancy. <u>American Family Physician</u> 29(5):273, May 1984.

Zlatnik FJ. Antepartum care (I): Common questions, our answers. <u>The Iowa Perinatal Letter</u> 3(4) July/August 1982.

RH SCREENING AND Rho-GAM

I. **Protocol for Routine Rh Screening and Administration of Rho-GAM.**
   A. Initial visit: draw blood for ABO group, Rh type, and antibody screening.
   B. 28 weeks: if patient is Rh negative and antibody negative, repeat antibody screen and inject Rho-GAM, 300 microgram.
   C. Following delivery: collect mother's blood and cord blood for fetal cell screen and ABO/Rh determination. If infant is not Rh negative, mother receives Rho-GAM, 300 microgram.

II. **Additional Rho-GAM Requirements:**
   A. If at anytime during pregnancy, fetal-maternal hemorrhage is suspected, a Kleinhauer-Betke test should be performed. If positive, 10 microgram of Rh immune globulin should be administered per milliliter of fetal blood calculated to have entered the maternal circulation.
   B. A 50 microgram dose of Rho-GAM is indicated for an Rh-negative woman after a 1st trimester terminated or miscarried pregnancy.
   C. A 300 mg dose of Rho-GAM is indicated for the Rh-negative woman who undergoes amniocentesis, or who undergoes a spontaneous or induced abortion later than 13 weeks gestation.
   D. The Kleinhauer-Betke test should be performed post delivery if a larger than usual fetal-maternal hemorrhage may have taken place, such as with placental abruption. More than the standard 300 microgram dose may be required, which protects only up to 14 cc of Rh positive red cells.

III. **Isoimmunization:** If the patient is Rh negative and the antibody screen is positive prior to Rho-GAM administration, obtain an antibody titer and consider referral to a specialist. Amniocentesis will be required if the titer is above a critical value to evaluate fetal hemolysis by amnionic fluid spectrophotometry. These infants are at risk for erythroblastosis fetalis.

References

Copelund CP. The proper use of RH immoglobulin. <u>The Iowa Perinatal Letter</u> 1(3), May/June 1980.

Driscoll CE, *et al*, eds. <u>Handbook of Family Practice</u>. Chicago: Year Book Medical Publishers, 1986.

HEPATITIS SCREENING IN PREGNANCY

I. **Recommended Screening**

   A. Women from high risk populations and/or locations: Asia, Pacific Islands, Alaska (Eskimo), even if born in continental U.S., American Indians, immigrants from: South Pacific, Caribbean, Haiti, Sub-Sahara Africa. Also consider immigrants from the Middle East, Eastern Europe, Central and South America.

   B. Women with histories of: Acute or chronic liver disease, work or treatment in a hemodialysis unit, work or residence in an institution for the mentally retarded, rejection as a blood donor, receiving blood transfusion on repeated occasions, frequent occupational exposure to blood in medical-dental settings, household contact or intimate sexual contact with an HBV carrier or hemodialysis patient, multiple episodes of sexually-transmitted diseases, percutaneous use of illicit drugs.

II. **Infants Born to HBSAg Positive Mothers**:

   A. Administer hepatitis immune globulin, .5cc IM within 12 hours after birth.

   B. Administer hepatitis B vaccine .5cc IM within the first 7 days of life. Repeat vaccination at one and six months.

Reference

Johnson CA. Prenatal screening. <u>American Family Physician</u> 37(5):175, May 1988.

ALPHA-FETOPROTEIN

I. **Overview**: the measurement of alpha-fetoprotein in maternal serum between 16 and 20 weeks gestation may be used as a screening test to detect fetal neural tube defects. Values are partially dependent on maternal weight and length of gestation. Elevated values should be rechecked and an ultrasound should be performed to ensure correct dating, and to rule out multiple gestation or fetal demise. Women with elevated values on recheck should be referred for amniocentesis. It is important that the test be run by a laboratory familiar with AFP screening and with well-established reference ranges.

II. **Disorders Associated with Elevated AFP**
   - open neural tube defects (meningomyelocele, anencephaly).
   - fetal nephrosis.
   - fetal GI obstruction.
   - prematurity/low birth weight.
   - abdominal pregnancy.
   - fetal demise or distress.
   - multiple gestation.

III. **Disorders Associated with Low AFP Levels**
   - missed abortions, molar pregnancies and chromosomal abnormalities.

IV. **Projected Outcome**
   A. Approximately 5% of screening AFPs will return elevated. On recheck, 60% of these will remain elevated.
   B. Of the 3% with confirmed elevated AFP, half will have normal ultrasound and amniocentesis will generally show normal amniotic fluid AFP. 4% will have elevated amniotic fluid AFP and have other laboratory evidence for abdominal wall defect or spina bifida.
   C. Of the other half of pregnancies with confirmed elevated serum AFP, ultrasound will show underestimated gestational age, multiple gestation, fetal demise, and anencephaly (in that order of frequency).

V. **Risks**: Psychological stress, false positives, false reassurance, and potential fetal trauma secondary to amniocentesis.

References

Campbell TL. Maternal serum alpha-fetoprotein screening: benefits, risks and costs. Journal of Family Practice 25(5):461, Nov. 1987,

Evans MI, *et al*. The variation in maternal serum alpha-fetoprotein reports in one metropolitan area: concerns for the quality of prenatal testing. Obstetrics and Gynecology 72:342, 1988.

Pritchard JA, *et al*, eds. Williams Obstetrics, 17th edition. Connecticut: Appleton-Century-Crofts, 1985.

Schwager EJ and Weiss BD. Prenatal testing for maternal serum alpha-fetoprotein. American Family Physician 35(4):169, April 1987.

Williamson R. Maternal alpha-fetoprotein screening. Iowa Perinatal Letter 7(1), Jan/Feb 1986.

ANTENATAL FETAL SURVEILLANCE

I. **Ultrasound**
   A. Indications:
      1. Determine the presence or absence of an intrauterine pregnancy.
      2. Determine fetal maturation and predict the date of confinement.
      3. Measure fetal growth, and identify intrauterine growth retardation.
      4. Identify multiple gestation pregnancies.
      5. Detect fetal anomalies.
      6. Detect oligo- or polyhydramnios.
      7. Demonstrate an abnormal placenta, such as in molar degeneration.
      8. Demonstrate fetal positions.
      9. May identify maternal uterine and pelvic anomalies.
   B. Timing: Will depend on the indication for ultrasound. In general, the earlier in pregnancy, the better the EDC can be predicted by sonography. Fetal anomalies may not become apparent until after 20 wks. Amniotic fluid determination is helpful in the decision to induce or follow postdates pregnancies.

II. **Amniocentesis**
   A. Indications.
      1. Identify selected inherited disorders in the following population: (generally done at 16-18 wks gestation).
         a. Pregnancies in women age 35 or older.
         b. Previous pregnancy resulting in the birth of a child with a chromosome abnormality.
         c. Downs or other chromosome abnormality in either parent or close family member.
         d. Mother is a carrier of any X-linked disease.
         e. Neural tube defect in either parent or a first degree relative.
         f. Previous child born with a neural tube defect.

g. Elevated serum AFP.
h. Either parent is a carrier of a genetically transmitted metabolic disease.
i. Pregnancy after three or more spontaneous abortions.

2. Determine fetal maturity late in pregnancy.
   a. Lecithin to sphingomyelin (L/S) ratio. If L/S > 2.0, then there is a low risk of respiratory distress secondary to prematurity.
   b. Phosphatidylglycerol (PG). Phosphatidylglycerol first appears at 35 wks gestation, and increases in concentration until 40 wks. If present, it provides reassurance of fetal lung maturity.

3. Detect isoimmunization.

III. Indications for NST/CST/Biophysical Profile

- Hypertension disorders.
- Diabetes mellitus.
- Multiple gestation.
- Suspected oligohydramnios/IUGR.
- Maternal heart or renal disease.
- Hemoglobinopathy.
- Postdate pregnancies.
- Previous unexplained fetal demise.
- Maternal perceptions of decreased fetal movement.

IV. Non-stress Testing (NST)

A. Equipment: External fetal heart rate monitor and a hand on the abdomen which palpates fetal movements.

B. Indications: High risk pregnancies when uteroplacental insufficiency may occur. Examples: diabetes, hypertension, preeclampsia, IUGR, or postdates pregnancies. Timing should be the earliest point at which an intervention would be performed if a clearly abnormal result is obtained (generally 32-34 weeks).

C. Interpretations: A reassuring NST demonstrates three or more fetal movements accompanied by a fetal heart rate acceleration of 15 beats per minute or more lasting 15 seconds during a 20 minute period. Lack of fetal movement is unsatisfactory for testing. A repeat NST should then be performed after a meal. Lack of movement for short periods of time may be due to fetal sleep, however absence of movement for prolonged periods of time may be ominous. The NST is abnormal when the criteria for a reassuring NST are not met or late or variable decelerations are present. A CST and/or ultrasound examination are then indicated.

V. Contraction Stress Testing (CST)

A. Equipment: External fetal heart rate monitor, external uterine tocographic transducer, nipple stimulator or intravenous oxytocin to stimulate uterine activity.

B. Indications: Same as for NST. May be evaluation of 1st choice in some high risk pregnancies. Otherwise, generally the follow-up to an abnormal NST.

C. Possible Contraindications: Threatened preterm labor, incompetent cervix, placenta previa, hydramnios, multiple gestation, previous preterm labor, previous classical C-section.

D. Interpretations/Management:

1. Negative: (Reassuring) At least three maternal uterine contractions in 10 minutes are identified, each lasting 40 seconds. No contractions associated with late decelerations of the fetal heart rate. Repeat in one week unless otherwise indicated.

2. Suspicious: A late deceleration is identified, but not with every contraction. Cannot assure fetal health for one week. Repeat the next day.

3. Unsatisfactory: Fewer than three contractions in ten minutes are noted, or the tracing is not acceptable. Cannot assure fetal health for one week. Repeat CST or other evaluation advised.

4. Positive (Non-reassuring): Consistent and persistent late decelerations of the FHR are identified.

    a. FHR reactive: Up to 50% are false positive. Generally good outcome. Delivery with intrapartum FHR monitoring, if mature. If immature, consider daily monitoring or continuous FHR recording.

b. FHR non-reactive: ominous. Rarely false positive. Consider immediate delivery by C-section regardless of maturity.

 5. Hyperstimulation: Occurs when uterine contractions are more frequent than every two minutes or more than 5 in 10 minutes, last longer than 90 seconds, or persistent uterine hypertonus is present. Decelerations in this setting cannot be interpreted, and the CST should be repeated.

VI. Biophysical Profile

A. Equipment: Real time ultrasonography.

B. Indications: Potentially same as NST.

C. Interpretation: Five parameters are examined and given a score of zero or two. The total score ranges from zero (ominous) to ten (very reassuring).

D. Management of pregnancy according to biophysical profile results (Table 8-1).

Table 8-1. Management Protocol.

Score	Interpretation	Recommended management
10	Normal infant, low risk for chronic asphyxia	Repeat testing at weekly intervals; repeat twice weekly in diabetic patients and patients $\geq$ 42 wk
8	Normal infant, low risk for chronic asphyxia	Repeat testing at weekly intervals; repeat twice weekly in diabetic patients and in patients $\geq$ 42 wk; indication for delivery oligohydramnios
6	Suspected chronic asphyxia	Repeat testing within 24 hr; deliver patient if repeat test is 6 or less or if oligohydramnios is present
4	Suspected chronic asphyxia	$\geq$ 36 weeks and favorable cervix, delivery; if < 36 wk and lecithin/sphingomyelin ratio < 2.0, repeat test in 24 hr; indication for delivery-repeat score $\leq$ 6

Table 8-1 (continued)

Score	Interpretation	Recommended management
		oligohydramnios > 36 weeks and favorable
0-2	Strong suspicion of chronic asphyxia	Extend testing time to 120 min; indication for delivery-persistent score ≤4, regardless of gestational age

Adapted from Niswander KR, ed. Manual of Obstetrics: Diagnosis and Therapy, 3rd edition. Boston/Toronto: Little, Brown & Company, 1987.

References

Antepartum fetal surveillance. ACOG Technical Bulletin 107, Aug. 1987.

Crvikshark DP. Genetic diagnosis by amnioscentesis. Iowa Perinatal Letter 1(5), July/August 1980.

Jack BW, et al. Routine obstetric ultrasound. American Family Physician 35(5):173, May 1987.

Niswander KR, ed. Manual of Obstetrics: Diagnosis and Therapy, 3rd edition. Boston/Toronto: Little, Brown & Company, 1987.

Norman CA and Karp LE. Biophysical profile and antepartum fetal assessment. American Family Physician 34(4):83, April 1986.

Pritchard JA, et al, eds. Williams Obstetrics, 17th edition. Connecticut:Appleton-Century-Crofts, 1985.

Zlatnik FJ. Antepartum fetal surveillance. Iowa Perinatal Letter 5(2), March/April 1984.

HYPEREMESIS GRAVIDARUM

I. **Definition**

   Severe nausea and vomiting in the first trimester of pregnancy.

II. **Etiology**

   The etiology of this syndrome is unknown. There is thought to be a relationship to serum HCG levels. The incidence of hyperemesis gravidarum is increased in multiple gestation and molar pregnancies.

III. **Management**
   A. Outpatient Treatment.
      1. Reassurance. Condition will improve with time.
      2. Saltine crackers before rising.
      3. Small, frequent meals.
      4. Antiemetics.
         a. Phosphorated carbohydrate solution (Emetrol).
         b. Diphenhydramine (Benadryl): frequently ineffective.
         c. Dimenhydrinate (Dramamine): sedating.
         d. Bendectin: 10 mg doxylamine succinate and 10 mg pyridoxine. Removed from market, although large studies have not shown evidence of teratogenicity. Doxylamine succinate can be purchased in 25 mg tablets (Unisom) over the counter.
         e. Promethazine (Phenergan) and prochloperazine (Compazine) non-teratogenic phenothiazines which can be used orally or per rectum.
      5. Consider hospitalizing the patient if severe symptoms, weight loss, signs of dehydration, ketones in urine, or high urine specific gravity are present.
   B. Hospital Management.
      1. Correct hypovolemia, ketosis, and electrolyte imbalances with IV fluids.

2. Monitor fluid intake and output.
3. Give nothing by mouth for 24-48 hours.
4. Antiemetics as above. Also consider parenteral antiemetcis if needed.

References

Niebyl JR. Using medictions in pregnant women. Syllabus from The University of Iowa Refresher Course for Family Physicians, March 1989.

Zlatnik F. From morning sickness to hyperemesis gravidurum. <u>Physiology and Pathology</u> 3(2), Mar/April, 1987.

DIABETES IN PREGNANCY

I. **Gestational Diabetes Mellitus** (GDM), (Class A Diabetes)
   A. Definition: Excessive carbohydrate intolerance during pregnancy in women who did not have diabetes mellitus previously. The incidence varies from 3-12%.
   B. Risk Factors.
      1. Obesity.
      2. Maternal age > 25.
      3. Positive family history of diabetes.
      4. History of gestational diabetes, macrosomic infant or stillbirth.
      5. Symptoms or signs of diabetes; and glucosuria.
   C. Evaluation.
      1. Glucose challenge test (GCT).
         a. Timing: A GCT is frequently performed as a routine screen for GDM in all pregnancies at 24-28 weeks gestation. It should be performed earlier if symptoms are present. Some sources recommend screening at the first prenatal visit if there are risk factors.
         b. Procedure: A blood glucose level is obtained one hour after a 50 gm glucose load.
         c. Interpretation: A level of 140 mg % or greater is abnormal. This value has a high negative predictive value, but there are many false positives. It should be followed by a fasting 3 hour glucose tolerance test.
      2. Glucose tolerance test (GTT).
         a. Timing: Recommended follow-up of normal GCT.
         b. Procedure: The patient must eat a diet containing at last 150 gm carbohydrate for 2 days. The patient has a serum glucose level obtained after an overnight fast, and then ingests 100 gms of glucose solution. Serum glucose levels are then obtained at one, two, and three hours.
         c. Interpretation (Table 8-2)

Table 8-2. Venous Samples

	Fasting	1 hour	2 hour	3 hour
Upper limits normal	105	190	165	145

D. Potential Morbidity.
   1. Infants born to diabetic mothers have 5 times the normal risk for respiratory distress syndrome.
   2. Macrosomia, and associated birth trauma are related to maternal hyperglycemia.
   3. Increased incidence of neonatal hypoglycemia, hypocalcemia, and jaundice.
   4. Congenital anomalies are at increased incidence with first trimester hyperglycemia.

E. Management of gestational diabetes.
   1. Dietary adjustment is the mainstay of therapy.
      a. Caloric intake should be 30-35 kcal/kg/day. Intake should be reduced to 24 kcal/kg/day if patient is obese.
      b. The patient should avoid cakes, candy, and other fast acting carbohydrates.
      c. Dietary composition should be 50-60% carbohydrate, 20-25% protein, and 20% fat, with high fiber content.
   2. Obstetric surveillance.
      a. Early ultrasound for accurate gestational dating.
      b. Follow every 2 weeks until 36 weeks, then weekly.
      c. Check fasting blood glucose and review home monitoring each visit. If fasting glucose levels are > 105, (or postprandial values are 120-130), then the patient should be hospitalized to ensure adherence to diet.
      d. If fasting glucose remains $\geq$ 110, the patient becomes "class B," and insulin therapy is indicated.
      e. The patient should also check a double voided urine specimen daily to rule out ketonuria, which reflects inadequate caloric consumption.

328   Obstetrics

    f. If macrosomia is suspected, ultrasound examination is performed to obtain the fetal abdominal and biparietal diameters. If the AD/BPD is > 1.5 or estimated fetal weight $\geq$ 4000 gm, a cesarean section is recommended at term. Amniocentesis is helpful in documenting fetal lung maturity prior to cesarean section.

    g. Antepartum NST is often initiated on a weekly basis at 34-35 weeks gestation. If euglycemia can be documented, consider delaying monitoring until 38 weeks. After 40 weeks gestation, fetal surveillance is initiated, and delivery recommended if there is any evidence of fetal jeopardy.

    h. Maternal fasting and 2 hour postprandial serum glucose is checked 6 weeks postpartum to rule out overt diabetes mellitus. She is counseled that she has an approximate 35% risk of developing diabetes at some point in her life.

II. Diabetes Mellitus

A. White's Classification (Table 8-3).

Table 8-3.

Class	Description
A	Gestational diabetes. Glucose intolerance during pregnancy, normal fasting glucose.
AB	Gestational diabetes with elevated fasting glucose or 2 hour postprandial glucose > 120.
B	Overt diabetes developing after age 20, duration < 10 yrs.
C	Overt diabetes developing before age 20 or duration > 10 yrs.
D	Overt diabetes developing before age 10 or greater than 20 yrs duration.
E	Overt diabetes with calcified pelvic vessels.
F	Overt diabetes with nephropathy.
R	Overt diabetes with retinopathy.
RF	Overt diabetes with retinopathy and nephropathy.

B. Morbidity.

    1. Classes C, D, F, and R are associated with an abortion rate up to 30%.

2. The incidence of major anomalies (cardiac, neural tube, genitourinary, gastrointestinal, and musculoskeletal) is several times higher than the general population and is associated with first trimester hyperglycemia.
3. Vascular disease in particular is associated with IUGR and a greater incidence of fetal demise.
4. Ketoacidosis may carry a 50% fetal mortality.

Management: The care of pregnant diabetic individuals is best managed by a coordinated team of specialized health care providers, and is beyond the scope of this chapter.

References

Board PJ, *et al*. Gestational diabetes: definition, diagnosis, and treatment strategies in practical diabetology. 5(6):1, 1980.

Creasy RK and Resnik R, eds. Maternal-Fetal Medicine Principles and Practice. Philadelphia: W.B. Saunders Company, 1984.

National Diabetes Data Group. Classification and diagnosis of diabetes mellitus in other categories of glucose intolerance. Diabetes 28:1039, 1979.

Niswander KR, ed. Manual of Obstetrics: Diagnosis and Therapy, 3rd edition. Boston/Toronto: Little, Brown & Company, 1987.

Werner CP. The diagnosis and management of gestational diabetes. The IA Perinatal Letter 3(5), Sept/Oct, 1987.

HYPERTENSION IN PREGNANCY

I. **Pregnancy-Induced Hypertension** (PIH)
   A. Hypertension Alone.
      1. BP $\geq$ 140/90.
      2. Systolic BP rise of $\geq$ 30 mmHg.
      3. Diastolic BP rise of $\geq$ 15 mmHg.

II. **Preeclampsia/Eclampsia**
   A. Preeclampsia is defined as the triad of pregnancy-induced hypertension, proteinuria and edema. Preeclampsia may be divided into mild and severe categories.
      1. Criteria for mild preeclampsia.
         a. Hypertension as defined above, but not meeting criteria for severe hypertension.
         b. Proteinuria, 5 gm/24 hrs.
         c. Mild edema, signaled by weight gain > 2 lbs/week or > 6 lbs/month
         d. Urine output > 500 cc/24 hrs.
      2. Criteria for severe preeclampsia.
         a. BP > 170/110.
         b. Systolic BP rise $\geq$ 60 mmHg.
         c. Diastolic BP rise $\geq$ 30 mmHg.
         d. Proteinuria > 5 gm/24 hrs.
         e. Massive edema.
         f. Urine output < 500 cc/24 hrs.
         g. Any of the changes in mild preeclampsia plus pulmonary edema, headaches, visual changes, right upper quadrant pain, elevated liver enzymes, or thrombocytopenia.
   B. Eclampsia--rare. Defined as preeclampsia with the addition of convulsions.
   C. Risk factors for PIH: First pregnancy, multiple gestation, polyhydramnios, hydatidiform mole, malnutrition, positive family history of PIH, underlying vascular disease. Suspect molar pregnancy if preeclampsia occurs early in gestation.

Hypertension in Pregnancy

III. Evaluation Of PIH/Preeclampsia

A. History: Document risk factors and any symptoms outlined above.

B. Physical: Look for evidence of edema (particularly of the hands and face), BP changes, retinal changes, hyperreflexia, RUQ tenderness.

C. Initial Laboratory Studies.

1. Blood: CBC with platelets, electrolytes, BUN and creatinine, uric acid, liver function tests, (SGOT, SGPT, LDH) and coagulation studies (PTT and fibrinogen).

2. Urine: 24 hr collection for protein, and creatinine clearance.

3. HELP Syndrome: Hemolysis, Elevated liver function test, Low Platelets.

IV. Management Of PIH/Preeclampsia

A. Ambulatory Management.

Controversial. For pregnancy-induced hypertension without significant proteinuria: home bedrest and sodium restriction are recommended. Home blood pressure monitoring, weight, and urine protein checks are helpful. It is generally recommended that these patients be evaluated twice weekly, and that antepartum surveillance (NST) begin early. Lab tests should be repeated weekly, or more frequently if symptoms arise. An ultrasonic exam should also be performed periodically to ensure adequate amniotic fluid.

B. Hospital Management.

1. Indicated for women with pregnancy-induced hypertension and 2+ or greater proteinuria, and those who fail outpatient management. Bedrest with bathroom privileges is allowed. The goal of IV fluids in severe cases is to replace urine output plus insensible losses. Alternatively, D_5W can be administered at 125 cc/hr. Phenobarbitol (30-60 gm im or po q6 hr), Secobarbitol (100 mg hr), or hydroxyzine (50-100 mg po) are useful for sedation.

2. Laboratory evaluation and weights are performed daily to every other day. Antepartum surveillance in-

cluding NST's and amnionic fluid determinations via ultrasound is essential.

3. Delivery is the treatment of choice and delivery should be accomplished when the fetus is mature, but may be required early if maternal health is in danger, or if there is evidence of fetal distress. Electronic FHR monitoring during labor is indicated.

C. Antihypertensive Therapy.
  1. Indicated only if BP persistently $\geq$ 160/110
  2. Aim for a diastolic BP 90-100. Avoid over-correction, as normal blood pressures can result in placental hypoperfusion.
  3. Diuretics are never indicated. These patients are already hypovolemic.
  4. Long term medications (if the fetus is immature) include aldomet, atenolol, and labetolol. During labor, IV hydralazine is used. It is given in 5-10 mg doses every 20 to 30 minutes until a satisfactory BP is achieved, then in 5-25 mg doses IV every 3-6 hours as needed. Side effects include headache, palpitations, and lupus-like syndrome.

D. Anticonvulsive Therapy.
  1. Seizure prophylaxis is indicated in ALL preeclamptic patients during labor and delivery, and for 24 hours postpartum. Seizures may occur in the absence of hyperreflexia, and increased DTR's may be present in the normal population; therefore, hyperreflexia is not a useful predictor of risk.
  2. Magnesium sulfate is the drug of choice.
     a. Prophylactic: Loading dose is 5 gm IM in each buttock or 4 gm IV over 10-15 minutes. Maintenance is 5 gm IM q4h or 1-2 gm/h IV.
     b. Treatment of seizures: 1 gm/minute IV until seizure controlled up to 4-6 gm max.
     c. Serum levels: Therapeutic level is 3-8 mg/dl (2.5-6.7 mEq/L). Serum levels of magnesium sulfate should be monitored until stable, and then every 12 hours.

d. Magnesium toxicity may be signaled by excessive drowsiness and absence of patellar reflexes. Respiratory depression must be avoided. If necessary, 10% calcium gluconate may be administered intravenously to reverse the effects.

V. Chronic Hypertension

A. Risks.
   1. Maternal: If no superimposed preeclampsia occurs, then there is no additional maternal risk. In the presence of superimposed preeclampsia (20%), there is increased maternal mortality, frequently from intracranial hemorrhage.
   2. Fetal: There is an increased incidence of perinatal death, IUGR, and fetal distress.

B. Management.
   1. Treatment of chronic hypertension can decrease maternal, and to some extent, fetal morbidity, but cannot reduce the risks of superimposed preeclampsia. Appropriate medications include methyldopa, hydralazine, and propranolol. Diuretics are not indicated.
   2. Laboratory evaluation is performed early in pregnancy.
   3. Obstetric visits are scheduled every other week at 24 weeks, and weekly after 30 weeks.
   4. Early ultrasound is obtained for dating, and repeated periodically to look for evidence of IUGR.
   5. Antenatal surveillance (NST's) should begin at 34 weeks.
   6. The pregnancy should not be allowed to go beyond 40 weeks. Delivery may be required earlier if there is evidence of IUGR or fetal distress or if hypertension cannot be controlled by bedrest and medication.
   7. Intrapartum monitoring is required during labor.
   8. If there is evidence of IUGR, C-section is preferable to a prolonged induction.

9. Complicated cases or women with superimposed preeclampsia should be handled at an appropriate referral center.

References

Creasy RK and Resnick R, eds. <u>Maternal-Fetal Medicine Principles and Practice</u>. Philadelphia: W.B. Saunders Company, 1984.

Hacker N and Moore JG, eds. <u>Essentials of Obstetrics and Gynecology</u>. Philadelphia: W.B. Saunders Company, 1986.

Pritchard JA, *et al*, eds. <u>Williams Obstetrics, 17th edition</u>. Connecticut: Appleton-Century-Crofts, 1985.

Varner MW. Hypertension in pregnancy. <u>IA Perinatal Letter</u> 7(6), Nov/Dec, 1986.

EARLY ANTEPARTUM HEMORRHAGE

I. **Definition:** Vaginal bleeding at < 20 wks gestation

II. **Differential Diagnosis**

   A. Benign vaginal or cervical lesions; the pregnant cervix is very vascular and friable. This diagnosis is made by speculum exam--bleeding will not be from the os.

   B. Abortion.

   1. Threatened abortion: The early symptoms of pregnancy may be present. Vaginal bleeding has occurred, with or without cramping. No history of passage of tissue or amnionic fluid is obtained. On exam, the patient is afebrile, the abdomen is soft and non-tender. The uterus is appropriate for gestational age and non-tender. The internal cervical os is closed.

   2. Inevitable abortion: Symptoms are the same as for threatened abortion. Menstrual cramping is often present and evidence of ruptured membranes may be noted. The internal os is dilated. (Do not confuse with an incompetent cervix, which is not associated with cramping and is potentially treatable).

   3. Incomplete abortion: Cramping and bleeding have occurred, and the patient reports passage of tissue. (Blood clots may be mistaken for tissue however.) Speculum examination reveals a dilated internal os and tissue present within the endocervical canal or vagina. Bleeding may be heavy.

   4. Complete abortion: Cramping and bleeding have occurred and a history of passage of tissue has been obtained. On examination, the uterus is firm, and smaller than one would expect for gestational length of pregnancy.

   5. Septic abortion: Consider if temperature of 38°C is present with symptoms and signs of abortion in any stage. Abdominal and uterine tenderness are present as well as purulent discharge and possibly evidence of shock.

   C. Ectopic pregnancy: Vaginal bleeding occurs in 50-94% of patients with ectopic pregnancies. Pelvic pain is generally present. Abdominal tenderness is present in 97% of cases. Rebound tenderness may be present. The uterine size is suggestive of early pregnancy and the cervix is typically tender on motion. An adnexal or cul-de-sac mass can be palpated in 40% of cases. Risk of ectopic pregnancy is increased if there is a history of tubal infection or surgery, endometriosis, prior infertility problem, or if pregnancy occurred while on a progestin-only BCP or IUD.

D. Molar pregnancy: Placenta undergoes trophoblastic proliferation and typically resembles a cluster of grapes. Occurs more often in women <20 or >40 years of age and almost always cause some degree of vaginal bleeding. Hydatidiform moles are associated with hyperemesis gravidarum and onset of preeclampsia prior to the third trimester. The uterus is larger than expected for gestational age in 50% of the cases. Ovarian enlargement may occur secondary to thecal lutein cysts. Ultrasonic findings typically leave the "snow storm" pattern.

III. **Management**-(See Figure 8-1)

References

Deutschman M. The problematic first-trimester pregnancy. <u>American Family Physician</u> 39(1) :185 , Jan. 1989.

Niswander KR, ed. <u>Manual of Obstetrics: Diagnosis and Therapy, 3rd edition</u>. Boston/Toronto: Little, Brown & Company, 1987.

Rayburn WF and Lavin JP, eds. <u>Obstetrics for the House Officer</u>. Baltimore:Williams & Wilkins, 1984.

Early Antepartum Hemorrhage

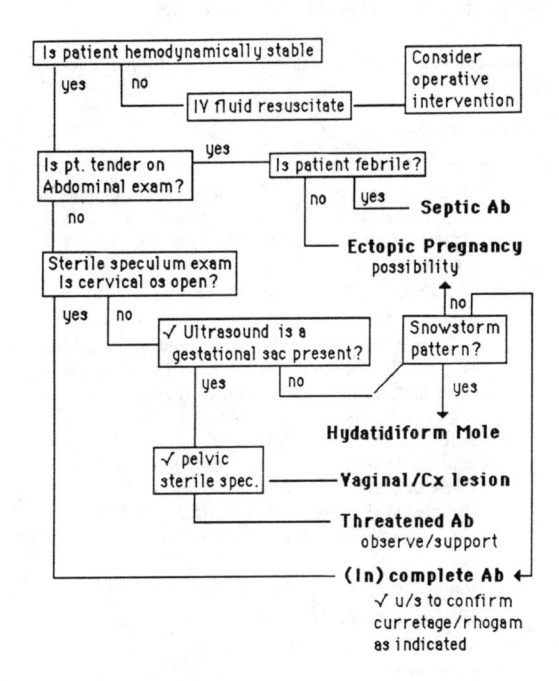

Fig 8-1. Early Pregnancy* - Vaginal Bleeding
* Pregnancy confirmed with β-HCG

LATE ANTEPARTUM HEMORRHAGE

I. **Definition**: Vaginal bleeding that occurs after 20 weeks gestation

II. **Differential Diagnosis:**
   A. Placenta Previa.
      1. Incidence: Occurs in 1 of 200 deliveries. The diagnosis of placenta previa is very common in the 2nd trimester, but more than 95% of these do not have previa at delivery.
      2. Classification: Placenta previa may be marginal, partial, or total.
      3. Diagnosis: Vaginal bleeding is typically bright red and painless. The blood loss is not massive, but tends to recur and become heavier as the pregnancy progresses. Diagnosis may be aided by ultrasound. A speculum exam is debatable. Digital examination is contraindicated other than in a double setup situation when delivery is desirable and can be rapidly accomplished by C-section. Maternal risk factors include increasing age, multiparity, and prior uterine scar.
   B. Placental abruption.
      1. Incidence: Placental abruption occurs in 10% of all deliveries. Severe abruption is rare.
      2. Classification:
         a. Mild: Slight vaginal bleeding (< 100 cc), no FHR abnormalities are present, there is no evidence of shock or coagulopathy.
         b. Moderate: Moderate vaginal bleeding (100-500 cc), and uterine hypersensitivity with or without elevated tone. Mild shock and fetal distress may be present.
         c. Severe: Extensive vaginal bleeding (> 500 cc), tetanic uterus, and moderate to profound maternal shock are present. Fetal demise and maternal coagulopathy are characteristic.

3. Diagnosis: The diagnosis of placental abruption is clinical. Although vaginal bleeding is present in 80% of the cases, it may be concealed in the remainder. Thus, the maternal hemodynamic situation may not be explained by observed blood loss. Pain and increased uterine tone are typically present. Risk factors include prior history of abruption, maternal hypertension, cigarette or cocaine use, increasing maternal age or multiparity. Abruption may be associated with preterm premature rupture of membranes, twin gestation following delivery of first infant and trauma.
- C. Uterine rupture: Very rare. May mimic severe abruption. An abdominal film may show free intraperitoneal air or an abnormal fetal position. Hysterectomy is required.
- D. Other: Vasa previa (velamentous insertion of the cord - rare), cervical dilatation with loss of mucous plug may be confused with other causes of vaginal bleeding, cervical or vaginal lesions (polyps, condylomata).

III. **Laboratory Evaluation.** Laboratory evaluation should include a CBC, type and cross, coagulation studies, urinalysis, and ultrasound.

IV. **Management of Placenta Previa and Placental Abruption**
- A. Placenta previa.
    1. Term gestation. If pregnancy 37 weeks or greater, or if fetal maturity has been documented, a Cesarean section is indicated unless only a minimal degree of placenta previa present.
    2. If bleeding is sufficient to jeopardize the mother or fetus despite transfusion, Cesarean section may be indicated regardless of gestation.
    3. In the preterm gestation, expectant management is indicated. Most patients require inpatient observation. Physical activity is restricted. Nothing is allowed in the vagina, including examining fingers. The hematocrit is maintained at 30% or greater. Once 36-37 wks gestation is reached with fetal maturity demonstrated by amniocentesis, the patient is readied for elective double setup examination.

4. Remember that placenta accreta may complicate placenta previa in women with history of previous C-section. Hemorrhage can necessitate hysterectomy.

B. Placental abruption.

1. If placental abruption is mild and the fetus is immature, expectant management may be indicated, with fetal heart rate monitoring and serial laboratory/ultrasound examination. Occasionally a small separation occurs without further problem. These patients have no uterine symptoms. Observation is required but if no fetal distress occurs in the next 2 days, the patient may be sent home.

2. In all other cases, delivery is indicated. A vaginal delivery is preferred when fetal distress is not present or the fetus is no longer viable. A C-section is indicated if fetal distress is present. A C-section is also performed when there is a threat to the mother's life or a failed trial of labor.

3. Shock must be treated with adequate replacement of blood loss. Fresh whole blood is preferable. While awaiting blood, colloid may be used (3 cc colloid for every cc estimated blood loss.) Urine output must be maintained at 25-30 cc/hr. A central venous pressure line or Swan-Ganz catheter will assist in monitoring hemodynamic status.

4. Coagulopathy should be treated with fresh whole blood. Fresh frozen plasma is used alternatively. One unit of FFP increases fibrinogen concentration by 25 mg/dl. Platelet transfusion is required if the count is less than 50,000. Heparin is not used in DIC secondary to placental abruption.

References

Niswander KR, ed. Manual of Obstetrics: Diagnosis and Therapy, 3rd edition. Boston/Toronto: Little, Brown & Company, 1987.

Varner M.W. Third-trimester bleeding. Iowa Perinatal Letter 5(6), Nov/Dec 1987.

Zlatnik F. Third-trimester bleeding. Iowa Perinatal Letter 10(2), March/April 1989.

INTRAUTERINE GROWTH RETARDATION (IUGR)

I. **Definition**

   IUGR is a presumptive diagnosis in utero that the fetus weighs less than the tenth percentile for its gestational age.

II. **Risk Factors**

   A. Chronic maternal disease: chronic maternal HTN, pregnancy induced HTN, diabetes, cyanotic heart disease, collagen vascular disease, severe maternal anemia, renal disease.

   B. Genetic disorders or birth defects: trisomies and other chromosomal abnormalities, fetal malformations.

   C. Intrauterine infections: rubella, herpes, toxoplasmosis, syphilis, CMV.

   D. Previous history of SGA baby, smoking, drug or alcohol abuse.

   E. Abnormalities of the placenta.

III. **Diagnosis**

   One should be suspicious when the fundal height does not exhibit the predicted 1 cm/week growth between 20 and 36 weeks gestation. Serial ultrasonic scanning may confirm the diagnosis.

IV. **Management**

   The development of IUGR makes the pregnancy high risk. Close antepartum surveillance is required and the decision on when to deliver the infant is complicated. These pregnancies are typically handled by physicians experienced in high risk obstetrics and neonatal care.

References

Losh DP and Durhing JL. Management of the postdate pregnancy. American Family Physician 36(2):182, Aug. 1987.

Niswander KR, ed. Manual of Obstetrics: Diagnosis and Therapy, 3rd edition. Boston/Toronto: Little, Brown and Company, 1987.

VAGINAL BIRTH AFTER CESAREAN

I. Definition

Attempted vaginal delivery in a woman who has undergone previous cesarean section.

II. Decision To Attempt VBAC

A. Advantages.
   1. Rising maternal preference.
   2. Reduced expense relative to C-section.
   3. Overall reduced complications in terms of operative and postoperative problems.

B. Disadvantages.
   1. Requires closer intrapartum monitoring than a low risk delivery.
   2. If unsuccessful, a C-section after a trial of labor has increased infectious morbidity compared to that of an elective cesarean.

C. Contraindications.
   1. History of previous classical, t-shaped, or unknown uterine incision.
   2. Multiple gestation.
   3. Estimated birth weight > 4000 gms.
   4. Non-vertex presentation.
   5. Inadequate facilities or personnel for emergency cesarean delivery.
   6. Patient's refusal to consent.

D. Probability of Success.

Depends primarily upon the indication for the previous C-section. If the primary C-section was for breech position, abruption, placenta previa, cord accident, antepartum hemorrhage, hypertensive disorder, or fetal distress, then a 74%-94% chance of success can be anticipated. If the primary C-section was for "cephalopelvic disproportion" (CPD) or "failed induction," then a 35%-77% chance of success can be expected. This range reflects the difficulty of a clinical diagnosis of CPD, which may inappropriately include ineffective uterine contractions.

III. **Risks**

   A. Usual maternal and fetal risks of vaginal delivery.

   B. Uterine Rupture: Very rare. Incidence increased if prior C-section was classical.

   C. Cesarean section: Increased risk of C-section morbidity relative to elective C-section. However, risks comparable to primary C-section.

IV. **Management**

   A. Preparations.

   1. Type and screen for two units of whole blood, intravenous line should be inserted.

   2. The anesthesiologist, surgeon and physician caring for the newborn infant must be notified in advance and be available.

   B. Labor.

   1. Electronic fetal monitoring is recommended.

   2. Oxytocin may be used to augment labor, and close monitoring of uterine contractions (using intrauterine catheters) is necessary.

   3. The same expectations of normal progression during labor should be applied to patients with a prior C-section.

   4. An experienced physician should be in attendance throughout labor and delivery.

   C. Postpartum: Exploration of the uterus after delivery of the placenta is beneficial to assess scar integrity, although its prognostic significance is uncertain.

References

Clark SL, et al. Effect of indication for previous cesarean section on subsequent delivery outcome in patients undergoing a trial of labor. J Reprod Med 19(1):22-25, 1984.

Flamm BL. Vaginal birth after cesarean section: controversies old and new. Clin Obstet Gynecol 18(4):735-744, 1985.

Laurence C. Vaginal birth after cesarean delivery. American Family Physician 37(6):167-171, June 1988.

Lavin JP, et al. Vaginal delivery in patients with a prior cesarean section. Obstet Gynecol 59(2):135-148, 1982.

Nielsen TF. Cesarean section: a controversial feature of modern obstetric practice. Gynecol Obstet Invest 21(2):57-63, 1986.

Rayburn WF and Lavin JP, eds. Obstetrics for the House Officer. Baltimore/London: Williams & Wilkins, 1984.

Zlatnik F. Vaginal birth after cesarean, new guidelines. IA Perinatal Letter 6(3), May/June, 1985.

PRETERM LABOR

I. Definition

Onset between 20 and 37 weeks gestation of contractions occuring at least every 10 minutes and lasting 30 seconds. Discrimination from "false labor" is difficult without cervical dilation; however, postponement of treatment until this occurs may lower the chances of success.

II. Cause

Frequently unknown. Several factors have been associated with preterm labor.

A. Maternal Factors: infections (general, urinary tract, amnionitis), uterine anomalies, fibroids, retained IUD, cervical incompetency, overdistended uterus (polyhydramnios, multiple gestation), rupture of membranes.

B. Fetal Factors: congenital anomalies, intrauterine death.

III. Risk Factors (Table 8-4)

Table 8-4. System for determining risk of spontaneous preterm delivery

Points assigned	Socioeconomic factors	Previous medical history	Daily habits	Aspects of current pregnancy
1	Two children at home Low socioeconomic status	Abortion x 1 Less than 1 yr since last birth	Works outside home	Unusual fatigue
2	Maternal age <20 yr or >40 yr Single parent	Abortion x 2	Smokes more than 10 cigarettes per day	Gain of <5kg by 32 wk
3	Very low socioeconomic status Height <150cm Weight <45kg	Abortion x 3	Heavy or stressful work that is long and tiring	Breech at 32wk Weight loss of 2kg Head engaged at 32 wk Febrile illness

Table 8-4 (continued)

Points assigned	Socioeconomic factors	Previous medical history	Daily habits	Aspects of current pregnancy
4	Maternal age <18 yr	Pyelonephritis		Bleeding after 12 wk Effacement Dilation Uterine irritability
5		Uterine anomaly Repeated second-trimester abortion Diethylstilbestrol exposure Cone biopsy		
6		Preterm delivery Repeated second-trimester abortion		Twins Abdominal surgical procedure

Adapted from Creasy RK, et al. A system for predicting spontaneous preterm birth. Obstet Gynecol 55:692, 1980.

IV. Management

A. Initial Examination.

1. Estimate fetal weight and gestational age.
2. Ultrasound for position, r/o placental or fetal anomalies.
3. Document FHR and uterine activity with external monitoring.
4. Pelvic examination: Attempt to limit to one examiner. Rule out ruptured membranes. Obtain cervical culture for group B strep and possibly other pathogens. If membranes ruptured, pooled amnionic fluid can be used to determine fetal maturity by looking at the c/s ratio, otherwise amniocentesis may be necessary.
5. Obtain urinalysis and urine culture.

B. Determine tocolysis score (Table 8-5).

Preterm Labor

Table 26-1. Tocolysis score.

Factor	1	2	3	4
Contraction	Irregular	Regular, <10-min intervals	?	
PROM		High or questionable	?	Low
Bleeding	Spotting, moderate bleeding	Severe bleeding (>100ml)	?	
Cervical dilatation	1cm	2cm	3cm	≥4cm

Adapted from Niswander KR. Manual of Obstetrics: Diagnosis & Therapy, 3rd edition. Boston/Toronto: Little, Brown & Company, 1987.

C. Decision to inhibit labor.
1. Contraindications: Evidence of fetal distress, fetal anomalies, abrupto placenta, placenta previa with heavy bleeding, severe maternal disease.
2. Risks of Treatment: If membranes are ruptured, there is increased risk of cord prolapse with amnionitis. Fetal mortality is increased if labor is suppressed when there is IUGR. Mother may experience tachycardia, nervousness, or pulmonary edema secondary to medication.
3. Tocolysis will most likely be ineffective if there is a tocolysis score of greater than 5-7. Preparation should be made to deliver in the optimal setting.
4. Delay of labor beyond one week is generally not recommended after premature rupture of the membranes, unless the fetus is very small (<1250 gm), weekly cervical cultures and c/s determinations are recommended.

D. Protocol.
1. Bedrest in left lateral decubitus position. Effective alone in 50% of patients.
2. Sedation (100 mg secobarbital or 50 mg hydroxyzine).
3. Hydration, but avoid large boluses.

4. Antibiotics: Controversial. Do not use for > 2 days, to limit incidence of resistance.
5. Fetal HR and uterine activity monitoring.
6. Steroids may be helpful in accelerating fetal by maturity.
7. Pharmacologic intervention.

E. Sympathomimetics (smooth muscle relaxation).
   1. Ritodrine.
      a. Monitor maternal vital signs, fetal heart rate and activity, and uterine activity.
      b. Initial Dose: 50-150 micrograms/minute. Increase by 50 micrograms every 10 minutes until contractions stop or unacceptable side effects. Maximum dose is 350 micrograms/minute.
      c. Discontinue if labor persists at maximum dose. If labor arrests, continue infusion for at least 12 hours before attempt in conversion to oral therapy.
      d. Oral Therapy: Initiate with 10 mg 30 minutes before stopping infusion, then 10 mg every 2 hours (or 20 mg every 4 hours) for 24 hours. If labor remains in arrest 10-20 mg every 4-6 hours until suppression is no longer indicated. Maximum dose is 120 mg/day.
   2. Terbutaline.
      a. Give .25 mg subcutaneously every six hours x 2 doses, then 3 hours after 2nd dose add 2.5 mg PO.
      b. Continue 2.5 mg po every 2-4 hours. Up to 5.0 mg doses can be used.

F. Magnesium Sulfate: M_gSO_4 also decreases uterine contractility, but is not useful long term. It can be an adjunct to oral terbutaline.

G. Other: Antiprostaglandins and progesterone are under investigation.

References

Creasy RK and Resnik R, eds. <u>Maternal Fetal Medicine Principles and Practice</u>. Philadelphia: W.B. Saunders Company, 1984.

Driscoll CE, *et al*, eds. <u>Handbook of Family Practice</u>. Chicago: Year Book Medical Publishers, 1986.

Eggelston MK. Management of preterm labor and delivery. <u>Clinical Obstetrics & Gynecology</u> 29(2): June 1986.

Gonik B and Creasy RK. Preterm labor: its diagnosis and management. <u>Am J Obstet Gynecol</u> 154:3-8, Jan. 1986.

Niswander KR, ed. <u>Manual of Obstetrics: Diagnosis & Therapy, 3rd edition</u>. Boston/Toronto: LIttle, Brown & Company, 1987.

PREMATURE RUPTURE OF MEMBRANES (PROM)

I. Definitions
- "Premature" rupture of membranes occurs if there is a delay of greater than one hour until onset of labor.
- "Preterm premature" rupture of membranes occurs prior to 37 weeks gestation.

II. Diagnosis
A. History of fluid gush.

B. Sterile speculum exam.
1. Pooling of fluid in vaginal vault.
2. pH Determination: Amniotic fluid typically turns nitrazene paper blue. Contamination with vaginal/cervical mucus, blood, or urine may lead to false interpretation.
3. Fern Test: Allow a sample of fluid to air dry on a glass or slide. Examination of amniotic fluid under the microscope reveals a characteristic "fern" pattern.

C. Gestational age.

D. Cervical digital examination: Controversial. Increases risk of amnionitis. Avoid if possible unless patient is in labor and delivery is inevitable.

III. Management
A. Term PROM: Some literature suggests that if the patient does not spontaneously go into labor, she can be managed conservatively. However, this entails close observation for development of chorioamnionitis and possibly additional hospitalization. Many sources recommend induction and delivery within 24-36 hours after admission.

B. Preterm PROM: Fetal maturity must be considered. Manage conservatively until the fetus is mature unless chorioamnionitis or fetal distress develop, or labor cannot be inhibited with tocolysis. Positive cervical cultures should be treated, but do not necessitate induction without other signs of chorioamnionitis. Follow maternal and fetal vitals, including temperature every 6 hours and daily WBC. Use of antibiotics for prophylaxis is under investigation.

C. Amnionitis: Indicated by maternal or fetal tachycardia, maternal fever, uterine tenderness, foul cervical discharge, uterine contractions, leukocytosis, presence of leukocytes or bacteria in amniotic fluid.

References

Driscoll CE, *et al*, eds. Handbook of Family Practice. Chicago: Year Book Medical Publishers, 1986.

Nagey DA and Saller DN. An analysis of the decisions in the mangement of premature rupture of the membranes. Clinical OB & Gyn 29(4), Dec 1986.

POSTDATE PREGNANCY

I. **Definitions**
   A. Prolonged Pregnanacy: Longer than 40 weeks.
   B. Postdates Pregnancy: Longer than 42 weeks gestation.
   C. Postmature Pregnancy: Longer than 42 weeks gestation with evidence of placental dysfunction.

II. **Etiology**
   A. Most Common: Error in estimating EDC.
   B. Risk Factors.
      1. History of prolonged gestation (50% risk).
      2. Older age.
      3. Anencephaly or fetal endocrinopathy.

III. **Potential Morbidity**
   A. Maternal.
      1. Birth trauma secondary to macrosomic infant.
      2. Increased incidence of operative delivery and secondary infection hemorrhage.
   B. Neonatal.
      1. Meconium aspiration.
      2. Polycythemia.
      3. Hyperbilinanemia.
      4. Hypoglycemia.
      5. Anoxic organ damage.

IV. **Management** (Figure 8-2)

Reference

Losh DP nd Dutring JL. Management of the postdate pregnancy. American Family Physician 36(2):184, Aug. 1987.

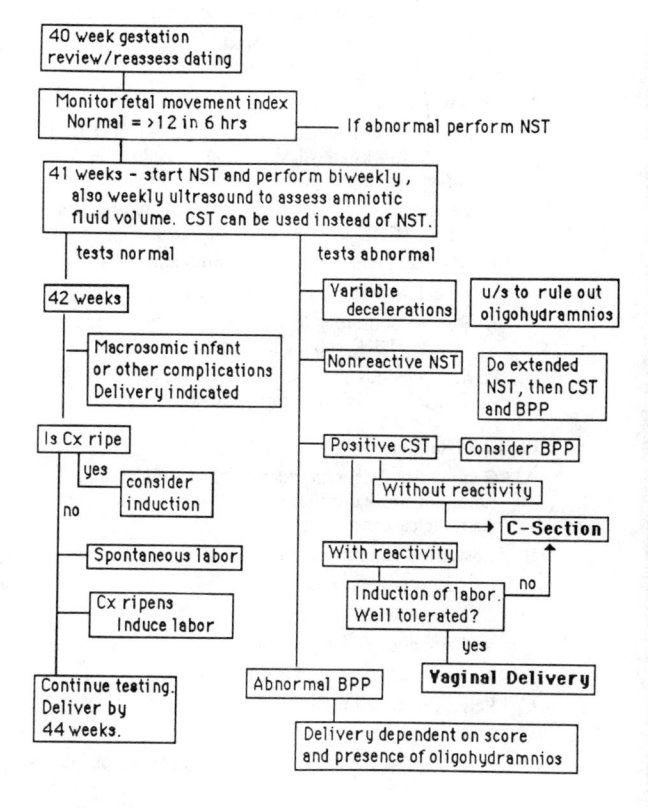

Fig 8-2. Postdate Pregnancy Management

Abbreviations:

BPP = Biophysical profile, CST = Contraction stress test, NST = Non stress test.

EVALUATION OF LABOR

I. **History**
   A. Defining labor:
      1. Contractions: onset, frequency, duration, intensity.
      2. Membranes ruptured or intact.
      3. Fetal movement.
   B. Review prenatal course.
      1. Accuracy of estimated data of confinement (EDC) - usually 40 wks after LMP. May be modified by other parameters in pregnancy such as an early ultrasound.
      2. Length of gestation - calculated by comparing date of labor to EDC, using EDC as "40" weeks.
      3. Ask about coexisting medical problems.
      4. Calculate weight gain during pregnancy.
      5. Review laboratory data: blood type, Rhogam requirements, VDRL, rubella immunity, hematocrit.
   C. Review previous pregnancies: number, gestation, fetal size, duration of labor, complications.

II. **Physical Examination**
   A. General: Vital signs, fundoscopy, thyroid palpation, chest examination, examination of the extremities, brief neurological exam.
   B. Obstetrical abdominal examination.
      1. Assess fetal position.
      2. Fundal height.
      3. Estimation of fetal weight.
      4. Auscultation of fetal heart tones.
   C. Pelvic examination.
      1. Inspection.
         a. Look for herpetic lesions, condylomata, lacerations.
         b. Speculum examination may reveal pooling of vaginal fluid, consistent with rupture of membranes. A nitrazine test or swab of vaginal fluid on a glass slide may be necessary to prove

the presence of amniotic fluid in the vagina. The basic pH of this fluid will turn the nitrazine paper blue. Care must be taken to avoid the cervical mucus, which is also basic and may give a false positive test. If an air dried sample of fluid reveals a "fern pattern," then the presence of amniotic fluid is confirmed.

2. Palpation of the cervix.

   a. Dilation of the cervical os. Dilation may range from 0 to 10 cm.

   b. Effacement--the degree of thinning of the cervix. The cervix may range from 3cm long (thick or zero % effaced) to paper-thin (100% effaced).

3. Palpation of the presenting part.

   a. Identification - head, foot, buttock, other.

   b. Station - Station is described as the relationship of the fetal presenting part to the level of the ischial spines in the maternal pelvis. Station may range from -3 to +3. Zero station occurs when the lower most presenting part is palpable at the level of the ischial spines.

   c. Position - Position is described as the orientation of the presenting part in regard to the maternal pelvis. Vertex presentation with the vertex positioned either to the right or left anteriorly is the most common.

III. **Normal Pattern of Labor** (Table 8-6)

IV. **Management of Abnormal Labor Patterns** (Figure 8-3)

Reference

Niswander KR, ed. *Manual of Obstetrics: Diagnosis and Therapy, 3rd edition.* Boston/Toronto: Little, Brown & Company, 1987.

Obstetrics

Table 8-6. Stages of Labor

	Latent First Stage	Active First Stage	Second Stage	Third Stage	Fourth Stage
Definition	Onset of labor until complete cervical dilation. Mild contractions, variable effacement. Dilation up to 4 or 5 centimeters.	Stronger, regular contractions, occurring every 3-5 minutes and steady dilation of cervix and descent of presenting part.	Complete cervical dilation to delivery. "Pushing stage".	Interval after delivery of infant until placenta delivered.	Interval after placenta delivered until one hour postpartum.
Usual rate of progression					
primagravida	Usually some progress occurs within 6-8 hrs	Cervical dilation $\geq$1.2cm/hr fetal descent $\geq$1.0cm/hr	30 min to 2 hrs	Placenta usually separates within 5 minutes	
multipara		cervical dilation $\geq$1.5cm/hr fetal descent $\geq$2cm/hr	5-30 min	10 min	
Protraction disorder					
primagravida	20 hours	cervical dilatation <1.2cm/hr fetal descent <1.0cm/hr	2 hrs. Some centers allow 3 hrs if epidural anesthesia has been given		
multipara	14 hours	cervical dilatation <1.5cm/hr fetal descent <2cm/hr	2 hours		
Arrest disorder		deceleration phase > 3 hr			
Primagravida		No dilation over > 2 hr No descent over > 1 hr			
Multipara		deceleration phase > 1 hr No dilation over > 2 hr No descent over > 1 hr			

Evaluation of Labor 357

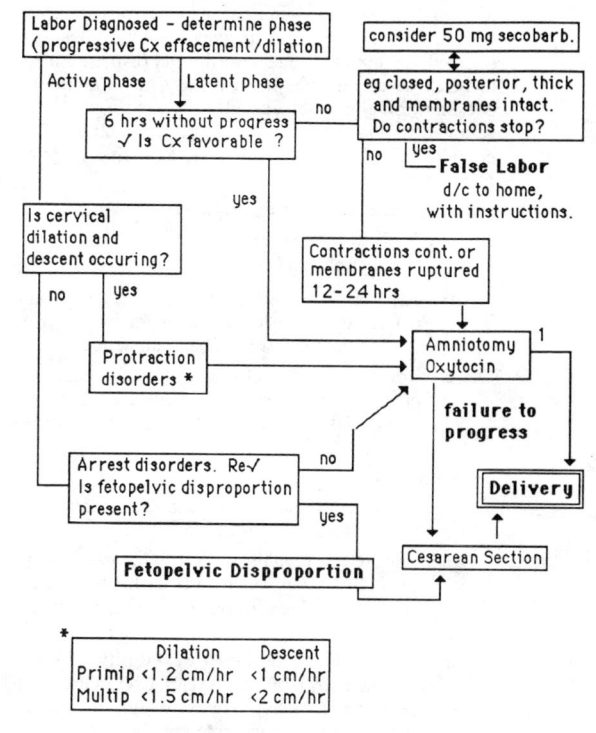

```
┌─────────────────────────────────────┐     ┌──────────────────────────┐
│ Labor Diagnosed - determine phase   │     │ consider 50 mg secobarb. │
│ (progressive Cx effacement/dilation)│     └──────────────────────────┘
└─────────────────────────────────────┘                  ↑
    Active phase  │  Latent phase           ┌──────────────────────────┐
                  ↓                    no   │ eg closed, posterior,    │
          ┌────────────────────┐ ──────────→│ thick and membranes      │
          │ 6 hrs without      │            │ intact. Do contractions  │
          │ progress           │            │ stop?                    │
          │ √ Is Cx favorable? │            └──────────────────────────┘
          └────────────────────┘               no │    │ yes
                                                  │    └─ **False Labor**
   ┌──────────────┐         yes                   │       d/c to home,
   │ Is cervical  │                               ↓       with instructions.
   │ dilation and │                    ┌──────────────────────┐
   │ descent      │                    │ Contractions cont. or│
   │ occurring?   │                    │ membranes ruptured   │
   └──────────────┘                    │ 12-24 hrs            │
      no │  yes                        └──────────────────────┘
         ↓                                        │
   ┌──────────────┐                               ↓
   │ Protraction  │ ─────────────────→  ┌──────────────────┐ 1
   │ disorders *  │                     │  Amniotomy       │──┐
   └──────────────┘                     │  Oxytocin        │  │
                                        └──────────────────┘  │
                                              ↗               │
                                  **failure to progress**     │
                                          ↗                   ↓
   ┌────────────────────────┐    no                    ┌──────────┐
   │ Arrest disorders. Re-√ │ ───────────              │ Delivery │
   │ Is fetopelvic          │                          └──────────┘
   │ disproportion present? │                                ↑
   └────────────────────────┘                                │
         │ yes                             ┌────────────────────┐
         ↓                                 │ Cesarean Section   │
   ┌──────────────────────────┐            └────────────────────┘
   │ **Fetopelvic Disproportion** │
   └──────────────────────────┘
```

	Dilation	Descent
Primip	<1.2 cm/hr	<1 cm/hr
Multip	<1.5 cm/hr	<2 cm/hr

Fig 8-3. Management of Abnormal Term Labor.

Notes: With amniotomy and oxytocin, internal monitors for uterine contractions and fetal heart rate may be required. Upright position may be helpful.

INTRAPARTUM MONITORING AND MANAGEMENT

I. **Fetal Heart Rate:** Electronic fetal heart rate monitoring may be performed via an external doppler, or direct scalp lead when membranes are ruptured.

   A. Indications: Meconium staining, use of oxytocin, delivery of an anticipated premature, postmature, Rh sensitized, or growth retarded infant, medical complications associated with uteroplacental insufficiency (hypertension, diabetes, severe anemia, heart disease, renal disease), presence of abnormal auscultatory findings, prior cesarean section (VBAC), other intrapartum obstetrical complications (failure to progress, excessive vaginal bleeding).

   B. Fetal heart rate tracing interpretation:

   1. Baseline fetal heart rate.
      a. Normal 120-160 bpm.
      b. Tachycardia > 160 bpm. Etiology: fetal hypoxia, maternal fever, maternal hyperthyroidism, parasympatholytic or sympathomimetic drugs.
      c. Bradycardia < 120 bpm. Etiology: fetal asphyxia, anesthetics, fetal cardiac conduction defect. Usually benign if good variability is present.

   2. Variability
      a. Short term variability - beat to beat variations is normally 5 to 10 bpm.
      b. Long term variability - refers to the waviness of the FHR tracing, which normally has a frequency of 3-10 cycles/min and an amplitude of 10-25 bpm.
      c. Decreased variability - variability may be decreased by fetal sleep cycles, CNS depression secondary to hypoxia or drugs, parasympatholytic agents, extreme prematurity, or congenital anomalies. Loss of variability with an otherwise non reassuring FHR tracing is as-

sociated with a high incidence of fetal acidosis and low apgar scores.

3. Common Periodic Patterns.

   a. Accelerations - Reassuring if associated with fetal movement. May be compensatory before or after deceleration.

   b. Early decelerations - Occur coincidentally with uterine contractions and are associated with fetal head compression. These are vagally mediated and not ominous if occur late in labor.

   c. Late decelerations - Characterized by a latency period between the onset of uterine contraction and the beginning of the deceleration. Late decelerations are indicative of uteroplacental insufficiency, and are always considered potentially ominous.

   d. Variable decelerations - Characterized by variable duration, timing, and intensity. This is a reflex pattern, typically secondary to cord compression. Poor prognostic signs are:

- association with poor FHR baseline variability.
- lack of pre- and post-deceleration accelerations.
- level ascending limb (slow return to baseline).
- biphasic shape (W = knot in cord).
- failure to return to baseline.

   e. Prolonged decelerations; isolated decelerations > 120 seconds can be seen with maternal hypotension, maternal hypoxia, tetanic contractions, prolapsed umbilical cord, fetal scalp procedures (vagal), and paracervical or epidural anesthesia. A prolonged deceleration after severe variable deceleration may signal impending fetal demise.

C. Management of abnormal FHR pattern/fetal distress (Fig 8-4).

1. Turn patient onto side to alleviate vena cava compression.

2. Discontinue intravenous oxytocin.

3. Apply 100% oxygen to mother by face mask.

4. Correct maternal hypotension.
5. Vaginal examination to rule out prolapsed cord.
6. Consider fetal scalp sampling for pH determination.
7. Consider immediate delivery.

Normal (120-160bpm)
— beat to beat variability +/- 8bpm —

Early Decels (fetal head compression)
Uniform/symmetric - early timing

Late Decels (Uteroplacental - vascular insufficiency)
Uniform/symmetric - late timing

Variable Decels (Cord compression)
Variable shape/variable timing

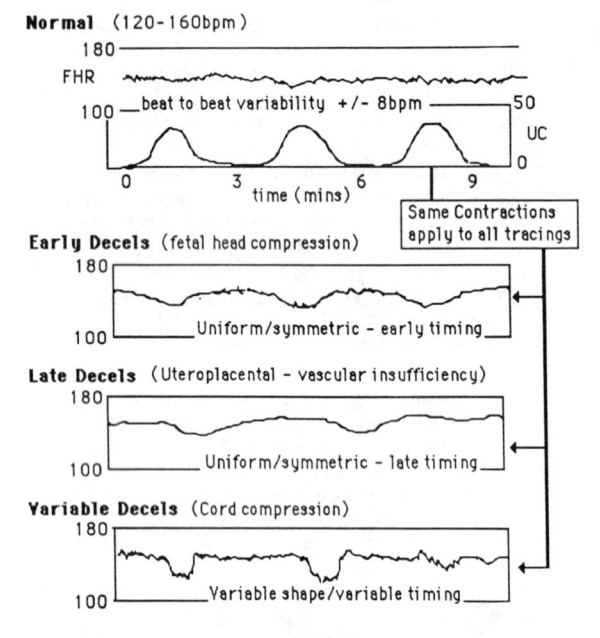

Same Contractions apply to all tracings

Fig 8-4. Fetal Heart Rate Patterns

II. **Uterine Activity**: May be determined by an indirect (external) pressure monitor, or by an intrauterine pressure transducer when more accurate estimations are required.

Intrapartum Monitoring and Management 361

- A. Contractility: Effective contractions should have an amplitude of 50-75mm Hg, duration of 45-90 seconds, and frequency of 3-5 minutes.
- B. Resting tone: Spontaneous labor 5-10 mm Hg. Induced labor 15-20 mm Hg.
- C. Rhythmicity: Presence of coupling or tripling may represent hyperstimulation.
- D. Configuration: Typically bell-shaped. May become rectangular during pushing. The area under the curve when an internal transducer is used may be calculated to determine the adequacy of uterine contractions.

III. **Fetal Scalp PH**

- A. Procedure for obtaining scalp pH - (see Hospital Procedures section).

References

Driscoll CE, *et al*, eds. Handbook of Family Practice. Chicago: Year Book Medical Publishers, 1986.

Klavan M, *et al*. Clinical Concepts of Fetal Heart Rate Monitoring. Massachusetts: Hewlett-Packard Co., 1977.

Krebs AB, *et al*. Intrapartum fetal heart rate monitoring I classification and prognosis of fetal heart rate patterns. Am J of Ob/Gyn 133(7):762, 1979.

Niswander KR, ed. Manual of Obstetrics: Diagnosis & Therapy, 3rd edition. Boston/Toronto: Little, Brown & Company, 1987.

Pritchard JA, *et al*, eds. Williams Obstetrics, 17th edition. Connecticut: Appleton-Century-Crofts, 1985.

PELVIMETRY

I. **Pelvic Inlet**

   A. Transverse Diameter: Average 13.5 cm; cannot be measured clinically.

   B. AP Diameter: Most important. Can be estimated clinically by determining the distance between the lower margin of the symphisis pubis and the sacral promontory. This value is known as the diagonal conjugate. The obstetrical conjugate (or true AP diameter) is 1.5 to 2.0 cm shorter. If the obstetric conjugate is 10 cm or greater, one may assume that the pelvic inlet is of an adequate size for childbirth.

II. **Pelvic Midplane**

   The specific diameters of the midpelvis are not measured clinically. Contraction of the midpelvis is suspected if the ischial spines are quite prominent, the pelvic sidewalls converge, or the sacral concavity is quite shallow.

III. **Pelvic Outlet**

   A. Transverse diameter of the pelvic outlet should be equal to 8.0 cm. This can be estimated by placing a fist on the perineum between the two ischial tuberosities.

   B. The AP diameter is estimated by noting the angle made by the pubic rami. The effective outlet diameter may be decreased by a narrow pubic arch. Although a contracted outlet is rarely the sole cause of dystocia, it may be associated with contraction of the midpelvis.

IV. **X-ray Pelvimetry**

   A. Indications.

      1. History of previous injury to maternal pelvis.

      2. Breech presentation of fetus in which vaginal delivery is anticipated.

   B. Advantages: Allows direct measurement of the AP diameters, as well as the transverse inlet of the pelvis.

   C. Potential Hazards: There is a possible increase in the incidence of malignancy in the fetus secondary to radiation exposure. CT pelvimetry drastically decreases radiation exposure to fetus.

D. Parameters (Table 8-7).

Table 8-7. X-ray Pelvimetry Chart

Diameters	Average normal (cm)	Average total (cm)	Low normal (cm)
Pelvic inlet		25.5	22.0
Anteroposterior	12.5		
Transverse	13.0		
Midpelvis		22.0	20.0
Anteroposterior	11.5		
Transverse (bispinous)	10.5		
Pelvic outlet		18.0	16.0
Anteroposterior (posterior sagittal)	7.5		
Transverse (bituberal)	10.5		

Adapted from Niswander KR, ed. Manual of Obstetrics: Diagnosis & Therapy, 3rd edition. Boston/Toronto: Little, Brown & Company, 1987.

Reference

Pritchard JA, *et al*, eds. Williams Obstetrics, 17th edition. Connecticut: Appleton-Century-Crofts, 1985.

INDUCTION OF LABOR

I. **Indications and Contraindications**
   A. Indications for Induction of Labor.
      1. Pregnancy-induced hypertension.
      2. Premature rupture of membranes.
      3. Chorioamnionitis.
      4. Postdate pregnancy.
      5. Isoimmunization.
      6. Other evidence of hostile intrauterine environment.
      7. Diabetes mellitus.
      8. Other selected maternal diseases.
      9. Fetal demise.
   B. Contraindications.
      1. Placenta previa.
      2. Cord presentation.
      3. Floating presenting part.
      4. Abnormal fetal lie.
      5. Active genital herpes.
      6. Invasive cervical carcinoma.
      7. Pelvic structural deformities.
      8. Prior classical uterine incision.
      9. Oxytocin stimulation would be relatively contraindicated in conditions which predispose to uterine rupture (high parity, advanced maternal age, fetopelvic disproportion, uterine overdistention, prior uterine scar).

II. **Risks**
   A. Amniotomy.
      1. Cord prolapse.
      2. Injury to fetal part (unlikely with blunt instruments).
   B. Oxytocin.
      1. Hyperstimulation.
      2. Uterine rupture.

3. Water intoxication (hyponatremia may result if excessive oxytocin is administered with large volumes of non-electrolyte containing IV fluids).

III. **Methods**

A. Determine indications for induction of labor, weighing the relative contraindications and risks.

B. Assess the inducibility of the cervix (Table 8-8).

Table 8-8. Bishop Score to Assess Likelihood of Successful Induction of Labor

Physical Findings	Rating 0	1	2	3
Cervix				
Position	Posterior	Mid	Anterior	-
Consistency	Firm	Medium	Soft	-
Effacement (%)	0-30	46-50	60-70	≥ 80
Dilatation (cm)	0	1-2	3-4	≥ 5
Fetal head				
Station	-3	-2	-1	+1

Adapted from Driscoll CE, et al. Handbook of Family Practice. Chicago: Year Book Medical Publishers, 1986.

C. Decide whether to use amniotomy alone, or with oxytocin. Amniotomy in the face of a ripe cervix (high Bishop's score) may be sufficient. Oxytocin is indicated in arrest disorders of active labor if inadequate uterine activity is the etiology, rather than fetopelvic disproportion. Oxytocin is also indicated for a prolonged latent phase, in conjunction with complicating factors such as premature rupture of membranes or a postdates pregnancy.

D. Guidelines for Amniotomy.

1. Cervix should be dilated enough to allow reaching the membranes with the amniotomy hook.
2. The fetus should be vertex (unless breech delivery is planned) with the presenting part well engaged and well applied to the cervix.
3. The umbilical cord should not be palpable.
4. Membranes are hooked, and a gentle tug should cause release of amnionic fluid.

5. Assess fluid for presence of meconium.
6. Monitor fetal heart tones prior to and after the procedure.

E. Guidelines for Oxytocin Administration.
1. The patient should have intravenous access and fetal heart rate/uterine contraction monitoring.
2. Place 10 units of oxytocin in 1000 cc of $D_5$1/2 NS or D_5LR.
3. Begin with a low dose of oxytocin: 0.5 to 2 milliunits per minute. (Each ml of the above solution contains 10 milliunits).
4. Various protocols exist regarding the rate for increasing the dose and the maximum dose. If little uterine response is observed, the dose can be increased by 1-2 mU/min every 30 minutes. Most patients respond to rates of 20 mU/min or less. The faster the increase, the more likely the risk of hyperstimulation. The rate of administration is held steady when a good labor pattern (strong contractions every 2 or 3 minutes) is achieved.
5. If at any point the fetal heart rate indicates distress, the patient should be placed on her side, oxygen administered, and oxytocin discontinued. Reinstatement of oxytocin drip requires reassessment of the situation.

References

Induction and augmentation of labor. ACOG Technical Bulletin. No. 110. Nov. 1987.

Zlatnik, FJ. The most valuable obstetric drug. IA Perinatal Letter. 5(4) July/August, 1984.

VAGINAL DELIVERY

I. **Normal Spontaneous Vaginal Delivery**
   A. Cardinal Movements (for vertex presentation).
      1. Engagement: occurs late in pregnancy for primigravida, at the onset of labor for multigravida.
      2. Flexion: of the neck so that the smallest diameter possible presents. (If the neck does not flex, it may actually extend during labor, producing a brow or face presentation).
      3. Descent: progressive with thinning of the cervix and lower uterine segment. Depends upon the force of contractions, pelvic and presenting part configuration.
      4. Internal rotation: occurs during descent. Vertex rotates from transverse to either posterior or anterior position to pass the ischial spines.
      5. Extension: occurs as the head distends the perineum and the occiput passes beneath the symphysis.
      6. External rotation: occurs after delivery of the head with the head rotating back to a transverse position as the shoulders internally rotate to an anteroposterior position.
   B. Management of vertex delivery.
      1. Preparations for delivery should be made when the presenting part begins to distend the perineum, sooner for multigravida. Anesthesia should be administered at this time (local or pudendal). Episiotomy is not performed until delivery is imminent.
      2. Delivery of the head.
         a. Controlled so that there is no forceful, sudden expulsion (which may produce injury to mother or baby). As the vertex appears beneath the symphysis, the perineum is supported by direct pressure from a draped hand over the coccygeal region. This will protect the perineum and assist in extension of the head as the vertex passes the symphysis.

- b. As the head is delivered, it will rotate to a transverse position, at which time the baby should be checked for the presence of umbilical cord about the neck. If present it should be gently slipped over the infant's head (or double clamped and cut if this cannot be done easily).
- c. The mouth and nose should be cleared of secretions with a bulb syringe or DeLee suction trap.

3. Delivery of the shoulders. Shoulders should be rotated to an AP position in the pelvic outlet as the head externally rotates. Gentle traction downward on the head will assist in bringing the anterior shoulder beneath the symphysis. Gentle elevation of the infant head toward the symphysis will release the posterior shoulder.

4. Delivery of the body. The rest of the body will generally deliver spontaneously and quickly after delivery of the shoulders. Care must be taken to control the delivery of the body to prevent unnecessary injury.

5. Immediate care of the infant includes double clamping and cutting of the umbilical cord. The clamp closest to the umbilicus should be just distal to the skin reflection. A clear airway must be assured and body temperature maintained by drying and wrapping or placing under a radiant heater.

II. Forceps delivery: Forceps are generally used to shorten the second stage of labor when in the best interests of the mother or the fetus. A fully dilated cervix and experienced physician are required. Advantages must be weighed against the increased risk of maternal lacerations.

A. Indications:

1. Prolonged second stage.
   a. primigravida with regional anesthesia: > 3 hours.
   b. primigravida without regional anesthesia: > 2 hours.
   c. multigravida with regional anesthesia: > 2 hours.

Vaginal Delivery

- d. multigravida without regional anesthesia: > 1 hours.
 2. Fetal distress.
 3. Maternal exhaustion.
B. Requirements:
 1. Fetal head engaged and in vertex/face presentation.
 2. Position of head known exactly.
 3. Membranes ruptured.
 4. Cervix fully dilated.
 5. No clinical evidence of cephalopelvic disproportion.
C. Definitions.
 1. Outlet forceps. The fetal scalp is visible at the introitus. The head is at or on the perineum, and the sagittal suture is in the AP plane or rotated up to 45 degrees.
 2. Low forceps. The leading point of the skull is at least at +2 station.
 3. Midforceps. The leading point of the skull is engaged but is above +2 station. (Mid forceps delivery should only be attempted in extreme situations while simultaneously preparing for cesarean delivery.)
D. Technique:
 1. Ensure adequate anesthesia.
 2. Empty bladder by straight catheterization.
 3. The posterior blade is inserted first, followed by the anterior one. If the vertex is in the AP position, the maternal left blade is lubricated and held in the left hand, with the handle 90 degrees in the air (almost vertical). The right hand is placed between the blade and left vaginal wall. The blade is then gently slipped into place on the fetal head. The maternal right blade is held in the right hand and inserted in the same manner.
 4. Application is checked. The superior borders of the blades should be equidistant from the lambdoidal suture lines. The sagittal suture should be midline. The posterior fontanelle should be no more than 1cm above the shank.

5. Blades are locked and application rechecked.
6. Episiotomy is performed.
7. Traction is applied in the appropriate manner. Forceps are removed after delivery of the fetal head.

E. Indications for selected forceps:
- Simpsons--good for primigravida with prolonged 2nd stage (molded fetal head).
- Elliots-better if multigravida, less molded fetal head.
- Tucker-McLane--have sliding lock, good for asynclitic fetal head.
- Keelar--have minimal pelvic curve, often used for rotation.
- Piper--used in breech extractions.

III. **Vacuum extraction**. A safe, effective alternative to forceps delivery. A term, vertex fetus is required. Delivery should not be one that will require rotation or excessive traction. Prior scalp sampling is a contraindication.

A. Advantages.
- Simpler to apply, with fewer mistakes in application.
- Less force applied to fetal head.
- Less anesthesia necessary (local anesthetic may suffice).
- No increase in diameter of presenting head.
- Less maternal soft tissue injury.
- Less fetal injury.
- Less parental concern.

B. Disadvantages.
- Traction applied only during contractions.
- Proper traction necessary to avoid losing vacuum.
- Possibly longer delivery than with forceps.
- Small increase in incidence of cephalohematomas.

C. Technique.
1. Ascertain that the cervix is fully dilated and the vertex is in low or outlet position.
2. The vertex is then wiped clean, the labia spread, and the cup compressed and inserted. Pressure is applied inward and downward, until contact is made with the fetal scalp. The cup should be placed over the posterior fontanelle.

3. A finger is swept around the cup to make sure no maternal tissue is within the cup. Suction pressure is raised to 100 mmHg, and the location of the cup is rechecked.

4. With the onset of a contraction, suction pressure is raised to 380 to 580 mmHg. (Negative pressure should not exceed 600 mmHg.) Traction is applied perpendicular to the cup, in line with the maternal axis.

5. Should the cup dislodge, the fetal scalp is to be checked before the cup is reapplied.

6. When the contraction subsides, the suction pressure is reduced to 100 mmHg.

7. The sequence is repeated with each contraction. More than three good attempts are not recommended unless progress is being made.

8. As the head crowns an episiotomy may be cut. Traction is then changed to a 45 degree angle upward as the vertex clears the symphysis.

9. Suction is released and the cup removed after delivery of the fetal head.

10. The procedure should be discontinued if one fails to achieve extraction after ten minutes at maximal pressure, extraction is not achieved within 30 minutes of initiation, the cup disengages three times, fetal scalp trauma is sustained, or no progress is made after three pulls.

References

Committee on obstetrics: Maternal & fetal medicine. No. 59, Feb. 1988.

Epperly TD and Bretinger ER. Vaccuum extraction. American Family Physician 38(3):205, Sept. 1988.

Niswander KR, ed. Manual of Obstetrics: Diagnosis & Therapy, 3rd edition. Boston/Toronto: Little, Brown & Company, 1987.

Pritchard JA, et al, eds. Williams Obstetrics, 17th edition. Connecticut: Appleton-Century-Crofts, 1985.

BREECH DELIVERY

I. **Overview**

   A. Incidence: 25% of all pregnancies < 28 wks gestation, 3-4% of all pregnancies at or beyond 34 wks gestation.

   B. Etiology: Low birth weight, placenta previa, uterine and fetal anomalies, contracted pelvis, multiple fetuses all contribute to breech presentations.

II. **Types of Breech**

   1. Frank: Thighs/hips flexed, knees extended. 65% of cases are frank.

   2. Complete: Thighs/hips flexed, one or both knees flexed. 10% of cases.

   3. Incomplete/Footling: One or both thighs extended, one or both knees below the buttocks. 25% of cases.

III. **Breech Delivery--Buttocks, Extremities and Shoulders**

   A. Criteria for vaginal delivery and breech presentation.

   1. Frank breech presentation.

   2. Fetal weight 2500-3800 gm.

   3. Fetal head flexed.

   4. Gestational age at or beyond 36 weeks.

   5. Adequate maternal pelvis.

   6. No other maternal or fetal indicator for C-section.

   B. Technique:

   1. Do not assist delivery until buttocks have advanced through the introitus as this is the only way to assure that the cervix has dilated. A finger may be inserted into the anterior groin and gentle traction applied. The back must rotate into an anterior position behind the symphysis. After the buttocks have been delivered past the introitus, the extended legs must be disengaged by upward and outward pressure in the popliteal fossa. This flexes the knee and allows delivery of the foot.

   2. After delivery of the breech and legs, the torso will spontaneously deliver to the level of the shoulders. A

small amount of umbilical cord should be advanced out of the introitus to avoid traction on the cord. The infant is rotated in each direction so that in turn each shoulder is brought from a posterior position to a position beneath the symphysis. When the angle of the scapula is visible, the arm may be delivered by hooking the fingers in the antecubital fossa or by direct pressure on the lateral aspect of the angle of the scapula, which rotates the angle medially and brings the shoulder out beneath the symphysis. After delivery of one arm, the infant is rotated (with back towards the symphysis) so that the second shoulder is brought behind the symphysis and the arm delivered. The infant then should be in an occiput-anterior position for delivery of the head.

IV. **Breech Delivery--the Head**: May be attempted without instrumentation if the baby's condition is good. If there is evidence of distress, forceps should be used immediately without attempting the following maneuver.

A. Mauriceau-Smellie-Veit maneuver:

1. Have infant straddled over one forearm.

2. Using the same hand, place the middle finger in the infant's mouth, and the index and ring fingers on either side of the mouth, on the fetal maxillae.

3. With the opposite hand, place the middle finger over the infant's occiput to maintain head flexion, with the other fingers draped over the shoulders.

4. Apply gentle downward traction while an assistant provides suprapubic pressure.

5. If delivery does not occur quickly with gentle traction, forceps should be applied. Additional attempts at non-instrumented delivery are not attempted.

B. Piper forceps extraction

1. The infant's body is supported by an assistant with a towel sling. The arms must also be in the sling.

2. Forceps are introduced from below the infant's body and directed upward without rotating the blades. The left blade is inserted first to a position on the infant's face from chin to vertex.

3. Forceps are used primarily to maintain flexion of the head. Gentle traction should be combined with upward pressure on the handles so that the head flexes beneath the symphysis.

Reference

Hacker N and Moore JG, eds. *Essentials of Obstetrics and Gynecology*. Philadelphia: W.B. Saunders Company, 1986.

EPISIOTOMY

An episiotomy is deliberate incision in the perineum used to facilitate vaginal delivery.

I. Type/Advantages

A. Midline: Good anatomic end results, easy repair, low incidence of postpartum pain or dyspareunia. May extend through the anal sphincter and into the rectum.

B. Mediolateral: Less likely to extend through the sphincter, but more likely to cause pain during healing, dyspareunia, or excessive blood loss. Good anatomic results are more difficult to obtain.

II. Repair of Midline Episiotomy

(Note: The same process is used in repair of mediolateral episiotomies although reapproximation of the tissues requires greater diligence).

A. Approximate the vaginal mucosa and submucosa with 2 "0" or 3 "0" chromic gut, Dexon, or Vicryl sutures in running, locked stitches. Begin proximal to the apex of the incision in the vaginal wall. Approximate and pass under the hymenal ring. This suture may be tied off or held for future use.

B. For a moderate to deep episiotomy, deep interrupted sutures are placed in the fascia and muscle of the perineum. The suture used is of the same type and size as for the vaginal mucosa.

C. A continuous non-locking suture technique is used to approximate the superficial fascia. One may use the remainder of the suture from closure of the vaginal mucosa, starting from the fourchette and running toward the anus.

D. Once the posterior apex is reached, one may continue with the same suture material back up the perineum, using a subcuticular stitch.

E. When the anterior apex is reached and the episiotomy repair is completed, the needle is passed under the hymenal ring. A smaller stitch of vaginal tissue is taken to allow the stitch to be tied. The knot will thus be inside the vaginal introitus, and therefore, less irritating to the patient.

Reference

Pritchard JA, *et al*, eds. <u>Williams Obstetrics, 17th edition</u>. Connecticut: Appleton-Century-Crofts, 1985.

MALPRESENTATIONS

I. **Face**
   A. Incidence: 0.2%.
   B. Diagnosis: vaginal examination. Differentiated from a breech by the fetal mouth and malar prominences forming the corners of a triangle. In a breech, the anus forms a straight line with the fetal ischial tuberosities.
   C. Management: In the absence of pelvic contraction and with good uterine contractions, vaginal delivery is usually possible. Face presentations must be in the mentoanterior (MA) position to deliver. Fifty percent of mentoposterior (MP) presentations rotate to MA. Manual version should not be attempted.

II. **Brow**
   A. Incidence: rare.
   B. Vaginal delivery generally can not take place in a brow presentation. 50-75% will convert to a vertex or face presentation, allowing vaginal delivery.

III. **Transverse Lie/Shoulder Presentation**
   A. Incidence: 0.3%.
   B. Etiology:
      1. Excessive relaxation of maternal abdominal wall secondary to grandmultiparity.
      2. Prematurity.
      3. Placenta previa.
      4. Contracted pelvis.
   C. Management. Labor with shoulder presentation increases both maternal and fetal risk. Cesarean section is indicated.

IV. **Compound Presentation**
   A. Definition: A fetal extremity prolapses along side the presenting part. This may be associated with fetal prematurity or cord accidents; fetal morbidity is increased.

B. Management: A Cesarean section is indicated if there is evidence that the extremity is preventing normal labor, if there is evidence of fetal distress, or if the extremity is a leg (non frank breech presentation).

References

Hacker N and Moore JG. <u>Essentials of Obstetrics and Gynecology</u>. Philadelphia: W.B. Saunders & Company, 1986.

Pritchard JA, *et al*, eds. <u>Williams Obstetrics, 17th edition</u>. Connecticut: Appleton-Century-Crofts, 1985.

SHOULDER DYSTOCIA

I. **Incidence:** Directly related to fetal size: >2500gm 0.15%, >4000gm 1.7%, >4500gm 10.0%.

II. **Diagnosis:** Suspect shoulder dystocia if there is reason to suspect macrosomia (gestational diabetes, history of large infants, large maternal size, prolonged gestation), or if second stage is prolonged. Consider C-section. In vaginal deliveries, suspect dystocia if the head pulls back against the perineum after delivery, and external rotation is difficult.

III. **Management**
   A. Ensure adequate maternal anesthesia and cut a very generous episiotomy.
   B. Attempt McRobert's maneuver. The mother's thighs are hyperflexed, bringing her feet "to her ears."
   C. Have an assistant apply suprapubic pressure. This causes the shoulder to move under the symphysis pubis. Attempt delivery with gentle downward traction.
   D. If the above measures are unsuccessful, attempt to gently rotate the posterior shoulder by pushing on the posterior scapula until the shoulder passes under the symphysis, and can be delivered as the anterior shoulder. This is known as the Wood's screw maneuver.
   E. If this is unsuccessful, try delivering the posterior arm first, then rotating the anterior shoulder into the oblique position for delivery.
   F. If all else fails, one may attempt deliberate fracture of the clavicle of the impacted shoulder. The thumb and forefinger are used to push the clavicle outward to avoid a pneumothorax. Although the fracture will heal, damage to cervical nerve roots may occur and cause permanent sequelae.

References

Harris BA. Shoulder dystocia. <u>Clinical Obstetrics & Gynecology</u> 17(1), March 1987.

Pritchard JA, *et al*, eds. <u>Williams Obstetrics, 17th edition</u>. Connecticut: Appleton-Century-Crofts, 1985.

CESAREAN SECTION

I. **Indications**
   A. Maternal/Fetal.
      1. Cephalopelvic disproportion.
      2. Failed induction of labor.
      3. Abnormal uterine action.
   B. Maternal.
      1. Maternal Diseases: Eclampsia/pre-eclampsia with noninducible cervix, diabetes mellitus (if macrosomic infant precludes vaginal delivery), cardiac disease, cervical cancer, active herpes progenitalis.
      2. Previous Uterine Surgery: Classic cesarean section, previous uterine rupture, full thickness myomectomy.
      3. Obstruction to the Birth Canal: Fibroids, ovarian tumors.
   C. Fetal.
      1. Fetal distress.
      2. Cord prolapse.
      3. Fetal malpresentations (breech, transverse lie, brow).
   D. Placental.
      1. Placenta previa (unless marginal).
      2. Abruptio placentae.

II. **Procedure**
   A. Anesthesia: Epidural, spinal, general.
   B. Abdominal Incision: Vertical vs. Pfannenstiel (low transverse).
   C. Layers: Skins, fascia, rectus abdominus muscles, peritoneum, vesicouterine peritoneum, uterus.
   D. Hysterotomy Incision: Typically low transverse. Low vertical may be indicated in extreme prematurity, transverse lie, or some cases of placenta previa. A classical incision (vertical to fundus) is associated with higher risk of uterine rupture during a subsequent labor.

III. Risks

A. Maternal: Infection, hemorrhage, injury to urinary tract, adverse reactions to anesthesia, prolonged recovery.

B. Fetal: Depend on gestational age and indications for C-section. Less birth trauma, although injury can be sustained during operative delivery. May have increased incidence of respiratory distress syndrome.

Reference

Hacker N and Moore JG. eds. <u>Essentials of Obstetrics and Gynecology</u>. Philadelphia: W.B. Saunders & Company, 1986.

POSTPARTUM CARE

I. **Examples Of Orders After Routine Vaginal Delivery**
   A. Immediately Postpartum.
      1. Bedrest, and vitals q15 minutes for 1 hour postpartum.
      2. Consider NPO for 1-2 hours postpartum.
      3. Ice pack to perineum immediately postpartum.
   B. Therafter.
      1. Ambulate as tolerated when stable.
      2. Diet: general or other.
      3. Vitals: q4 hours.
      4. Tucks to perineum prn.
      5. Sitz baths tid & hs prn.
      6. IV (if present) : discontinue when vitals stable and uterine bleeding normal.
      7. Urethral catheterization if unable to void in 6-8 hours.
      8. Breast binder if not nursing.
      9. Masse breast cream if nursing.
      10. CBC following a.m.
      11. Type and cross for Rhogam if indicated.
      12. Medications.
         a. Vitamins: Continue prenatal vitamins; additional $FeSO_4$ if anemic.
         b. Pain: Ibuprofen 400-600 mg po q4-6 hours for cramping/pain.
         c. Laxatives: Dulcolax supppository prn if no 3rd or 4th degree laceration. If 3rd or 4th degree laceration, Colace 100 mg po BID with water. MOM 30 g po Qd prn.
         d. Lactation: Parlodel (bromocriptine) can be given to inhibit lactation in non-nursing mothers, but it is expensive, must be given for 2 weeks, and some women have rebound symptoms when it is discontinued.

II. Hospital Care

A. Physical Examination.

1. Monitor uterine changes. The fundus should be firm and at or below the umbilicus. Gradual involution occurs over the next 6 weeks.

2. Lochia (uterine drainage) is initally red or bloody, gradually becoming serosanguinous. By 2-3 weeks it should be white. Tampons are contraindicated.

3. Breasts are examined for signs of infection, presence of milk, and skin problems. Water colostrum is present initially. Milk production should occur by the 3rd to 5th day. Breast feeding should not be allowed for greater than 15 minutes on each side per feeding initially to help prevent soreness.

4. Legs should be examined for evidence of thrombophlebitis.

B. Parental Education.

1. Newborn care.
2. Breast feeding if applicable.
3. Preventation of lactation/engorgement if applicable.

III. Discharge

A. Discharge Instructions.

1. Rubella vaccination, if indicated, prior to discharge.

2. Instruct regarding signs of puerperal infection, postpartum hemorrhage, mastitis.

3. Counsel on avoidance of intercourse, tampons x 4-6 weeks.

4. Contraception (Barrier methods vs. oral contraception). OCP's can be started early, if desired. Low dose or progestin only pills have less impact on lactation.

5. Nutrition: especially if breastfeeding.

6. Medications: vitamins, iron, stool softener, when appropriate. Counsel of medications to avoid during breastfeeding.

7. Discuss need for rest, possible stresses that can occur with new infant at home.

B. Follow-up
   1. Postpartum check at 4-6 weeks
   2. Newborn checkup typically at 2 weeks.

Reference

Niswander KR, ed. Manual of Obstetrics: Diagnosis & Therapy, 3rd edition. Boston/Toronto: Little, Brown & Company, 1987.

POSTPARTUM HEMORRHAGE

I. **Definition**

Postpartum hemorrhage is most often defined as greater than 500 cc blood loss in the first 24 hours after delivery. However, blood loss after spontaneous vaginal delivery is frequently up to 600 cc, and between 1-1.5 liters after instrumental or operative delivery. Therefore, clinical experience is necessary to determine when bleeding is occurring too rapidly, at the wrong time, or is unresponsive to appropriate treatment. Blood loss will be less well tolerated if the patient has not had the normal expansion of blood volume during pregnancy, such as in cases of preeclampsia.

II. **Diagnosis**

   A. Risk Factors.

   Multiparity (>5 babies), previous postpartum hemorrhage, manual removal of the placenta, placental abruption or previa, polyhydramnios, prolonged labor, precipitant labor, difficult forceps delivery, prolonged oxytocin administration, breech extraction.

   B. Etiology.
   1. Uterine atony accounts for most cases.
   2. Other causes include retained placenta, cervical or vaginal tear, coagulopathy.

   C. Physical Examination.
   1. Vital signs (BP and pulse may underestimate the degree of blood loss).
   2. Uterus should be palpated for evidence of atony, tenderness.
   3. Vaginal exam may reveal evidence for laceration (generally bright red blood) or atony (darker blood). Bimanual exam may reveal mass (suggesting broad ligament or paravaginal hematoma).
   4. A hematocrit is only helpful in comparison to the value prior to delivery. It will not adequately reflect acute blood loss.

III. **Management**

   A. Evaluate promptly once excessive bleeding is detected. Reliable IV access must be obtained with 2 large bore IVs. Monitor vitals and maintain circulatory status with fluids. If the patient shows evidence of symptomatic hypovolemia, blood should be sent for type and crossmatch patient. Coagulation profile should also be obtained.

   B. Review clinical course for probable cause (see predisposing factors listed above).

   C. Perform bimanual examination in recovery area/delivery room.

   1. If uterus is found to be boggy, initiate stimulation with massage or oxytocin (40 units in 1,000 ml crystalloid-infuse at 200 ml/hr or 10 units oxytocin IM). If no response promptly, give Hemabate 0.2 mg IM.

   2. If placental fragments detected within uterus on exploration or on ultrasound, return to delivery room for curettage.

   3. Laceration or hematoma should be repaired in delivery room.

   D. If cause is not identified or fails to respond to the above measures, notify obstetric physicians, anesthesia and operating room personnel of potential need for surgical intervention.

   E. Inform patient of the problem and what measures are being taken to correct it. Get an appreciation of her desires regarding further childbearing and hysterectomy.

   F. If hemorrhage is unresponsive to the above measures, administration of prostaglandins should be considered. Prostaglandin E2 (20 mg) vaginal suppositories, and prostaglandin F2 (1 mg) intramyometrial injection have been used. A synthetic derivative, Prostin 15/M may be used. The drug is given intramuscularly at a dosage of 250 micrograms, and can be repeated in 15 minutes. A response should be obtained by the second dose. This method is reported to be effective in at least half of the cases of persistent uterine atony.

   G. If uterine bleeding persists, then surgery must be considered. Packing is a temporary measure and is rarely effective. Surgical alternatives include: uterine artery and hypogastric artery ligation. Hysterectomy is the treatment of last resort when the patient desires future fertility, but may be preferred if sterility is desired.

References

Hacker N and Moore JG, eds. Essentials of Obstetrics & Gynecology. Philadelphia: W.B. Saunders Company, 1986.

Herbert WNP and Cefalo RC. Management of postpartum hemorrhage. Clinical Obstetrics and Gynecology. 27(1), March 1984.

Johnson SR. Postpartum hemorrhage. The IA Perinatal Letter. 7(2), March/April, 1986.

Pritchard JA, et al, eds. Williams Obstetrics, 17th edition. Connecticut: Appleton-Century-Crofts, 1985.

PUERPERAL FEVER

I. **Definition**

Temperature > 38.4 in first 24 hours or > 38.0 for two consecutive days in the following 9 days postpartum.

II. **Differential Diagnosis** (Table 8-9)

Table 8-9. Differential diagnosis of puerperal febrile morbidity.

Diagnosis	Risk Factors	Clinical features
Endomyometritis	Chorioamnionitis, prolonged rupture of membranes and labor, multiple vaginal examinations, cesarean section, retained products, contact with group A streptococci carrier, carriage of group B streptococci, indigent patient, internal monitoring (?), manual placental removal (?)	Fever malaise, abdominal pain, uterine tenderness, purulent lochia, leukocytosis; usually within 48 hours of delivery
Pelvic abscess	Pelvic infection with delayed anaerobic therapy	Continued fever, pain, ileus; pelvic mass; usually after day 5
Septic pelvic thrombophlebitis	Pelvic cellulitis	Continued spiking fever, with or without pain; unresponsive to antibiotics; possible tender mass; diagnostic response to intravenous heparin
Wound infection	Cesarean section in labor, emergency surgery, electrocautery, open drains, obesity, diabetes	Fever; tender, erythematous or fluctuant incision; drainage of blood or pus; usually after day 5
Pulmonary atelectasis	Recent general anesthesia, abdominal incision, narcotic analgesics	Fever usually within 48 hours; poor inspiratory effort; dullness, decreased breath sounds or rales
Pyelonephritis	Unrecognized bacteriuria, bladder trauma, catheterization	Fever, malaise, costovertebral angle tenderness, pyuria
Deep vein thrombosis	Traumatic delivery, cesarean section, delayed ambulation, varicose veins	Fever; lower-extremity pain, swelling, and pallor

Table 8-9 (continued)

Diagnosis	Risk factors	Clinical features
Mastitis	Usually breast-feeding, contact with Staphylococcus aureus carrier	Usually 3-4 weeks postpartum; fever, malaise; swollen, tender, indurated breast

Adapted from Niswander KR, ed. Manual of Obstetrics: Diagnosis & Therapy, 3rd edition. Boston/Toronto: Little, Brown & Company, 1987.

III. Endometritis

A. Etiology.

1. Infection is initially caused by multiple aerobic organisms followed by anaerobic bacteria. In particular, high fever within the first 25 hours after delivery may be caused by gram negative sepsis, Group B streptococcal disease, clostridial sepsis, or toxic shock syndrome.

2. Risk factors include: chorioamnionitis, prolonged rupture of membranes, multiple vaginal exams, cesarean section, retained products, indigent patient, possibly internal monitoring.

B. Treatment.

1. Cultures of the cervix and blood may help identify the causative organism.

2. Therapeutic regimens.

   a. Beta-hemolytic strep.

- PCN G, 4-5 million units IV q6h, or
- Ampicillin, 1-2 gm IV q4-6h, or
- Cefazolin, 1 gm IV q6h

   b. Polymicrobial (following vaginal delivery)

- Ampicillin 2 gm IV q4-6h, or
- Cefazolin 1 gm q6h, and
- Aminoglycoside (e.g., gentamicin, 2 mg/kg IV loading followed by 80-100 mg IV q8h).

   c. Clinical failure.

- Add clindamycin, 600 gm IV q6h, or
- Metronidazole 15 mg/kg IV loading and 7.5 mg/kg q6h.

   d. Following C-section.

- Clindamycin 600 mg IV q6h and
- Aminoglycoside (as above).
    e. Clinical failure
- Add ampicillin 2 gm IV q4h

References

Niswander KR, ed. <u>Manual of Obstetrics: Diagnosis & Therapy, 3rd edition</u>. Boston/Toronto: Little, Brown & Company, 1987.

Puerperal infections. <u>IA Perinatal Letter</u> 5(1), January/February, 1984.

9/ GENERAL SURGERY

Ann Stein, M.D.

WOUND MANAGEMENT

I. **General Principles.** Goal of wound management is primarily restoration of function, which requires minimizing risk of infection and repair of injured tissue, with minimum of cosmetic deformity.

II. **Significant History**
   A. Mechanism of injury.
      1. Blunt trauma: split or crush type injuries will swell more and tend to have more devitalized tissue and higher risk of infection.
      2. Sharp trauma: clean edges, little cellular injury and little risk of infection.
      3. Bite injury: consider type of animal for risk of severe infection.
      4. Consider also the risk of an underlying fracture or retained foreign body with the increased risk of infection. X-ray suspicious injuries. When obtaining an x-ray for a foreign body, remember that wood or low lead glass may not show and that wound exploration is necessary.
   B. Time of injury: After 3 hours, the bacterial count in a wound increases dramatically. After 8 hours most wounds should be left open to close by secondary intention or delayed primary closure. Wounds up to 24 hours old on the face may be closed after good cleaning. The blood supply in this area is much better and the risk of infection therefore much less. The wound should be rechecked for infection between 24 and 48 hours if you are closing a wound of this sort. The risk of infection may also be reduced on theses wounds by using tape closures.

C. Tetanus status (Table 9-1):

Table 9-1. Tetanus status

Last tetanus booster	Clean wound	Dirty wound
Unknown or never immunized	0.5 cc tetanus toxoid; repeat 6 wks & 6 mos to 1 yr	0.5 cc tetanus toxoid and repeat at 6 wks & 6 mos to 1 yr. 250u human tetanus immuned globulin.
< 10 years > 5 years	none (consider 0.5ml tetanus toxoid)	0.5 cc tetanus toxoid
10 years	0.5 ml tetanus toxoid	0.5 cc tetanus toxoid

D. Allergy history: check specifically for iodine, tape, lidocaine, and antibiotics.

E. Other medical illnesses.

1. Diabetes: small vessel disease and immune suppressed; both increase risk of infection. Antibiotics should be used for lower extremity injuries with frequent rechecks.

2. Chemotherapy or steroid dependence: immune suppressed. Need to use antibiotics orally for prophylaxis for any contaminated wound. Slowed healing may require sutures to remain in 1.5 to 2 times normal healing time. After suture removal, reinforce wound with wound tapes to avoid dehiscence.

3. Peripheral vascular disease: increased risk of infection and delayed healing; watch wound carefully.

F. Social.

1. Type of work patient does may increase risk of infection or delay healing with large amount of dirt, grease, or excessive use of the involved part. May need to splint, increase protective bandaging, or give temporary work release.

2. Personality will affect patient's interest and motivation in caring for the wound. May require additional wrapping, splinting, or more frequent rechecks.

III. **Physical Exam**

A. Vascular injury: direct pressure is the first choice for controlling bleeding. If a fracture is involved, immobilization will help control bleeding. A tourniquet proximally may be required for uncontrollable bleeding. Tourniquet may be left in place up to 2 hours without damage to the tissue. Do not clamp vascular structures until you can determine if this is a significant vessel to surgically repair. If the anatomy is suspicious for injury to major vascular structures, obtain angiogram. Capillary refill should be checked distally and be less than 2 seconds. Bleeding on the scalp is best controlled by suturing the wound. For extremities, inflating a blood pressure cuff above systolic pressure assists in wound inspection, eventually in repair.

B. Neurologic: check distal muscle strength and sensation. For hand and finger lacerations check 2 point discrimination which should be less than 1 cm at the fingertips. A crush injury may also decrease 2 point discrimination and may take several months for recovery. A lacerated nerve may be repaired immediately or delayed; this depends on the surgeon's preference. Always check sensation prior to administering anesthesia. Numbness may also be the first sign of a developing compartment syndrome.

C. Tendons: most significant in forearm and hand injuries, but applies throughout the body. This can be evaluated by inspection, but individual muscles must also be tested for full range of motion and full strength.

D. Bones: check for open fracture or associated fractures. X-ray if any question. An open fracture is an indication for surgical debridement and repair except in the case of a distal phalanx fracture where copious irrigation and oral antibiotics are acceptable treatment if the injury can be watched carefully for infection. Even an obvious fracture should be x-rayed in case comparison is needed in the future for fracture healing or development of osteomyelitis.

E. Foreign bodies: inspect and x-ray the area. Glass may penetrate at an angle and be buried deeper than the wound appears to be. During exploration spread the tissue; do not cut tissue and risk neurovascular injury. Remember that glass must have high levels of lead to be radio-opaque. Wound markers should be used during x-ray and views obtained in two planes to help localize the object for recovery.

Wound Management

IV. **Repair**
   A. Wound healing:
      1. Collagen formation peaks at day 7. Wound has 15-20% of full strength at 3 weeks, 60% full strength at 4 months. Epithelialization occurs in 48 hours under optimal conditions. The wound is completely sealed then.
      2. Scar formation: requires 6-12 months for a mature scar. Scars should not be revised until 12 months have past. Skin tension leads to a wider scar; increased tension with loss of tissue, if perpendicular to the direction of maximal skin tension, or if in areas of excessive motion. Contractures can develop when a scar intersects perpendicular to a joint crease. Z-plasty or W-plasty may be required to revise in the future. Close approximation of portions of wounds gives the most pleasing scar and frequently debriding jagged edges widens a scar or makes edges uneven and difficult to close.
   B. Anesthesia: (see Hospital Procedures section for local, regional and field blocks)
      1. Local: distorts edges of wound. Small gauge needle (27 or 30 gauge), slower infiltration and deeper infiltration decreases the pain of infiltration. Subdermal injection may require 5 to 6 minutes for anesthesia to pinprick. Is simple, effective and quick.
      2. Regional: especially good for fingers, hands, feet, toes, mouth and face.
      3. Topical anesthesia: TAC (0.5% tetracaine, 1:2000 adrenalin, 11.8% cocaine); requires approximately 30 minutes for onset. Use only in clean wounds as the vasoconstriction decreases the resistance to infection.
      4. Anesthetics: true allergies to local anesthetics are rare and generally seen only with esters. Most "allergic" reactions are actually vasovagal or other adverse response.
         a. Lidocaine most frequently used with onset 2-5 min., duration 60 min. Can use 3-5 mg/kg with not more than 300 mg total. Can repeat dose after 30 minutes.

b. Mepivacaine (Carbocaine) has onset 5-10 min., duration of 90-120 min.
c. Bupivacaine (Marcaine) has onset 5-10 min., duration of 90-120 min.

C. Wound prep:
1. Debridement: devitalized tissue should be removed. Heavily contaminated tissue in sites free of critical tissue should be removed. Irrigation is the most effective means of cleansing a wound using a 35 cc syringe and a 19 gauge needle. Scrubbing does not cleanse the wound as well and using any disinfectant in the wound damages healthy cells needed for healing and resisting infection.
2. Skin disinfection can be performed with povidone-iodine or chlorhexidine. Shaving the area increases the risk of infection. However, hair can be clipped in the area if necessary. Never shave eyebrows as they are needed for alignment of the wound.

D. Wound Closure:
1. Time of closure related to risk of infection. Linear, clean face wounds may be safe for closure up to 24 hours after occurrence. However, within 3 hours of injury significant bacterial contamination occurs and most wounds should not be primarily closed after 4 to 8 hours. Heavily contaminated wounds (with feces, saliva, grease, or dirt) may have high enough infectious risk to close by secondary intention or by delayed primary closure. Wounds on the lower extremities and stellate wounds also carry a higher risk of infection.
2. Tape Closure: carries a lower risk of infection than suturing and may be a consideration for higher risk wounds. This may also be considered for small children to avoid a frightening surgical procedure. Often the child will not play with a tape closure if attention is not drawn to the wound.
3. Open wound care: saline wet to dry dressings with gauze or antibiotic ointment dressings will keep the tissue moist and gentle washing of the wound 2 to 3 times per day will remove bacterially contaminated

secretions. Gauze dressing (especially larger pore size) will help gently debride dead infected tissue. Avoid iodine dressings as this damages healthy tissue and will slow granulation. When clean tissue is apparent, closure with wound tapes can then be attempted.

4. Suturing: precision point cutting needle should be chosen for skin when a cosmetic closure is important. Conventional cutting needle for routine skin or dermal skin closure. Noncutting needle should be used for subcutaneous tissue. Sutures for subcutaneous tissue should be selected by the time for healing required and the importance of strength and function. Extensor tendons are slow healing and should have permanent suture of small size chosen. Muscle fasciae layers may require permanent suture if under high tension. The majority of subcutaneous or dermal suturing may be performed with an intermediate duration absorbable suture. Skin suture should be chosen by the smallest size adequate for skin tension. Nonabsorbable monofilament suture gives the lowest risk of infection and lowest suture reactivity leading to scars. See table 9-2.

5. Dressings: consider antibiotic ointment to decrease infection until skin surface closes. Immobilize if motion of a joint is going to increase skin tension and delay healing.

V. **Follow Up Care**

A. Risk of infection highest 24-48 hours, so if high risk wound recheck during this period. Consider antibiotic use for:

1. Patients prone to endocarditis.

2. Hip prostheses.

3. Lymphedema.

4. Contaminated foot wound in diabetics or others with peripheral vascular disease.

5. Wounds contaminated by feces, saliva, or vaginal secretions which are primarily closed.

6. Human bites should always have antibiotic treatment.

B. Suture removal; general guidelines:
- Face 3-5 days with tape reinforcement after suture removal.
- Scalp 7-10 days.
- Trunk 7-10 days.
- Arms 7-10 days.
- Legs 10-14 days.
- Joints, dorsal surface 14 days.
- Increase length for diabetics or steroid-dependent patients who may require several weeks to heal.

VI. Bite Wounds

Good irrigation is mandatory for puncture wounds. All these wounds are much more prone to infection.

A. Human bites: multiple organisms involved, including anaerobes. Osteomyelitis, septic arthritis and tenosynovitis are common complications. Any wound involving a joint should be irrigated in the operating room and intravenous antibiotics used. Facial wounds are the only wound that should be considered for closure and must have antibiotics used in conjunction. Augmentin is first choice followed by a cephalosporin.

B. Cat bites: higher risk of infection than dog bites, particularly with Pasturella multicida as the major pathogen present. Antibiotics should be used on all bites. Augmentin or tetracyclines (in PEN allergic patients).

C. Dog bites: less prone to infection and may be treated without antibiotics if irrigated well, seen soon after injury, and not complicated by devitalized tissue. If antibiotics are advisable Augmentin or Tetracycline (if PEN allergic).

D. Rabies treatment:
1. Domestic dog or cat in healthy condition and available for 10 days observing: no treatment.
2. Domestic dog or cat in rabid condition or suspected: human immune globulin and human diploid cell vaccine.
3. Domestic dog or cat condition unknown: consult public health in area.

Table 9-2. Sutures

Nonabsorbable	Strength	Reaction	Ease of use	Infection resistance	Note
Nylon monofilament	+++	++	++	+++	Good for skin, double throw first knot.
Prolene monofilament	++++	+	+	++++	Good for skin, increase # of knots.
Ethibond braided/coated	+++	++ 1/2	+++	+++	Rarely needed
Stainless steel wire monofilament	++++	+	+	+	Difficult but good for tendons
Silk	+	++++	++++	++	Mostly used with napes, nipples & intraoral
Absorbable					
Gut	++	+++	++	+	Rarely used as loses strength rapidly
Chromic treated gut	++	+++	++	+	Intraoral lacerations
Dexon braided polymer	+++	+++	++++	++++	Subcutaneous & intraoral
Vicryl braided polymer	+++	+	++++	+++	Subcutaneous & intraoral
Polychoxanone monofilament	++++	+	Excellent	Uncertain	Not widely available

Adapted from Barkin R and Rosen P, eds. Emergency Pediatrics. St. Louis: C.V. Mosby Company, 1986.

4. Wild animal: skunk, bat, fox, coyote, raccoon, carnivores: regard as rabid unless negative by lab tests.
5. Livestock, rodents, rabbits, hares: consult public health in area.

References

Driscoll CE, *et al*, eds. Handbook of Family Practice. Chicago: Year Book Medical Publishers, 1986.

Dushoff IM. A stitch in time. Emergency Medicine pp 1-16, January 1973.

Edlich RF, *et al*. Principles of emergency wound management. Annals of Emergency Medicine 17(12):1284, December 1988.

Goldstein EJ and Richwald GA. Human and animal bite wounds. American Family Physician 36(10:101, July 1987.

Simon B, ed. Emergency Medicine - Concepts & Clinical Practice. St. Louis: C.V. Mosby Company, 1988.

PREOPERATIVE CARE AND EVALUATION

I. **Admit Orders**
   A. Admit to ward/Primary Physician.
   B. Diagnosis and planned procedure.
   C. Condition.
   D. Vitals: for elective procedure; routine. For emergency procedure; increased frequency if unstable or if attempting to adjust fluids prior to surgery.
   E. Activity: bedrest if unstable vitals, otherwise encourage activity to avoid DVT, muscle atrophy, pneumonia.
   F. Nursing: monitoring neuro checks, monitoring lines (CVP, Swan-Ganz), pre-op teaching, PCA pump, pulmonary toilet.
   G. Diet: determined by rest of medical history and the preparation required for surgery. Period of NPO prior to surgery dependent upon age of patient (infants may have clear liquids up to 4 hours before surgery, adults should be NPO at least 6-8 hours).
   H. I&O's: fluids for rehydration (NS or LR), maintenance and correction of electrolyte imbalance. Blood products if needed. Monitoring of fluids and fluid status (CVP/Swan-Ganz, Foley).
   I. Special Tests. CXR: current to within one month unless likelihood of acute changes. Also depends on emergency surgery, age, chronic illness. EKG: older than 40 y.o. baseline EKG, or if risk factors for CAD or history of arrhythmias. Tests for specific surgery that might help avoid problems during surgery (e.g., IVP to localize ureters for pelvic surgery) or to identify concurrent problems (cholelithiasis and PUD, UGI and LGI bleeding sources).
   J. Special Meds.
      1. Patient's routine meds, change meds to IM or IV as needed.
      2. Increased steroids pre-op if steroid dependent.
      3. Pain medications as needed, including those regularly taken, assuming diagnosis made or decision to

operate made. Consent needs to be signed prior to narcotics.
4. Antibiotics as indicated for infection/sepsis or prophylaxis of endocarditis, indwelling hardwear or graft placement.
5. Prep for surgery: bowel preps, DVT prophylaxis with s.q. heparin.
6. Premeds per anesthesia to lower anxiety, lower secretions, and to interact with narcotics for sedation.

K. Labs:
1. Minimal: CBC with platelets, UA, SCP (black, Puerto Rican).
2. With any acute illness, medications affecting fluid/electrolyte balance, major surgery: electrolytes, BUN, creatinine, glucose.
3. Consider: calcium, total protein and albumin, PT/PTT, RPR, liver enzymes, amylase, drug levels, marker levels prior to surgery (acid phosphatase, CEA).
4. Pulmonary history: ABGs and spirometry.
5. Type and cross as indicated for procedure.

II. Medical History of Major Importance

A. Neurologic:
1. TIAs: for minor surgery without anticipated BP changes continue medication. For major surgery consider arteriogram as may need concurrent endarterectomy.
2. Seizures: some anticonvulsants are oral only. May need to change meds if patient will by NPO for long period of time.

B. Hematologic disorders:
1. Positive sickle cell screen: needs Hgb electrophoresis. If majority is Hgb S will need partial exchange transfusion prior to surgical procedure.
2. Clotting disorders: may need evaluation, transfusions.
3. Anemia: ideally hct > 30%, with Hgb > 10 by time of surgery.

C. Integument disorders:

1. Active infections or open wounds in area may delay elective surgeries due to post operative infection risk.
2. Chronic skin disorders should be optimally controlled for post op healing.
3. Keloid formers: may need to consider different closure techniques.

D. Nutritional status:
1. For elective or semi-elective surgery consider optimizing nutritional status if patient has chronic disease.
2. Obesity: weight loss to improve cardiopulmonary status and decrease problems with healing.

E. Cardiac:
1. Congenital disease, rheumatic fever, unevaluated murmurs, CABG within 6 months, status post valve replacements: consider need for prophylactic antibiotics. Aortic stenosis at high risk if markedly decreased valve area.
2. Hypertension: diastolic should absolutely be less than 110 and optimally in normal range.
3. Atherosclerotic disease:
    a. Angina: mild stable; eligible for minor elective surgery. More than this needs further evaluation. Urgent procedures may want to have intra-aortic balloon pump availability.
    b. History of MI < 3 weeks has 25% mortality; urgent procedure only. At 3 months 10% mortality; semi-urgent procedures. At 6 months 5% mortality: elective. At 1 year, same risk as asymptomatic patient.
    c. Increased risk of MI within first 48 hours; patient should have increased monitoring postoperatively.
4. Arrhythmias:
    a. Increased risks with > 5 PVCS/minute, coupled PVCS, V-tach, PVCs on QRST, history of cardiac arrest, 2nd or 3rd degree heart block, bradyarrhythmias.

b. Consider if pre-op pacemaker or post operative cardiac monitoring is appropriate.

5. Congestive heart failure: optimize control and fluid balance. Consider preoperative Swan-Ganz catheter and evaluation of cardiac output with different PCWPs to find optimal balance for post operative control.

F. Pulmonary.

1. COPD: optimize pulmonary toilet. Check for any change in sputum production or color indicating active infection; delay elective or semi-urgent procedures.

2. Baseline spirometry and ABGs may help with post operative management.

References

Condon RE and Nyhus LM, eds. Manual of Surgical Therapeutics, 4th edition. Boston: Little, Brown & Company, 1978.

Driscoll CE, et al, eds. Handbook of Family Practice. Chicago: Year Book Medical Publishers, 1986.

Nussbaum, MS, ed. The Mont Reid Handbook. Chicago: Year Book Medical Publishers, 1987.

POSTOPERATIVE CARE

I. **Orders**

   A. Vital Signs: q30 minutes first few hours then reduce as stable.

   B. Activity: Bedrest until fully awake; up walking that night or next morning depending on surgery.

   C. Nursing.

   1. Encourage turning, coughing, deep breathing and incentive spirometry.

   2. Dressing changes.

   3. Parameters to notify doctor such as urine output (< 1/2 cc/kg/hr), fever, hyper- or hypotension, tachy- or bradycardia, inability to void within 8 hours of beginning surgery, or unusual drainage on dressings.

   D. Diet: NPO until nausea resolves or resumption of bowel activity as determined by bowel sounds, passing gas, or having bowel movement. Start with clear liquids and advance as tolerated.

   E. I & O's.

   1. Record I & O's q shift or more frequently if patient's condition is unstable.

   2. IV fluids: with surgeries involving third spacing for 24 hours replace with isotonic solutions or colloid. NG losses should be replaced with 0.45 NS and if in exceptionally large amounts then replace losses cc for cc. Maintenance fluids should generally be 0.2 NS or 0.45 NS. Avoid K+ in fluids until it is clear that the urine output is adequate and there is no evidence of hypotension. If hypotension and oliguria are both present, the cause is most likely volume depletion and a bolus of 500 or 1000 cc isotonic fluid may be tried. Urine output should be 0.5 cc/kg/hr minimum.

   3. Instructions for care of all tubes and drains including a Foley catheter and nasogastric tube.

   F. Medications.

   1. Pain medications: oral, IV (via PCA or injection), IM. Adequate doses improve mobility. High doses lead to hypoventilation and atelectasis.

2. Antiemetics: first consider if medications may be causing nausea, if tubes are plugged, or if this is post-anesthetic nausea.
3. Antibiotics: for infection or for prophylaxis.
4. Routine medications that need to be renewed.
5. Prn medications such as laxatives, sleeping medications, and antacids, etc.

G. Special test such as follow up chest x-rays or serial EKG's. Patients intubated should have daily chest x-rays. Serial EKG's should be performed for high risk cardiac patients as the first three days have the highest risk of post operative MI.

H. Laboratory: follow up CBC for possibility of hemorrhage or for large amount of blood loss. If patient continues on IV fluid, check daily electrolytes.

II. Post Operative Fevers

A. Respiratory:
- initial may be secondary to aspiration.
- 24-48 hours post op most commonly due to atelectasis.
- After 48 hours most likely developing pneumonia.

B. Wound infections:
- first 24 hours suggests Clostridium
- 48 to 72 hours most commonly due to Strep species
- 4 days consider enteric aerobes and anaerobes and Staph.

C. Thrombophlebitis: occurs intraoperatively and fever usually begins after 24 hours.

D. Urinary tract infections: usually related to instrumentation or indwelling Foley catheter and occurs after 24 hours.

E. Less common causes:
1. Transfusion reaction: immediate.
2. Malignant hyperthermia: starts intraoperatively.
3. Drug reaction.
4. Endocrine including thyroid crisis or adrenal insufficiency.

5. Thrombophlebitis from IV site.

Reference

Condon RE and Nyhus LM, eds. <u>Manual of Surgical Therapeutics, 4th edition</u>. Boston: Little, Brown & Company, 1978.

ABDOMINAL PAIN

I. **History**

A. Location: the area of the pain, including its origin and pattern of radiation, are one of the keys to diagnosis (Table 9-3).

Table 9-3.

Location	Diagnoses	Secondary or radiation area
RUQ	congestive hepatomegaly	to back or midline
	perforated duodendum ulcer	
	cholecystitis	to high midline back & right scapula
	cholangitis	
	hepatitis or hepatic abscess	to right shoulder
	pancreatitis	straight through to back
	subphrenic abscess	in midline to shoulder of affected side
	pneumonia	
	pulmonary embolus	in other affected areas of chest also substernal,
	myocardial pain	left shoulder may have
	appendicitis	mobile, highriding color
Midepigastric	pancreatitis	to midline back
	duodenal ulcer	posterior ulcer to upper midline back
	gastric ulcer	posterior ulcer to midline back may involve pancreas
	cholecystitis	right scapula & upper midline
	pancreatic carcinoma	midline back or L flank
	hepatitis	to right shoulder
	intestinal obstruction	spreads to generalized discomfort
	appendicitis (early)	later shifts to right lower quadrant
	subphrenic abscess	to shoulder of affected side
	pneumonia	
	pulmonary embolus	other affected areas of chest as well
	myocardial pain	substernal, left shoulder

Abdominal Pain

Location	Diagnoses	Secondary or radiation area
Periumbilical	diverticulitis	can be more generalized
	pancreatitis	to midline back
	pancreatic carcinoma	to midline back
	intestinal obstruction	spreads to be more generalized
	aortic aneurysm	to low back - also common 1° site
	appendicitis (early)	later shifts to RLQ
	intestinal angina	becomes more severe and more generalized
	mesenteric thrombosis	
Left lower quadrant	regional ileitis	
	rectal disease	sacral region of back
	colonic tumor	prominant RLQ & LLQ
	diverticulitis	this can occur elsewhere, but is most common LLQ
	salpingitis	usually generalized lower abdominal
	cystitis	can feel low back as 1° or 2° site
	ovarian cyst	
	ectopic pregnancy	
	mittel schmerz	
	kidney/ureter disease	
	incarcerated hernia	flanks→groins→labia or testicles
Right lower quadrant	appendicitis	may spread midline or RUQ
	salpingitis	often generalized lower abdominal
	ectopic pregnancy	
	ovarian cyst	
	mesenteric adenitis	
	incarcerated hernia	
	Meckel's diverticulum	can spread to midline
	diverticulitis	
	regional ileitis	
	cecal tumor	
	cecal volvulus	generalized with persistent obstruction
	perforated foreign body at ileocecal valve	spreads to generalized pain
	ureteral calculus	flank→groins→labia or testicles

B. Chronology:
  1. Onset including date, location and quality of the pain at that time.

2. Pattern of the episodes including speed of onset, constant or varying nature during the pain, and time of resolution of an episode.
3. Frequency of reoccurrence.
4. Comparison of different episodes.
5. Severity.
C. Aggravating or relieving factors.
   1. Position.
   2. Eating or drinking: less than 45 minutes implies gastric origin, an hour or more implies pancreas, biliary tract, or small intestine.
   3. Activity or inactivity: are there certain movements that aggravate, do bumps in the road increase the pain, does sneezing or coughing affect it?
   4. Medications: either taken to try to affect it, or timing of medications as relates to development of pain.
   5. Defecation.
D. Associated symptoms.
   1. Weight loss: may be due to malignancy or decreased caloric intake secondary to pain. This can help identify significant intraabdominal disease with vague pains.
   2. Nausea and vomiting. It is most common with gastric, small intestinal, hepatic, or pancreatic disease. The development of nausea during the course implies a nonobstructing lesion that turned obstructive or caused an ileus due to irritation of the peritoneum or mesentery.
   3. Diarrhea and constipation mostly related to small intestine and colon. Either can occur with near obstruction. Diverticulitis is more related to constipation and inflammatory bowel diseases to diarrhea.
   4. Blood per rectum, melena, hematemesis; always double check with a hemoccult. Question foods or medicines taken that might confuse the observation.
   5. Jaundice: biliary tract, pancreas. Remember painless jaundice is the hallmark of pancreatic cancer. An episode of hemolysis such as with sickle cell disease or a massive GI bleed may confuse this finding.

Abdominal Pain

6. Reflux: characteristic of esophageal or gastric problems.
7. Change in appetite or taste: prominent with appendicitis and hepatic disease.
8. Dysuria, frequency, urgency, hematuria: renal problems often present as a complaint of abdominal pain.
9. Sexual activity, last period, birth control, history of venereal disease, vaginal discharge, spotting or bleeding. Patients often neglect these associated symptoms; most often related to the suprapubic/lower abdominal pains.

E. Past medical history.
1. Other major illnesses.
2. Prior surgeries.
3. Prior studies performed for evaluation of abdominal problems.
4. Family history of any similar complaints.
5. Medications: especially Digoxin, Theophylline, steroids, analgesics, antipyretics, antiemetics, barbiturates, diuretics.

II. Physical Exam

A. General appearance: position in bed, whether restless or still.
B. Vital signs
1. Pulse--increase due to pain, blood loss, dehydration.
2. Respiratory rate--increases with thoracic or upper abdominal source. Also check depth of respirations. Accompanies acidosis also.
3. Temperature--decreased temperature often with severe shock or toxemia. Appendicitis may start low (<101 degrees) and elevate with perforation. Normal temps may accompany perforated ulcer, ruptured ectopic or intestinal obstruction--initially not associated with bacterial spread.
4. Blood pressure--follows pulse change for dehydration, shock, or hemorrhage.

C. Signs of dehydration noted with mucous membranes and skin turgor.
D. Abdominal exam.
   1. Inspection: scaphoid/distended, movement, point of most severe pain, fullness of hernia sites, scars.
   2. Auscultation: bowel sounds (active, hyperactive, diminished, absent, high pitched), bruit.
   3. Palpation/Percussion: muscular rigidity (voluntary/involuntary), localized tenderness, masses, pulsation, hernias, peritoneal irritation (rebound, involuntary guarding, obturator, or psoas sign, hyperasthesia, Murphy's sign), liver dimension/spleen dimension.
   4. CVA tenderness.
   5. Pelvic: inspection cervix/vagina (bleeding, discharge) bimanual exam for masses and tenderness (cervical motion tenderness, dimension of uterus), bladder distension.
   6. Rectal: DO NOT NEGLECT. Localized tenderness, fluctuance, induration, masses, shelf, blood.

III. Laboratory

A. CBC with WBC and differential, platelet count, and urinalysis routinely done on most cases of abdominal pain.
B. Electrolytes with vomiting or diarrhea.
C. Liver function tests and liver enzymes, amylase for upper abdominal pain.
D. Other studies as indicated: Chest x-ray (upright) for pneumonia or free air. Abdominal flat plate and upright for bowel obstruction, ileus, free air, abnormal calcification. EKG--acute MI, ischemia, or arrhythmias. Paracentesis--may be important with fluid in the abdomen or in evaluation of abdominal trauma. Culdocentesis (non clotting blood for ruptured ectopic).

IV. Initial Treatment

A. Decide whether to:
   1. Admit and observe.

2. Operate.
- B. Keep NPO until diagnosis is clear.
- C. IV fluids--decide on expected fluid losses and current level of hydration.
- D. NG tube for vomiting, bleeding, or obstruction.
- E. Foley to monitor fluids.
- F. Serial exams for unclear diagnoses.
- G. Pain meds should be minimal until clear diagnosis.
- H. Serial labs may be helpful--especially CBC, lytes, cardiac enzymes.

V. **Diagnostic Studies**
- A. Ultrasound
  1. Upper abdominal for gallstones, common duct obstruction, pancreatitis, pancreatic psuedocyst.
  2. Kidney: may reveal obstruction if creatinine elevated; perinephric abscess.
  3. Pelvic: appendicitis, diverticulitis, mass, ovarian cyst, ectopic, PID with abscess.
- B. UGI: can use for questionable perforation if water soluble contrast used. Small bowel follow through may be useful for questionable obstruction.
- C. Lower GI for question of distal obstruction. Do not perform if suspicion of acute diverticulitis or any risk of perforation.
- D. IVP: masses, obstruction.
- E. CT scan: especially for abscesses, pancreatic mass or pseudocyst, dissecting aneurysm, rupture liver or spleen.

References

Condon RE and Nghus LM, eds. <u>Manual of Surgical Therapeutics, 4th edition</u>. Boston: Little, Brown & Company, 1978.

Nussbaum, MS, ed. <u>The Mont Reid Handbook</u>. Chicago: Year Book Medical Publishers, 1987.

APPENDICITIS

I. **Overview**: Appendicitis is a common cause of abdominal pain. However, the presentation is not always classical and a high index of suspicion is necessary. Affects any age group but is rare in infants, most common in adolescence and young adult years. Generally occurs from obstruction of the appendiceal lumen by lymphoid hyperplasia or fecalith.

II. **Clinical Presentation**

   A. History: classic history is that of periumbilical or epigastric pain which migrates to right lower quadrant. Anorexia, nausea and vomiting follow the onset of pain. Low grade fever is commonly present. Anorexia is less likely to be present in children. Presentation is more likely to be atypical in very young, very old, and pregnant patients.

   B. Physical exam: low grade temperature is common. High temperature is not common unless perforation has occurred. Abdominal exam should reveal right lower quadrant pain, possibly with rebound or guarding. Psoas sign may be present with worsening pain on passive extension of the right hip. Obturator sign is worsening of pain with internal and external rotation of the flexed right hip. Rectal exam may reveal localized tenderness or mass. Pelvic exam should be performed including speculum exam to evaluate the cervix.

   C. Laboratory: CBC with differential and UA should be obtained on all patients with lower abdominal pain. Also consider pregnancy test, cultures of cervix or urethra if indicated by history or physical. Mild to moderately elevated WBC with left shift is typical. UA may show ketonuria, but the presence of significant hematuria or pyuria suggests urinary tract as source of pain.

III. **Management**

   A. Classical presentation: consultation with surgeon on urgent basis for appendectomy. Pain relief should not be provided until surgeon has evaluated or decision to operate has been made. Patient should be kept NPO after arrival at emergency room or clinic.

B. Atypical presentation: in general, the history and physical exam are more reliable indicators of appendicitis than is the WBC. Surgeon should be consulted for suspected appendicitis if history and exam suggest the diagnosis. If minimal findings are present on exam, consider observation for several hours with repeated exams (including vitals and temperature), CBC with diff q 4 hours during observation period. Flat plate and upright X-rays of the abdomen may provide additional information. Ultrasound of appendix may be helpful. Patient kept NPO with IV fluids to maintain hydration until decision made to operate or discharge.

GALLBLADDER DISEASE

I. **Overview**: Asymptomatic cholelithiasis, choledocholithiasis, biliary colic, and acute cholecystitis are very common. Incidence of cholelithiasis increases with age and is more common in women. Other predisposing factors include obesity, pregnancy, diabetes, chronic hemolytic states.

II. **Asymptomatic Cholelithiasis**
   A. 80% of gallstones are asymptomatic, with a small percentage becoming symptomatic each year. Stones are composed of bile salts, cholesterol, phospholipids or unconjugated bilirubin. Calcification may occur and results in about 15% of the stones becoming radiopaque.
   B. Evaluation of the gall bladder:
      1. Lab tests may include liver function tests, amylase for evidence of pancreatic damage, WBC if symptoms acutely present. Alkaline phosphatase is possibly the most sensitive indicator of biliary disease.
      2. Plain x-rays may help as about 15% of stones are radiopaque.
      3. Ultrasound is often the initial exam used to evaluate for cholelithiasis. Can visualize stones, evaluate biliary ducts and pancreas. Obesity and overlying abdominal gas decrease the quality of the exam. Overall sensitivity is 90%, specificity 85%.
      4. Oral cholecystogram is performed by having patient ingest 3 grams of iopanoic acid about 12 hours prior to study. Failure of the gall bladder to opacify indicates gall bladder disease. Is not reliable in setting of significant hyperbilirubinemia or acute cholecystitis.
      5. Radionuclide excretion scan can be used in the setting of moderately elevated bilirubin and acute cholecystitis. Failure of gallbladder to visualize with presence of radioisotope in common bile duct 4 hours post-injection indicates acute cholecystitis.
   C. Management:
      1. Asymptomatic patients do not require surgery. However, the presence of pancreatitis, diabetes mellitus, or non-opacification of gallbladder on oral

cholecystogram are associated with possible increased risk of morbidity or mortality and surgery should be considered.

2. Gallstone dissolution may be considered in asymptomatic patients with normal gallbladder function or if patient refuses or is not a candidate for surgery. Recurrence rate is high if medication is not continued, dissolution rate is slow, side effects are common.

3. Lithotripsy dissolution is an option for treatment if available.

III. Biliary Colic

A. Caused by intermittent obstruction of the cystic duct by gall stones. History will generally include episodes of epigastric and RUQ pain which may radiate to back. Pain is usually constant, abrupt in onset and subsides slowly. Nausea is commonly associated. Attacks may be precipitated by ingestion of fatty foods.

B. Physical exam will reveal absence of fever, possible RUG or mid-epigastric tenderness without rebound. Gall bladder may be palpable.

C. Laboratory evaluation: CBC with differential should be obtained. WBC should not be significantly elevated. LFTs may be normal or slightly elevated.

D. Treatment: analgesics and anti-emetics should be provided acutely. Further evaluation may be obtained as convenient in the next few days with the patient instructed to avoid fatty foods. Cholecystectomy should be performed.

IV. Acute Cholecystitis

A. A significant percentage of patients with biliary colic will develop cholecystitis often due to a bacterial infection of the gallbladder. The vast majority of cases of cholecystitis are due to gall stones.

B. Presentation is similar to bilary colic with the additional features of low grade fever, leukocytosis, mild elevation of bilirubin, elevated alkaline phosphatase. Murphy's sign may be present (sudden increase in pain and inspiratory arrest with palpation of RUQ during deep inspiration).

C. Treatment: consultation with surgeon is required. Antibiotics may be indicated if signs of peritonitis are present. There are advantages and disadvantages to early or delayed surgery, although early surgery appears to generally result in lower morbidity, shorter hospitalizations. Surgeon will ultimately need to decide based upon the particular features of the case.

Evaluation of Breast Mass

I. History:
- Duration of mass.
- Pain (< 10% of cancerous lesions are painful).
- Nipple discharge (bloody more suspicious of cancer).
- Skin changes.
- Changes with menses.
- Axillary masses.
- History of trauma.
- Solitary vs. multiple masses (80% of solitary lesions are benign).
- Prior masses (Prior history of breast cancer increases risk five times; history of fibrocystic disease is 2.6 times risk).
- Family history (mother or sister with breast cancer 2-3 times risk; hx of premenopausal cancer 50 times risk).

II. Physical Exam
A. Inspection: dimpling, skin changes, nipple inversion, venous pattern.
B. Palpation.
   1. Mass: size, location (1/2 of all cancer in upper outer quadrant), consistency, fixation.
   2. Nipple discharge: identify if fluid from localized area.
      a. Bloody: intraductal papilloma.
      b. Milky: lactation, cancer, acromegaly.
      c. Clear: normal with menstrual cycle.
      d. Yellow: galactocele, cystic hyperplasia.
   3. Adenopathy: axillary, supraclavicular.

III. Mammography
A. Screening use only; not helpful for evaluating an obvious mass. False positive rate 11%, false negative rate 6%. Screen yearly after age 45. Start routine screening five years before the age female relatives were diagnosed with breast cancer.
B. Biopsy for:

1. Calcification: fine, focal or diffuse.
2. Masses: stellate or discrete.
3. Asymmetrical localized fibrotic area.
4. Altered subareolar ductal pattern.
5. Unrecognized skin edema.
6. Increased vascularity.

IV. **Evaluation** (Fig 9-1)

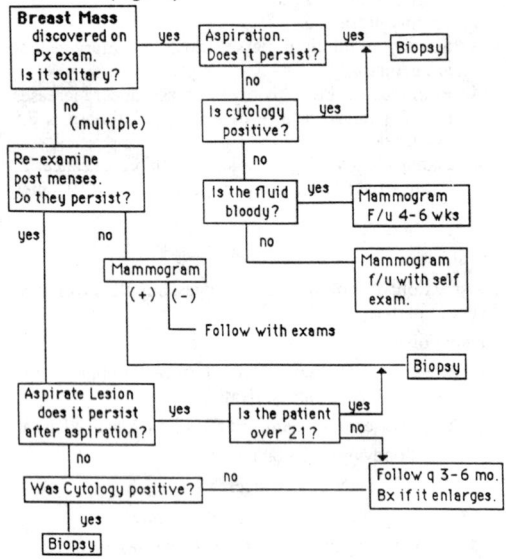

Fig 9-1. Breast Mass Management

References

Driscoll CE, *et al,* eds. Handbook of Family Practice. Chicago: Year Book Medical Publishers, 1986.

Nussbaum MS, ed. The Mont Reid Handbook. Chicago: Year Book Medical Publishers, 1987.

BURN INJURY

I. **Initial Assessment**

   A. Assess ABCs. Check for singed nares, cough, wheezes, hoarseness, facial burns, charred lips, carbonaceous secretions, or history of enclosed space fire. May need to intubate early as maximal edema occurs at 12 hours. Baseline ABGs and carbon monoxide level. CXR; may not show changes for 24-72 hours.

   B. Check fire history for chemicals that might have been inhaled and lead to pulmonary toxicity.

   C. Check for other injuries. EKG for electrical injuries.

   D. Fluid resuscitation for burns > 15-20% body surface area (BSA) in adults and > 10% BSA in small children. Estimate with Parkland formula % TBSA burn x weight (kg) x 4 cc/24 hours (one-half in first 8 hours, other half in next 16 hours). Do not use colloid in first 24 hours; use lactated ringers.

   E. NG tube for ileus if burn > 25%.

   F. Foley for fluid monitoring if significant burns.

   G. Pain medications.

   H. Cardiac monitoring for severe burns.

II. **Assessment of Burns**

   A. Surface area.

      1. Less than 10 y.o. use Lund-Bowdler chart.

      2. Greater than 10 years old: head and neck and each upper extremity are 9%, each lower extremity, anterior torso, and posterior torso are 18%, perineum 1%.

      3. Check with fluorescein for corneal burns.

   B. Depth.

      1. Superficial (first degree): epidermis only, painful and erythematous.

      2. Superficial partial thickness: epidermis and outer one half of dermis with sparing of hairs.

      3. Deep partial thickness: epidermis and destruction of reticular dermis. Can easily convert to full thickness

if secondary infection, mechanical trauma, or progressive thrombosis. (Partial thickness burns previously classified as second degree burns).

4. Full thickness: dry, pearly white, charred, leathery. Heals by epithelial migration from the periphery and by contracture. May involve adipose, fascia, muscle, or bone. (Full thickness burns previously classified as third degree burns).

C. Severity.

1. Minor: first degree and partial thickness < 15% BSA in adults and < 10% BSA in children < 6, full thickness < 2% BSA in adults.

2. Moderate: partial thickness 15% to 25% BSA in adults and 10-20% in children, full thickness burns < 10% BSA.

3. Major: (requires burn unit or burn center care) partial thickness burns > 20-25% BSA in adults and > 20% in children, full thickness burns > 10% BSA, burns of hands, face, eyes, ears, feet, perineum, inhalation burns, electrical burns, burns complicated by fracture or major trauma, all burns in infants or elderly, patients at poor risk secondary to prior medical conditions.

D. Cause of burn.

1. Thermal:

    a. Flame, especially with clothing, tends to be full thickness.

    b. Molten metal, tars, or melted synthetics lead to prolonged skin contact, should be cooled as rapidly as possible and should not be removed immediately after injury as this causes increased depth of injury. Tar may be softened with antibiotic ointments or cream.

    c. Liquid burns should be cooled rapidly and any clothing in contact with the area rapidly removed to decrease the contact time.

2. Electrical burns have a depressed, small, well-circumscribed entrance and an exit wound that may appear blown out. Underlying tissue necrosis can be very extensive.

3. Chemical agents:
    a. Strong acids are quickly neutralized or quickly absorbed. Large quantities may cause systemic acidosis. Use neutral solutions, not alkali to neutralize to minimize heat release of neutralization.
    b. Alkalis cause liquefaction necrosis and can penetrate deeply leading to progressive necrosis up to several hours post contact.
4. Radiation burns initially appear hyperemic and may later resemble third degree burns. Changes can extend deeply into the tissue. Sunburns are of this type and involve moderate superficial pain.

III. Treatment of Burns

A. Emergency room: cover wounds with cool normal saline soaked gauze for pain control until suitability for narcotics can be determined. Intravenous narcotics can help for initial wound care. Tetanus immunization status should be checked and the patient treated accordingly.

1. Clean with bland soap and water on 4 x 4s or a soft cloth.
2. Debride loose and foreign material. May leave blister intact if relatively small and patient is reliable for taking care of his wounds.
3. Rinse well with normal saline.
4. Wound dressing choices:
    a. Non-adherent inner layer of water soluble porous material followed by soft bulky absorbant gauze and covered with semi-elastic outer layer.
    b. Topical antibacterial agents such as 1% silver sulfadiazene, sulfamylon, or silver nitrate are applied, then covered with gauze pads. Dressings should be done daily with washing to remove old cream. Absolute contraindications to silver sulfadiazene: term pregnancy, premature infants, or less than 1 month old, hypersensitivity, G6PD deficiency. Relative: possible cross-sensitivity to other sulfonamides, pregnancy.

c. Heterograft, allograft or xerograft dressings can be used on an inpatient basis for partial thickness wounds. These should be examined daily and debrided as needed or removed if signs of infection develop.

5. Chemical burns should be washed with tap water at least 15 and preferably 30 minutes in duration, and should be started at the scene if possible. Alkali burns should be irrigated for one to two hours post injury. Chemical binding may be required for certain burns.

6. Tar burns need cooling, gentle cleaning, and application of a petrolatum base antibacterial ointment for 24 hours to help dissolve. After 24 hours the tar can be washed away and treated as a thermal burn.

7. Electrical burns should be cleaned as in thermal burns and mafenicle acetate applied as the topical antibacterial agent.

B. Follow up care.

1. Daily to twice daily dressing changes should be performed. Mild soap such as dish soaps can be used for cleaning. Necrotic debris and eschar may require debridement as healing occurs. Tub soaks can help loosen coagulum and speed separation of necrotic debris. Absolute sterility is not mandatory for dressing changes, however cleanliness and thorough cleaning of hands, sinks, tubs and any instruments used must be emphasized.

2. Contractures may not be apparent for weeks to months, therefore, range of motion exercises should be started during the early healing period. Any person with burns across joints should practice range of motion exercises frequently. If the hands are involved extensively, early excision and auto grafting may decrease the scarring of deep partial thickness and full thickness burns. Splinting and prolonged physical therapy may be required for rehabilitation. If the patient is prone to keloids, special garments may be used to reduce this scarring.

3. Pain medications may be necessary for sleep at night or for dressing changes. Codeine or hydrocodone is normally adequate after the initial ER visit. If the dose

is taken a half hour before the dressing change, it will facilitate cleaning and debridement.

4. All burns should be seen within 24 hours of initial treatment and if any signs of infection develop, cultures should be performed and hospitalization considered.

5. Prophylactic antibiotics should rarely be required but may be considered for immune compromised hosts, patients at high risk of endocarditis, or inpatients with artificial joints. Broad spectrum coverage with a first generation cephalosporin or with a penicillinase-resistant penicillin plus an aminoglycoside may be used if necessary.

6. In circumferential burns, extensive extremity burns, or electrical burns, watch for vascular or neurologic compromise indicating a developing compartment syndrome. Immediate escharotomy is then required. Extremities should be elevated to minimize swelling.

7. In extensive burns, nutritional support is extremely important. Metabolic rate may be increased 100-200% above normal. Electrolytes must be frequently checked to replace maintenance needs, loss through the burn wound, and loss secondary to elevated body temperature. Intravenous hyperalimentation may be required until the gastrointestinal tract is functioning.

References

Condon RE and Nyhus LM, eds. Manual of Surgical Therapeutics, 4th edition. Boston: Little, Brown & Company, 1978.

Emergency treatment of burn injury. Annals of Emergency Medicine 17(12):1305, December 1988.

Nussbaum MS, ed. The Mont Reid Handbook. Chicago: Year Book Medical Publishers, 1987.

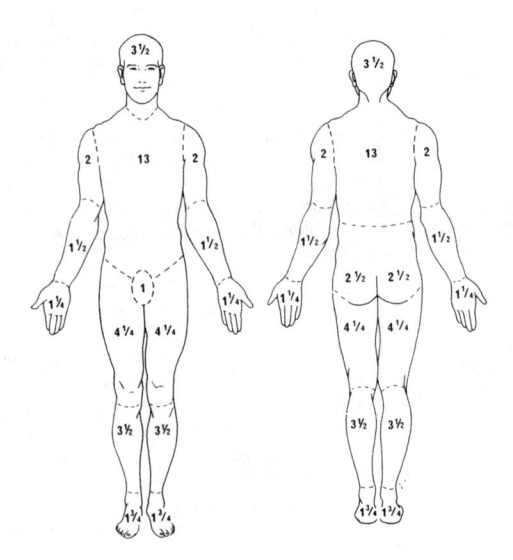

General Surgery

Age:	Birth-1	1-4	5-9	10-14	15	Adult	Partial thickness 2°	Full thickness 3°	Total
AREA									
Head	19	17	13	11	9	7			
Neck	2	2	2	2	2	2			
Anterior trunk	13	13	13	13	13	13			
Posterior trunk	13	13	13	13	13	13			
Right buttock	2½	2½	2½	2½	2½	2½			
Left buttock	2½	2½	2½	2½	2½	2½			
Genitalia	1	1	1	1	1	1			
Right upper arm	4	4	4	4	4	4			
Left upper arm	4	4	4	4	4	4			
Right lower arm	3	3	3	3	3	3			
Left lower arm	3	3	3	3	3	3			
Right hand	2½	2½	2½	2½	2½	2½			
Left hand	2½	2½	2½	2½	2½	2½			
Right thigh	5½	6½	8	8½	9	9½			
Left thigh	5½	6½	8	8½	9	9½			
Right leg	5	5	5½	6	6½	7			
Left leg	5	5	5½	6	6½	8			
Right foot	3½	3½	3½	3½	3½	3½			
Left foot	3½	3½	3½	3½	3½	3½			

Fig 9-1.

Adapted from Nussbaum MS, ed. The Mont Reid Handbook. Chicago: Year Book Medical Publishers, 1987.

10/ PEDIATRICS

Katherine M. Broman, M.D. and Eric Evans, M.D.

NEONATAL RESPIRATORY PROBLEMS

I. **Intrapartum Asphyxia**
   A. Cause: secondary to decreased transplacental gas exchange resulting in fetal hypoxia, acidosis.
   B. Signs: pallor, cyanosis, slow heart rate, apnea, flaccidity (low apgar score). Do not delay treatment to assess apgar.
   C. Treatment (see section on pediatric resuscitation):
      1. Apgar 8-10: no intervention needed.
      2. Apgar 5-7: stimulate infant by slapping feet or rubbing back, provide blow-by oxygen or place oxygen mask over baby's face.
      3. Apgar 3-4: if HR < 100 proceed with ventilations with bag-mask at 30 breaths/minute.
      4. Apgar 0-2: begin active ventilations and chest compressions if heart rate less than 60.

II. **Meconium Aspiration Syndrome**
   A. Overview: Occurs in 10% of cases with meconium stained amniotic (seen with fetal distress secondary to intrapartum asphyxia). The asphyxia may cause gasping in utero, but meconium usually doesn't go below cords until after birth.
   B. Diagnosis: meconium stained amniotic fluid and signs of asphyxia within 1-2 hours, peaks at 24-48 hours. X-ray will show patchy infiltrates.
   C. Treatment:
      1. When head on perineum (or at hysterotomy site), clear mouth, nares, and pharynx with De Lee suction or bulb suction.
      2. Hold finger in baby's mouth until pharynx cleared of meconium.
      3. Thin meconium: adequate suction on the perineum and after delivery are all that is usually required. Some

recommend laryngoscopy to visualize cords although it is not clear that thin meconium causes aspiration syndrome.
4. Thick meconium: visualize cords with laryngoscope. If meconium below cords, intubate and suction through ET tube.

III. Apnea

A. Definition: cessation of breathing for more than 15-20 seconds. Causes of apnea at birth differ from those associated with apnea later in the first few days of life.

B. Causes:
1. Apnea at birth: intrapartum asphyxiation, narcotics administered to mother during labor, congenital anomalies of the airway (choanal atresia, macroglossia, laryngeal atresia/cyst/web, diaphragmatic hernia).
2. Apnea later: prematurity, hypoglycemia, hypothermia, infection, CNS abnormality, gastroesophageal reflux.

C. Diagnosis: complete exam. Evaluation for sepsis, ABG, glucose.

C. Treatment: Resuscitate as needed. Determined by cause.

IV. Hyaline Membrane Disease

A. Overview: deficiency of surfactant with secondary generalized microatelectasis. Associated with prematurity (< 36 weeks), infants of diabetic mother, intrapartum asphyxia.

B. Diagnosis:
1. Clinical: tachypnea (rate > 50-60/min), intercostal retractions, grunting, nasal flaring, fine rales and decreased airflow per auscultation; disease peaks at 36-48 hours of age.
2. Lab: CXR shows "ground glass"; diffuse, fine reticulogranular infiltrates with air bronchograms. CBC, cultures to rule out sepsis, serial ABG's.

C. Treatment: monitor ABG.

1. If PaO_2 < 50 mmHg in 40% O_2, place UAC. May need ventilation if unable to maintain PaO_2 > 50 mmHg or if $PaCO_2$ > 55-60.
2. Maintain core temperature of 37 degrees.
3. Hydrate with $D_{10}W$ at 80-90 ml/kg/24 hours times 24 hours. Change to physiologic IV fluids after 24 hours.
4. Transfer to tertiary care nursery if necessary.

V. **Transient Tachypnea of the Newborn**

A. Overview: Self-limited tachypnea with no other or minimal signs of respiratory distress secondary to amniotic fluid aspiration. Occurs in term or near term infants, more frequent after C-section. Presents 2-4 hours after delivery; maximum severity within 24-48 hours.

B. Diagnosis:
1. Clinical: tachypnea (80-100/min), mild dyspnea evidenced by sternal retractions with coarse rales.
2. Lab: X-ray shows increase in perihilar markings, mild to moderate hyperinflation. Sepsis workup indicated if signs of respiratory distress, serial ABG's to adjust oxygenation if required.

C. Treatment: O_2 per hood as indicated. Rarely requires greater than 40%. If respiratory rate remains elevated, may require IV hydration. Many require no treatment other than observation.

References

Barken R and Rosen P, eds. Emergency Pediatrics, 2nd edition. St. Louis: C.V. Mosby, 1986.

Graef JW and Cone TZ, eds. Manual of Pediatric Therapeutics, 3rd edition. Boston: Little, Brown & Company, 1985.

Hen J. Current management of upper airway obstruction. Pediatric Annals 15(4):276, April 1986.

Wagener JS. Respiratory distress: exploring the causes in young children. Consultant, January 1986.

NEONATAL INFECTIONS

I. **Congenital: TORCHS**

   A. Evaluation: most infections asymptomatic. Consider screening if the following risk factors are present: known history of congenital infection, habitual abortion, infertility, contact with cats or mice, ingestion of raw meat, immunosuppressive therapy, rash, unexplained adenopathy, unexplained illness while pregnant, oral or genital lesion, occupational exposure (neonatal nurses, dialysis workers).

   B. Maternal diagnosis: Screen early for antibody to rubella and syphilis. Serology as indicated for HSV, CMV, HBV. Viral cultures for HSV, rubella, CMV, enterovirus. Vaginal cultures for gonorrhea, group B strep.

   C. Neonatal presentation:

   1. General: premature, intrauterine growth retardation, failure to thrive, hepatomegaly (elevated direct bilirubin), lethargy, thrombocytopenia, anemia, rashes, seizures.

   2. Toxoplasmosis: chorioretinitis, hydrocephalus, intracranial calcifications.

   3. Rubella: retinopathy, cataracts, patent ductus arteriosus, pulmonary artery stenosis, deafness, thrombocytopenia.

   4. Cytomegalovirus (CMV): microcephaly with periventricular calcifications, thrombocytopenia, hepatosplenomegaly.

   5. Herpes (HSV): skin vesicles, hepatitis, pneumonia, encephalitis, DIC.

   6. Syphilis: mucocutaneous lesion, osteochondritis, hepatomegaly, rash, persistent rhinitis, meningitis.

   7. AIDS: immunodeficiency. Sometimes dysmorphic features of microcephaly, hypertelorism, prominent boxlike forehead, flattened nasal bridge, triangular philtrum.

   D. Lab:

   1. TORCH screen, serum prior to transfusion, from baby and mother.

Neonatal Infections

2. IgM specific antibodies, acute and convalescent from baby and mother.
3. Viral cultures (HSV, rubella, CMV, enterovirus).
4. Tzanck prep smear from vesicles (infant and mother).
5. Urine cytology for CMV.
6. Placenta for histology.
7. Hepatitis B screen, HIV.
8. Liver enzymes, platelet count and clotting studies, RPR and FTA-ABS with titer.

E. Treatment and Prevention.
1. Toxoplasmosis: avoid cats and eating raw meat during pregnancy. Treatment depends upon severity as evidenced by rising titers, active disease. Antiprotozoal drugs.
2. Hepatitis A that develops near term: immune globulin 0.5 ml to infant.
3. Hepatitis B that develops during pregnancy: HBIG 0.5 ml at birth repeat at 3 and 6 months. Hep B vaccine starting at 3 months of age.
4. Rubella: prevented by adequate immunization of children and women of child bearing age, no treatment available.
5. CMV: no treatment available.
6. HSV: mothers with active genital lesions may require delivery by C-section. If primary HSV infections with positive cultures or vaginal delivery over active lesions or ROM > 4 hr, begin acyclovir (30 mg/kg/day IV divided tid) for 14 days. In the absence of genital lesions, obtain surface cultures of baby, observe 3-5 days before beginning treatment.
7. Syphilis: if mother has positive serology, obtain infant serology. If infant negative: no treatment. If infant positive: treat if symptomatic. If asymptomatic, treat if titer 3-4 times higher than mother's, FTA is 3-4 +, IgM greater than 20 mg/100ml. Procaine Pen G 50,000 units/kg IM q D x 10-14 days, or aqueous Pen G 50,000 units/kg/day q 12 hr IM x10-14 days.

II. Gonorrhea

A. Prevention: endocervical cultures during pregnancy at initial evaluation and at 36 weeks. Apply 1% silver nitrate or erythromycin to infant's eyes at birth.

B. Presentation: Ophthalmia presents within 3 days of birth. Other manifestations include rhinitis, anorectal infection, arthritis, sepsis, meningitis.

C. Mother with GC: obtain from infant gram stain, culture and sensitivities of eye, nasopharynx, ears, gastric, contents anorectum.

D. Treatment:

1. Asymptomatic: 1 dose 50,000 units aqueous Pen G IM and IV.

2. Symptomatic: 100,000 units/kg/day Pen G x10 days.

3. Ophthalmia: after silver nitrate or erythromycin, use saline irrigations and tetracycline or chloramphenicol eye drops. Many recommend systemic treatment also.

III. Neonatal Bacterial Sepsis

A. Etiology.

1. Predisposing factors include prolonged rupture of membranes (> 24 hours), premature labor, maternal fever, UTI, foul lochia, chorioamnionitis, IV catheters, intrapartum asphyxia, and intrauterine monitoring (pressure catheter or scalp electrode).

2. Organisms:

   a. Early infection: Group B strep, E. Coli, Klebsiella, Enterococcus, Listeria, Strep pneumonia, Group A strep, H influenzae.

   b. Late (> 5 days of age): Staph aureus, E. Coli, Klebsiella, Pseudomonas, Serratia, Staph epidermidis.

B. Presentation: may be subtle with irritability, vomiting, poor feeding, poor temperature control, lethargy. May progress to respiratory distress, poor perfusion, abdominal distention, jaundice, bleeding, petechiae.

C. Work-up: should include CBC (increased WBC, left shift, leukocytopenia, thrombocytopenia suggest infection), cultures of blood, urine and CSF. CXR. Latex agglutinations of blood, urine and CSF.

D. Treatment:
1. Begin antibiotics when sepsis suspected after cultures obtained.
2. Reevaluate therapy after 72 hour culture results available. If cultures positive, continue treatment for 7-10 days. If negative, continue antibiotics if patient demonstrated significant signs of sepsis. If patient did not demonstrate these signs and cultures are negative, may consider stopping antibiotics at three days and follow closely.

References

Barken and Rosen, eds. Emergency Pediatrics, 2nd edition. St. Louis: C.V. Mosby, 1986.

Graef JW and Cone TZ, eds. Manual of Pediatric Therapeutics, 3rd edition. Boston: Little, Brown & Company, 1985.

METABOLIC/HEMATOLOGIC DISORDERS OF THE NEWBORN

I. **Hypoglycemia**

   A. Defined as serum glucose < 30 mg/dl term, < 20 mg/dl premature.

   B. Cause:

   1. Decreased availability of glucose or inability to mobilize, IUGR, post dates, asphyxia, cold stress, sepsis, prematurity, polycythemia.

   2. Hypermetabolism, i.e. erythroblastosis.

   3. Hyperinsulinism in infant of diabetic mother.

   C. Diagnosis:

   1. Clinical: pale, cool, irritable, jittery, poor feeding, apnea, seizure, or no symptoms.

   2. Lab: low serum glucose.

   3. High index of suspicion in high risk infants.

   4. Most nurseries have a protocol in which they check serum glucose within 3-4 hours of birth.

   D. Treatment.

   1. Stable and 34 weeks gestation or more: 15-30 cc D5W po or enteral and advance to breast milk or formula. Serial serum glucose q 2-3 hours until 3 normals.

   2. Unstable or premature (less than 34 weeks): D10W at 100-150 ml/kg/24 hour IV. Advance to po feeds as tolerated, follow serial serum glucose levels.

   3. Symptomatic or serum glucose < 20 mg/dl: D10W 4 ml/kg IV over 5 min followed by constant infusion of D10 W 2-4 ml/kg/hr.

   4. Give glucagon 0.03 mg/kg/ IM if no immediate IV sites or no available IV glucose, then obtain IV access. (Glucagon is not effective if insufficient stores of glucogen are not present, as in IUGR or premature).

II. **Hypocalcemia**

   A. Overview: serum calcium < 7 mg/dl associated with asphyxia, prematurity, or infant of diabetic mother. Usually transient.

Metabolic/Hematologic Disorders of the Newborn 435

B. Diagnosis: jitters, irritable, seizures, low serum calcium, EKG--prolonged QT.

C. Treatment:
   1. Acute: calcium gluconate 100 mg (1 ml/kg of 10% solution) IV slowly.
   2. Maintenance: calcium gluconate 200-300 mg/kg/24 hour q 6-8 hr IV or po until on full feedings.
   3. If persistent, consider low magnesium or endocrine disorder.

III. **Neonatal Narcotic Withdrawal**

   A. Overview: passive addiction via maternal use.
   B. Diagnosis: jittery, irritable, large appetite, vomiting, sneezing, hypertonicity.
   C. Treatment: chlorpromazine 0.5 mg/kg/dose q 6-8 hr IV, IM, or po or phenobarbital 5 mg/kg/24 hour q 8-12 hr IV, IM, or po, gradually taper over 1-3 weeks, watch for apnea and bradycardia.

IV. **Polycythemia**

   A. Overview: defined as venous Hct > 65%. Associated with increased viscosity. Increased incidence with IUGR, Down's syndrome, infants of diabetic mothers. Etiology: increase in fetal rbc due to chronic in utero hypoxemia but normal blood volume, or increase in blood volume (cord milking at delivery, twin to twin transfusion).

   B. Diagnosis:
      1. Clinical: plethora, respiratory distress, hypoglycemia, irritable. May develop complications such as CHF, oliguria, cyanosis, gangrene, necrotizing enterocolitis.
      2. Lab: peripheral Hct > 65%, capillary Hct is usually 4%-7% higher than peripheral or central HcT.

   C. Treatment:
      1. Hct 65-70%: observe if asymptomatic. If symptomatic, partial exchange transfusion via umbili

cal vein, use FFP or 5% albumin in saline, volume of exchange

$$= \frac{[80 \times weight\ (kg)] \times (measured\ HCT - desired\ HCT)}{measured\ HCT}$$

2. Hct > 70%: partial exchange, monitor for complications.

V. Thrombocytopenia

A. Overview: may be a nonspecific sign of sepsis, hypoxia, prematurity, or DIC. Associated with Down's syndrome. Higher incidence with maternal factors of toxemia, ITP, platelet group incompatibility.

B. Diagnosis: laboratory (platelets < 50,000).

C. Treatment: treat underlying cause. Platelet transfusion indicated for:

1. platelets < 50,000 with bleeding.
2. platelets less than 30,000. Dose is 10 ml/kg/dose over 1-2 hour. Half-life 2-4 days, aim for platelet level between 50,000-100,000.

VI. DIC

A. Initiating factors in neonate:

1. Maternal: acute hemorrhage, dead fetal twin, amniotic fluid embolism.
2. Neonate: hypoxemia, sepsis, erythroblastosis, necrotizing enterocolitis, severe hyaline membrane disease.

B. Diagnosis: petechiae, purpura, underlying disease.

C. Treatment:

1. Treat underlying disease.
2. Transfuse FFP 10 ml/kg over 1-2 hr.
3. Transfuse platelets if platelet count < 30,000.
4. Vitamin K 1 mg IV.
5. If coagulopathy continues:
    a. Two volume (80-90 ml/kg) exchange transfusion with heparinized or CPD blood < 72 hours old via umbilical vein or packed RBC reconstituted in FFP in 5-10 ml increments to 50% Hct.

b. Consider heparin infusion of 100 units/kg/dose q 4 hr IV.

VII. Neonatal Jaundice

A. Non-Physiologic Jaundice-suggested by:
1. Clinical jaundice at less than 24 hours age.
2. Total bilirubin increasing by more than 5 mg/100ml in 24 hours.
3. Total bilirubin exceeding 12.9 mg/100 ml in full-term infant or 15 mg/100 ml in premature infant.
4. Direct bilirubin concentration exceeding 1.5-2 mg/100 ml.
5. Clinical jaundice persisting for more than 1 week in full-term infant or 2 weeks in premature infant.
6. Note: breast fed infants often present with physiologic jaundice between 5-10 days.

B. Evaluation of Pathologic Jaundice.
1. Serum bilirubin concentration, direct and total. If elevated:
2. Peripheral blood smear for red cell morphology and reticulocyte count. Blood type and Rh (on mother and infant), and direct Coombs test on infant as well as hematocrit or hemoglobin.

D. Treatment:
1. Adequate hydration may be all that is necessary if physiologic.
2. Treat underlying disorder if not physiologic.
3. Phototherapy for indirect bilirubin levels of:
   a. Baby < 2000 gm: 5x birth weight (in kg) = bilirubin level at which phototherapy necessary.
   b. 2000 gm: bilirubin 12-14--watch trend. If less than 1 wk old, bilirubin > 14--phototherapy.
4. Exchange transfusion indicated for:
   a. Term infant with bilirubin > 20 mg/dl.
   b. Premature with bilirubin > 10-15 mg/dl.
   c. Bilirubin > 10 mg/dl in first 24 hours of life.

E. Complications: Kernicterus. Exact level of bilirubin at which this occurs is not predictable; dependent upon multiple factors in addition to bilirubin level.

References

Graef JW and Cone TZ, eds. Manual of Pediatric Therapeutics, 3rd edition. Boston: Little, Brown & Company, 1985.

Maisels MJ. Jaundice in the newborn. Pediatrics in Review 3(10):305, April 1982.

FEVER

I. **Overview:**
   A. Definition: Oral temp > 37.8°C (100.0 F) or rectal temp > 38°C (100.4°F) for > 60 minutes.
   B. Keys.
      1. Must search for focus of infection causing fever. Attempts to reduce fever should not interfere with evaluation.
      2. Fevers need not be treated; some evidence to indicated slight fever helps fight infection. Unless > 41.1°C, fever does no specific harm to patient.
      3. Height of temperature elevation does not necessarily correlate with severity of cause.
      4. In neonates, hypothermia is as concerning as elevated temperature.
   C. Bacterial infections.
      1. Fevers in < 3 months old, likely organisms: gram negative bacteria, Group B beta-hemolytic strep.
      2. Fevers in 3 months - 24 months old, likely serious organisms: Strep pneumoniae, H. influenzae.
      3. Possible foci of infection: pneumonia, otitis media, UTI, septic arthritis, meningitis, bacteremia.

II. **Evaluation**
   A. History: (may be obtained by phone)
      1. Indications for immediate evaluation:
      - < 3 months old.
      - lethargy.
      - length of fever greater than 3 days.
      - fever of 105° F or greater.
      - stiff neck.
      - possible respiratory distress.
      - suggestion of dehydration (decreased urine output, significant vomiting or diarrhea).
      - limping, suggesting hip or knee pain.
      2. Other history: associated symptoms (cough, nasal congestion, foul smelling urine or new incontinence),

recent immunizations and immunization status, medications.

B. Exam:
1. Vitals, including temperature (rectal or tympanic usually more accurate), respirations and heart rate.
2. General appearance: level of activity/lethargy, weak cry, use of accessory muscles with respirations.
3. General exam focusing on areas of particular concern: upper respiratory tract including ears, lower respiratory tract, meningeal signs, extremities for evidence of arthritis.

C. Lab:
1. For child that appears seriously ill: plan admit, obtain CBC with differential, urine for analysis/culture and latex agglutinations (available for Group B strep, pneumococcus, Hemophilus, E.coli, meningococcus as indicated), CSF, CXR. Start empiric treatment for most common organisms in that age group or as indicated by physical/lab findings.
2. For child that does not appear seriously ill: consider obtaining CBC with differential. If no obvious source and WBC is > 15,000, or if temperature > 39.5°C, obtain blood cultures.

III. Treatment:

A. General principles.
1. ABC's if compromised.
2. Adequately hydrate patients (IV if po inadequate).
3. Dress appropriately for fever.
4. Antipyretics: acetaminophen, not aspirin, 10-15 mg/kg/dose, q4 hours.
5. Sponge bath with tepid water (not ice water or alcohol--do not want to induce shivering) after antipyretic given.

B. Antibiotics:
1. As indicated for identified source; otitis, pharyngitis.
2. If pneumonia suspected, admit for IV antibiotics if any evidence of respiratory distress. If child well-

hydrated and not in distress, may treat as outpatient with appropriate antibiotic. Follow-up in 24 hours.

3. If meningitis suspected, start appropriate parenteral antibiotics immediately (before CSF results if suspected on clinical grounds). Also consider use of steroids to reduce risk of sequelae.

4. If no source identified and child appears moderately ill, obtain blood cultures. May discharge to home if adequate hydration and reliable parents. Consider starting antibiotic empirically. Recheck in 24 hours (when preliminary culture results available).

References

Schmitt BD, ed. Pediatric Telephone Advice, 1st edition. Boston: Little, Brown & Company, 1980.

Soman M. Diagnostic workup of febrile children under 24 months of age: a clinical review. The Western Journal of Medicine 137(1) July 1982.

VOMITING/DIARRHEA

I. Overview

A. Either of these processes may be seen with most minor illness, including viral URIs, otitis, and pharyngitis. May also be seen in infants and toddlers after coughing ("post-tussive emesis"). In these situations, they do not tend to be most prominent symptom. In the setting of gastroenteritis, the child will frequently be otherwise well and vomiting and/or diarrhea is the only symptom.

B. Evaluation:
1. History: essential to obtain an estimate of the amount of fluid loss that is occurring, amount of intake, and urine output. Associated symptoms, especially fever (which increases fluid loss), should be sought.
2. Exam: in addition to evaluating for focus of infection, hydration status should be estimated. If fluid loss has been gradual, the following estimates are relatively accurate.
   a. dry mouth: about 5% volume depletion.
   b. decreased urine/tears, slightly decreased skin turgor: about 10%.
   c. sunken eyes, tenting of the skin: about 15%.
   d. thready pulses, mottling, significant oliguria or anuria: about 20%.
3. Lab: specific tests may be indicated by history and physical. If there is possible dehydration, urine specific gravity may be helpful in older children but electrolytes with BUN and Cr will be required in younger children.

C. Disposition:
1. Children age 1 or above should be admitted for severe dehydration (15-20%). For moderate dehydration (10%), may consider outpatient therapy with recheck in 24 hours. (This may include IV hydration in the emergency room or office). Mild dehydration (5%) can generally be treated as outpatient if serious infection is not present.

2. For infants (< 1 year), moderate and severe dehydration require admission for IV hydration. Mild dehydration may be treated as outpatient if adequate and prompt follow-up is assured.

II. **Vomiting**

   A. Evaluation:
   1. History: inquire as to frequency, volume, character (projectile), presence of blood, mucous or bile, dry heaves, and any attempts at treatment (medications, dietary modifications, etc.). With infants, need also determine how much is being fed (possible over-feeding), relation to position (possible reflux), choking or coughing with feeding (achalasia or T-E fistula).
   2. Exam: evaluate state of hydration. Careful attention to general exam searching for site of infection. Abdominal exam to rule out obstruction (pyloric stenosis, volvulus, intussusception).

   B. Treatment:
   1. Any associated infections should be treated accordingly. If exam suggests obstruction, surgeon should be consulted immediately.
   2. Dietary modifications are most important intervention. Patient should remain npo after vomiting for perhaps 2-8 hours (depending upon age). Then small amounts of clear liquids, preferably with some electrolytes present (such as ginger-ale, flat soda pops, Kool-Aid, jello water), are presented in gradually increasing amounts. Typical regimen would be:
   - two teaspoons (10 cc) every 10 minutes x 4, then if tolerated.
   - four teaspoons (20 cc) every 20 minutes x 4, then if tolerated.
   - three tablespoons (45 cc) every 40 minutes x 4, etc.
   - if vomiting occurs, begin again with period of npo.
   - once child is at usual level of intake, return to light diet x 24 hours, then to normal diet.
   3. Medications may be used for intractable vomiting:

- promethazine (Phenergan) available IM/IV or rectal suppository. Dose is 0.5 mg per pound, not to exceed 25 mg. May be repeated every 4 to 6 hours.

III. Diarrhea

A. Evaluation:
1. History: approximate volume and frequency of stools, character of stools including presence of blood, mucous. Associated symptoms of vomiting, fever, cough, etc.
2. Exam: estimate state of hydration, evaluate for other infectious processes.
3. Lab: as above for evaluating dehydration. Presence of blood in stools is indication for stool culture for enteric pathogens. Prolonged diarrhea is also indication for stool culture and stool for ova and parasites.

B. Treatment:
1. Diarrhea in the absence of vomiting is treated with large amounts of clear liquids given infrequently (to reduce the frequency of the gastrocolic reflex). Clear liquids should be used until diarrhea is resolving (24-48 hours), then BRAT diet may added (bananas, rice, apple sauce, toast). Regular diet may be resumed after 24-48 hours. If watery diarrhea occurs after reintroduction of milk, suspect secondary lactase deficiency and withhold lactose containing products for about 2 weeks (soy formulas may be used). Please see treatment of acute diarrhea (Chapter 4) for recommendations on use of anti-peristaltics.
2. Diarrhea with vomiting is treated as above for vomiting.

FEBRILE SEIZURES

I. **Overview:** Occur in age group 3 months to 5 years, average age 23 months. May be simple (nonfocal, less than 15 minutes) or complex (focal features, longer than 15 minutes, more than one in 24 hours). Usually are generalized with tonic and/or clonic features. 40% are less than 5 minutes, 75% are less than 20 minutes. 30-40% will have second febrile seizure within one year of the first. Temperature is usually $>39°C$ and commonly results from viral illnesses, otitis, and pharyngitis (which may be strep).

II. **Evaluation**
   A. History: carefully elicit details regarding duration, warning signs, number of seizures, post-ictal state, neurological development, previous personal or family history of seizures.
   B. Exam: thorough physical examination indicated to determine cause of fever and to evaluate neurologically. Mental status, evidence of focal neurological deficit, meningeal signs, anterior fontanelle should be evaluated.
   C. Lab:
      1. Lumbar puncture: definitely indicated if meningitis or sepsis suspected. Some recommend LP on all children with febrile seizures, others suggest necessary only if CNS infection suspected, seizure is complex (focal features, multiple, >15 minutes length), or if neurological exam is abnormal.
      2. CBC.
      3. Chemistries: glucose, lytes, BUN, calcium. These are generally not helpful in simple, classic febrile seizure, but required for prolonged seizure, especially if not responding to treatment. Bedside glucose determination should be done in this setting.
      4. UA as indicated for evaluation of fever.
      5. X-ray: head CT indicated for focal neurological signs.
      6. EEG: not recommended for simple febrile seizures.

III. **Treatment**
   A. Emergent:
      1. Diazepam, phenobarbital, and phenytoin may be used for status.
      2. Fever reduction and treatment of infection as indicated are the only treatment recommended for simple febrile seizures. Phenobarbital is not useful in preventing further seizures with the current febrile illness as therapeutic levels will not be attained for several days.
   B. Chronic:
      1. Phenobarbital, valproic acid may be used if the seizure is complex, the child has underlying abnormal neurological development or history of nonfebrile seizures, or if multiple seizures occur or child is < 1 yr old. Should be continued for 2 years or until child is 4 to 5 years old and then tapered over 2-3 months.

Reference

Kempe CH, Silver HK, and O'Brien D, eds. Current Pediatric Diagnosis & Treatment, 6th edition. Los Altos: Lange Medical Publishers, 1980.

PEDIATRIC MENINGITIS

I. **Presentation**
   A. Younger children have nonspecific signs including temperature instability, bulging fontanelle, irritability, nausea, vomiting, poor feeding, seizures, petechiae, respiratory distress. It is often difficult to distinguish a febrile seizure from a seizure secondary to meningitis in younger children.
   B. Older children may have above symptoms as well as nuchal rigidity, Kernig's sign (extension of legs causes pain), Brudzinski's sign (flexion of neck causes flexion of hips and knees), headaches. They often have otitis media.
   C. Past medical history may involve pneumonia, otitis media, sinusitis, trauma, prior surgery.
   D. VP or other shunt patients present with low grade symptoms including headache, nausea, low grade fever, malaise. 24% of these patients have infections associated with shunt alteration.

II. **Etiology**: related to age
   A. Bacterial.
      1. < 2 months: usually E.Coli or group B strep. May also see Listeria, H. flu, N. Meningitidis, S. pneumoniae.
      2. 2 months to 9 years: H. flu, N. Meningitidis, S. pneumoniae.
      3. 9 years: N. meningitidis, S. pneumoniae. Meningococcus peaks between 6 months and 2 years and again in young adults. 40% of patients are partially treated at time of diagnosis, usually with a penicillin, which affects gram stain and culture results. Thus latex agglutination can be quite helpful in diagnosis.
      4. VP shunts: often Staph epidermidis.
   D. Viral: enteroviral most common.
   C. Fungal and Mycobacterium tuberculosis: consider if endemic; rare.

III. **Complications**: Cerebral edema, septic chock and DIC (especially with N. Meningitidis) bacteremia with seeding of joints and myocardium, SIADH, subdural effusions, persistent fever (most patients afebrile by sixth day). Neurologic sequelae include cranial nerve deficits, hearing or vision deficits, mental retardation, learning disorders.

IV. **Evaluation:**
   A. Exam: physical findings as indicated above.
   B. Lab: lumbar puncture essential if meningitis suspected. Cell count, gram stain, cultures, chemistries should be obtained. In addition, latex agglutination for H. influenzae, S. pneumoniae, group B-strep, E. coli, N. meningitidis can be done on blood, urine, and CSF and can provide rapid identification of the organism involved. CBC with differential, electrolytes, serum glucose (to compare with CSF), and CXR. If focal neurological signs, obtain CT scan.

V. **Management**
   A. Stabilization: IV access, assessment of vital signs for hypoxia, dehydration, increased intracranial pressure, acidosis, DIC, electrolyte abnormalities.
   B. Bacterial: tailor antibiotics to result of gram stain, age, immunologic status, and then to result of C&S when available. Duration of therapy is 10 days for H. flu, S. pneumoniae; 14-21 days for group B strep and for gram negative enteric bacilli. Recent studies have suggested that use of steroids with antibiotics may reduce incidence of neurologic sequelae. Initial antibiotic:
      1. Less than 2 months of age: ampicillin 200 mg/kg/24 hours divided q 6 hours, and third generation cephalosporin 200 mg/kg/24 hour divided q 8-12 hours.
      2. 2 months to 9 years of age: cefuroxime or third generation cephalosporin 200 mg/kg/24 hours divided q 6-12 hours, or ampicillin 300 mg/kg/24 hours divided q 4-6 hours plus chloramphenicol 100 mg/kg/24 hours divided q 6 hours.
      3. Older than 9 years: PCN-G 250,000 units/kg/24 hours divided q 4 hours.

C. Viral: Supportive therapy, if any question about viral vs. bacterial, start antibiotics and await culture results. Hospitalize to ensure fluid intake, pain management, and monitor for worsening of condition. Monitor closely in following months for evidence of neurological sequelae.

D. Prophylaxis:
   1. N. meningitidis: prophylaxis indicated for intimate contacts of patient, including household members. Rifampin 10mg/kg (not to exceed 600 mg) po q 12 hours x 4 doses.
   2. H. influenzae: prophylaxis indicated for household contacts. All members should receive prophylaxis if there is a child less than 4 years of age in the household. Rifampin 10 mg/kg (not to exceed 600 mg) po q 12 hours x 8 doses.

Reference

Barkin R and Rosen P, eds. Emergency Pediatrics, 2nd edition. St. Louis: C.V. Mosby Co., 1986.

STRIDOR AND DYSPNEA IN THE YOUNG CHILD

I. **Epiglottitis**

   A. Etiology: infection of the epiglottis, most frequently by Hemophilus influenzae, type B.

   B. Clinical presentation: (see table 10-1) acute onset, low pitched inspiratory and expiratory stridor which sounds like a snore, frequently febrile, drooling, hoarseness. Generally do not cough.

   Table 10-1. Differential Diagnosis of Epiglottitis and Croup

Characteristic	Epiglottitis	Croup
Peak age	4 yr	12-24 mo
Onset	Rapid	Gradual
Posture	Sitting	Supine
Drooling	Yes	No
Fever	High	Low grade
Cough	Wet or absent	Barking
Voice	Muffled	Hoarse
Airway film	Enlarged epiglottis	Narrowed subglottic airway
Cause	Bacterial	Viral

   Adapted from Battaglia J. Severe croup/epiglottitis. Pediatrics in Review 7(8):227, Feb. 1986.

   C. Lab: (clinical presentation is all that is required to institute appropriate therapy). CBC with diff, blood and epiglottis cultures.(Invasive diagnostic tests that might distress the child should not be done until adequate airway is assured.) Soft tissue lateral neck x-ray will show characteristic enlargement of the epiglottis (thumb sign).

   D. Therapy:
   1. Airway: Endotracheal intubation is treatment of choice. Generally required for 12-24 hours. Attempts at visualizing epiglottis should be made in OR with preparations made for immediate intubation and surgical airway.

2. Antibiotic: cefuroxime or third generation cephalosporin. Chloramphenicol is second choice, 20-25 mg/kg q 6 hours.
3. Observation in ICU, with equipment at the bedside for intubation/tracheostomy if patient is not intubated. Humidified air and suctioning required.

II. **Laryngotracheobronchitis** (Croup)
   A. Etiology: viral (Parainfluenza), very common.
   B. Clinical presentation: gradual onset of cough, coryza 24-48 hours prior to stridor, mild fever, barking cough, high pitched stridor.
      1. Very mild: intermittent stridor, present when awake or excited, goes away when sleeping.
      2. Mild: continuous stridor when awake or asleep.
      3. Moderate: continuous stridor with sternal retractions; 5-10% will progress to upper airway obstruction.
      4. Severe: continuous stridor with evidence of respiratory failure; cyanosis, altered mental status.
   C. Lab: CBC with diff will usually be consistent with viral infection. Soft tissue AP of the neck will show subglottic narrowing (steeple sign).
   D. Therapy (often when riding into hospital cool air will improve symptoms and child is better on arrival):
      1. Humidified air.
      2. O_2 if evidence of respiratory distress.
      3. For moderate to severe disease, airway may be required urgently.
      4. Racemic epinephrine (nebulized) is often helpful but requires admission due to rebound effect.
      5. Corticosteroids (dexamethasone) may improve course and severity but don't exceed 1-2 doses IM. Usually reserved for patients with high risk of airway obstruction.

III. **Bacterial Tracheitis** (Atypical croup)
   A. Clinical presentation: history of croup, starting to improve but at 2-3 days condition worsens. High tempera-

ture, brassy cough, increased WBC with left shift. Trachea colonized with Staph aureus; secondary local infection.

B. Treatment: anti-staph antibiotics. May need intubation to remove thick secretions.

IV. Foreign Body Aspiration

A. Overview: Most frequent cause of death in children less than 1 year old. Usually death occurs immediately after aspiration, but it can occur 1-2 weeks out.

B. Clinical presentation: sudden onset of cough and stridor. If lodged in upper airway, may not be able to swallow or talk. If in lower airway, cough and wheeze.

C. Course: may have asymptomatic interval for lower airway foreign body. Late respiratory signs: pneumonia, abscess, bronchiectasis.

D. Treatment:
   1. If able to talk and breathe: removal by bronchoscopy by experienced individual.
   2. If unable to breathe:
      a. Immediate direct laryngoscopy for removal with Magill forceps (if equipment at hand).
      b. Heimlich maneuver. Repeat as necessary. Can scan mouth for object but do not probe blindly. Mouth to mouth resuscitation can convert total obstruction to partial.
      c. Cricothyrotomy may be only recourse if the above measures fail.

CHILDHOOD EXANTHEMS

I. **Chickenpox** (Varicella)
   A. Epidemiology: Causative agent is varicella-zoster virus. Age range is 2 to 8 years. Atypical presentation in very young children (less than 6 months) with higher incidence of complications. May occur year round but most commonly in late autumn, winter and spring. Highly contagious (attack rate near 95%). Period of contagiousness from 24 hours prior to eruption of rash until all lesions have crusted. Incubation is 14 days.
   B. Clinical Manifestations:
      1. Prodromal stage characterized by one day of fever, headache, malaise. May occur simultaneously with rash. Exanthem relatively profuse on trunk, sparse distally. First case in household tends to be least severe. Also, children with fair skin or recently damaged skin (burns, sunburn) will have more severe rash.
      2. Rash characterized by rapid progression from macule to papule to vesicle (6 to 8 hours). Typical vesicle is 2 to 3 mm "dew drop" on erythematous base. Drying of the vesicle begins centrally, producing an umbilicated appearance. Lesions appear in crops every few hours so that they are present in all stages simultaneously. Highly pruritic. Typical course is 5 to 10 days until all lesions have crusted.
   C. Treatment: symptomatic with antihistamines for itch, topical drying agents. Protect lesions from scratching (clip nails short, have child wear mittens if necessary) to lessen chance of secondary bacterial infection. There is an association with Reye's syndrome. Warn parents that if child develops vomiting, or lethargy towards the end of the illness, they should contact physician. No aspirin products should be used.

II. **Measles** (Rubeola)
   A. Epidemiology: Causative agent is a paramyxovirus. Age range is 2 to 14 years. Highly contagious, spread by direct contact with respiratory droplets. Occurs more frequently in winter months. Incubation is 10-14 days.

B. Clinical Manifestations.
1. Prodromal phase characterized by coryza, cough, conjunctivitis. Koplik's spots (small white spots on erythematous base) appear about 2 days after onset of prodrome. Begin in buccal mucosa, may spread. Rash appears 1-2 days after Koplik's spots. High fever is common.
2. Rash occurs 3-5 days after onset of prodrome, beginning on the face and about the ears. Over 24-48 hours spreads to rest of body. Erythematous, blotchy macular eruption that becomes maculopapular.
3. Potential complications include pneumonia, encephalitis and subacute sclerosing panencephalitis.

C. Treatment is symptomatic with acetaminophen for fever, antihistamines if needed for pruritus. Immunization is very effective.

III. **Rubella** (German Measles)

A. Epidemiology: Causative agent is rubella virus. Less contagious than chickenpox or measles. Probably spread by respiratory droplet. Period of contagiousness is from 1 week before the eruption to 1 week after its disappearance. Incubation period is 12-21 days. Highest incidence in the spring. Greatest concern is infection of women during early months of pregnancy which may result in stillbirth, miscarriage, or congenital defects.

B. Clinical Manifestation:
1. Prodromal phase is relatively mild and children may have none. Malaise, fever, and lymphadenopathy (including posterior cervical and occipital) may occur.
2. Rash consists of fine, faint, discrete macules appearing first on the face and spreading rapidly over trunk and extremities. Lasts 3-5 days.

C. Treatment: symptomatic, usually requires none. Rubella vaccine is effective and encouraged as the best means of preventing congenital rubella.

IV. Erythema Infectiosum (Fifth disease)

A. Epidemiology: Causative agent is human parvovirus. Commonly affects children and young adults, usually during spring months. Incubation is 7-14 days.

B. Clinical manifestations: Generally there is no prodrome. Rash is often first sign of the illness and may have associated malaise, fever. Confluent erythema of the face with circumoral pallor produces the "slapped cheek" appearance. 24 hours after rash erupts on face, a maculopapular rash appears on trunk and extremities with a reticular or "lacy" appearance. Lasts about one week. For several weeks afterwards the rash may flare with irritation of the skin from sun, heat, exercise. In adults, arthralgias or arthritis may accompany the illness and occasionally will persist for months.

C. Treatment: symptomatic.

V. Roseola Infantum

A. Epidemiology: causative agent believed to be human herpes virus 6. Incubation period is about 2 weeks. Affects infants and young children, age 3 months to about 3 years.

B. Clinical manifestations: Acute febrile illness with fever not uncommonly as high as 39.5 to 40.5° C. No other localizing signs are usually present. Laboratory investigation may reveal an initial leukocytosis (mostly lymphocytes) while later in the disease leukopenia may occur with relative lymphocytosis. Rash appears when abrupt defervesence occurs at about 3-4 days into the illness and is faintly erythematous, macular, and most prominent on trunk. Lasts from a few hours to 3 days.

C. Treatment: acetaminophen and fluids for fever.

VI. Scarlet Fever

A. Epidemiology: Causative agent is Group A beta-hemolytic strep that elaborates erythrogenic toxin. Epidemiology is the same as for strep pharyngitis.

B. Clinical Manifestation:

1. Prodromal phase is characterized by 12-48 hours of malaise, fever, sore throat.

2. Rash is characterized by a diffuse pink to red flush that blanches with pressure and has sand paper texture. Circumoral pallor, "strawberry tongue" and Pastia's lines (dark lines in skin creases) are also present. Rash may desquamate.

C. Treatment: penicillin or erythromycin as for any strep pharyngitis.

Reference

Kempe CH, Silver HK, and O'Brien D, eds. <u>Current Pediatric Diagnosis & Treatment, 6th edition</u>. Los Altos: Lange Medical Publishers, 1980.

BREAST FEEDING

I. Overview

A. Breast feeding is of proven nutritional value and emotional benefit (mother-child bonding). It is to be encouraged for all full term infants and most premature infants. (Protein content of breast milk may be inadequate for adequate growth of premature infants - premies who do not grow on breast milk may require protein supplementation).

B. Breast feeding should be encouraged and discussed during prenatal visits. Prenatal preparation of breasts ("toughening") by exposure to air, manipulation, application of emollients may help prevent later cracking and soreness.

C. Neonate should be allowed to breast feed as soon after delivery as possible. "Rooming in" to avoid separation of infant and mother is also helpful.

D. Infants should breast feed on demand rather than by a set schedule.

E. Breast milk is adequate source of nutrition for first 6-9 months of life assuming adequate volume of intake can by maintained. To assess adequacy of breast feeding, watch growth carefully - neonates should gain 1/2 ounce/day average over first 2 weeks of life if successfully breast feeding. Approximately 1 oz /day after 2 weeks. Schedule a 2 week visit to check for first-time breast feeding mothers and infants.

F. Expect up to a 10% loss in birth weight before weight gain commences.

G. Breast feeding can by supplemented by formula feeding.

H. Breast-fed infants pass colorless urine and soft, yellow, seedy stools after most feedings. Constipation with hard, dry stools is not observed in healthy, adequately breast fed infants.

I. Solid foods do not need to be introduced before 5-6 months of age. When introduced, solid foods should be offered after the baby has breast fed.

J. Breast feeding is not a reliable means of birth control!

K. Typical routine is 10 minutes on one breast and as long as infant desires to feed on second. Frequent short feedings are most effective for initiating breast feeding as nipple soreness is less likely and the more frequent stimulation will speed milk production. Begin each feeding on different side. Burp baby after each breast.

II. Nutritional Concerns

A. Failure to thrive in the breast fed infant.
   1. Infant causes:
      a. Inadequate intake because of poor suck, infrequent feeding or structural abnormality.
      b. Low net intake because of vomiting/diarrhea, malabsorption, or infection.
      c. Increased caloric need because of prematurity or small for gestational age, CHF.
   2. Maternal Causes
      a. Poor production because of inadequate diet (especially fluids), illness, fatigue.
      b. Poor let-down because of smoking, drugs, or psychological.
B. Iron stores: Necessity of iron supplementation in healthy full-term breast-fed infant is controversial. 10 mg/day is suggested. Premature infants outgrow iron stores more rapidly and will require supplementation, 2 mg/kd/day starting at age 8 weeks.
C. Fluoride: does not cross placenta and concentration in human milk is low. Exclusively breast-fed infants require fluoride supplementation; 0.25 mg/day for < 2 years; 0.5 mg/day for age 2-3. Supplementation may be discontinued when fluoride-supplemented tap water is used for preparing infant formula.
D. Vitamin D: 400 IU/day recommended until formula or vitamin-fortified cow's milk replaces breast feeding.

Reference

Neifert MR and Seacat JM. A guide to successful breast feeding. Contemporary Pediatrics 3:26, July 1986.

FAILURE TO THRIVE

I. Differential Diagnosis of Failure to Thrive

A. Inadequate intake:
- economic deprivation
- social deprivation.
- mechanical feeding problems.

B. Increased caloric requirements:
- chronic infection.
- malignancy.
- hyperthyroidism.

C. Failure to absorb calories:
- cystic fibrosis.
- celiac disease.
- milk allergy.
- parasites.

D. Failure to utilize nutrients:
- renal acidosis.
- hypercalcemia.
- renal or hepatic insufficiency.
- diabetes.
- other metabolic disorders.

II. General Groups

1. Normal head circumference, with weight reduced out of proportion to height. This is the most common type and represents inadequate caloric intake, malabsorption, or impaired utilization of nutrients.

2. The head circumference is normal or slightly large for age and weight is only moderately reduced, usually in proportion to height. This group generally suffers from structural dystrophies, dwarfism, or endocrine disease.

3. Normal or subnormal head circumference with weight reduced in proportion to height, due to CNS deficit.

4. Physical signs of neglect suggest malnutrition is the cause of the failure to thrive. These signs include:

dirty nails, diaper rash, skin infections, flat occiput and "bald spot".

III. Evaluation

A. History: Focus on diet history and parent-child interaction.

B. Physical exam for evidence of underlying disease process, including Denver Developmental Screening Test.

C. Initial labs: CBC, UA, electrolytes, BUN, stool for pH, ova and parasites, guaiac, and reducing substances.

D. Calculate the required fluid and caloric intake.

E. If the physical and laboratory are normal, hospitalize to observe feeding pattern, caloric intake and weight gain.

IV. Observation Period; Three different patterns of response to standard diet for age are seen.

A. Adequate intake with satisfactory weight gain in the hospital. This suggests faulty feeding technique, disturbed parent-infant relationship. Most common pattern.

B. Adequate intake but unsatisfactory weight gain. This suggests malabsorption (most common), increased caloric requirements or failure to utilize nutrients.

C. Inadequate intake due to mechanical difficulties with feeding. Causes include neuromuscular disorders, oropharyngeal structural abnormalities, fatigue with feeding from congestive failure or pulmonary insufficieny.

References

Graef JW and Cone TZ, eds. Manual of Pediatric Therapeutics, 3rd edition. Boston: Little, Brown & Company, 1985.

Hoekelman RA, ed. Principles of Pediatrics: Health Care of the Young. New York: McGraw-Hill, 1978.

CONSTIPATION

I. **Overview**: Constipation develops when children have difficulty with the character of the stool. This leads to pain and discomfort and finally decreased frequency.

II. **Diagnosis**

   1. Determine from history if stool pattern is actually abnormal (children do not need to have a stool EVERY day).
   2. Characteristics: consistency, size, frequency, fecal soiling.
   3. Anorexia, tenesmus, abdominal pain are common complaints (may be severe enough to mimic surgical abdomen).
   4. Physical exam: palpable mass, presence of hard stool in rectum or dilated rectal ampule.

III. **Etiology**

   A. Newborn: Usually anatomic.
   B. Older children: functional or dietary.
      1. Dietary: lack of fecal bulk or excessive cow's milk intake and early introduction of solids.
      2. Psychological: abnormal or problems with toilet training, voluntary retention or habit.
      3. Trauma: anal fissures or other lesions may result in retention to avoid pain.
      4. Overmedication: excessive use of suppositories, enemas, antihistamines, or other inhibitors of bowel motility.
      5. Congenital: atresia of rectum or colon, meconium plug syndrome in newborns (associated with congenital megacolon and cystic fibrosis), myelomeningocele or other neurological problems.
      6. Ileus: secondary to infection or inflammatory bowel disease.
      7. CNS diseases.

8. Metabolic: hypothyroidism, hypercalcemia, hypokalemia.

IV. Management

A. Simple constipation:
   1. Enemas and suppositories should be avoided. Exclude organic causes. Commonly, the stooling pattern is normal and parents need only reassurance. Otherwise, dietary manipulation often sufficient. If symptoms develop during toilet training, explore with the parents the possibility that excess pressure is being placed on the child.
   2. Treatment:
      a. Babies: 1-2 tsp karo syrup to each bottle. If older than 4 months, add fruit to diet, including fruit juices (prune).
      b. Older children: increase intake for fruit and vegetables (prunes, figs, raisins, celery, lettuce, beans, bran). Milk may be constipating, push other fluids temporarily. Milk of magnesia may be used, or docusate, 5-10 mg/kg/day, divided t.i.d. or b.i.d.

B. Long standing:
   1. Exclude organic causes.
   2. Fecal disimpaction: Pediatric enema after overnight mineral oil. May repeat one or two times and follow with dulcolax suppository b.i.d. x 2 days.
   3. In addition to the dietary changes, consider behavioral intervention (have child sit on stool for 10 minutes after each meal and before bed time) and continue mineral oil or milk of magnesia with dose increased to the point of producing daily soft stools.

Reference

Barkin R and Rosen P, eds. Emergency Pediatrics, 2nd edition. St. Louis: C.V. Mosby Co., 1986.

ANEMIA

I. **Definition**: Hemoglobin (Hb) concentration below the third percentile for patient's age. Remember term infants physiologic nadir of Hb is 10.5 g/dl at 2-3 months of age. Preterm infants may normally drop to 9 g/dl.

II. **Etiology**

　A. Iron deficiency: most common cause.

　　1. 6 months to 2 years: nutritional, secondary to excessive cow's mild intake and inadequate iron in diet.

　　2. Older than 2 years: need to investigate causes of chronic blood loss (such as parasites, a common cause).

　B. Other anemias (see Figure 10-1).

　　1. Impaired Hb production, maturation or release from bone marrow.

　　2. Destruction, sequestration, or acute loss of circulating red cells.

III. **Symptoms**

　A. Rapid onset: headache, dizziness, postural hypotension, tachycardia, hypovolemia.

　B. Chronic onset: (nutritional, leukemia) pallor, decreased exercise tolerance.

　C. Iron deficiency: may have behavior disturbances, learning problem, delayed motor development. If severe, may develop protein losing enteropathy with blood in the stools.

　D. Hemolytic: jaundice and splenomegaly.

IV. **Evaluation**

　A. Initial lab: CBC, WBC, platelet count, peripheral smear, reticulocyte count, RBC indices, stool for occult blood, O & P.

　B. Microcytosis suggests Fe deficiency. Obtain iron studies, FEP.

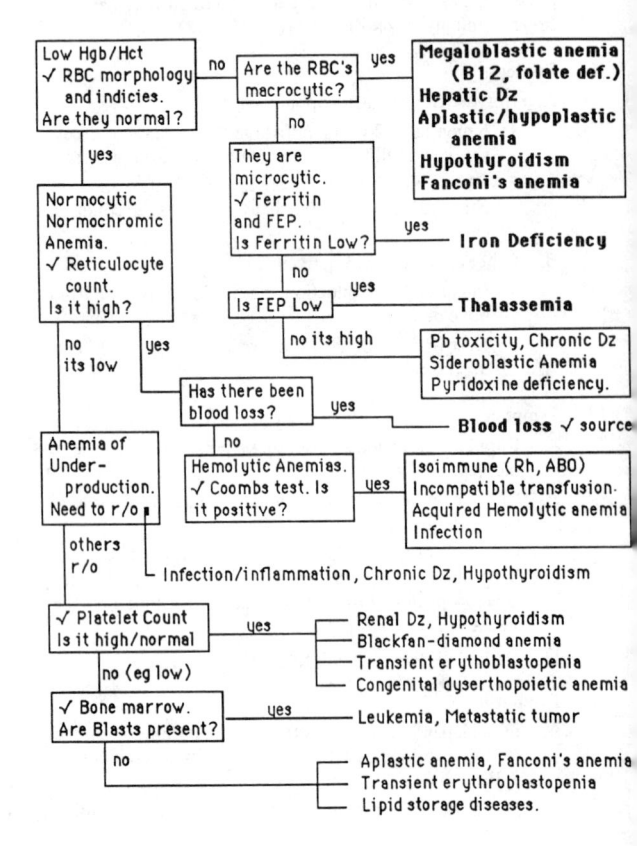

```
                    ┌─────────────────┐
Low Hgb/Hct    no   │ Are the RBC's   │ yes   Megaloblastic anemia
√ RBC morphology────│ macrocytic?     │─────  (B12, folate def.)
and indicies.       └─────────────────┘      Hepatic Dz
Are they normal?           │                 Aplastic/hypoplastic
                           │ no               anemia
                           ▼                 Hypothyroidism
                    They are                 Fanconi's anemia
                    microcytic.
                    √ Ferritin
                    and FEP.
                    Is Ferritin Low? ──yes──  Iron Deficiency
```

```
     yes                    │ no
      │              Is FEP Low ──yes──  Thalassemia
      ▼                     │
Normocytic                  │ no its high
Normochromic                ▼
Anemia.              Pb toxicity, Chronic Dz
√ Reticulocyte       Sideroblastic Anemia
count.               Pyridoxine deficiency.
Is it high?
```

```
  no          yes
  │            │
  │            ▼
  │      Has there been
  │      blood loss?  ──yes──  Blood loss √ source
  │            │
  │            │ no
  ▼            ▼
Anemia of    Hemolytic Anemias.          Isoimmune (Rh, ABO)
Under-       √ Coombs test. Is ──yes──   Incompatible transfusion.
production.  it positive?                Acquired Hemolytic anemia
Need to r/o                              Infection
  others
  r/o ──── Infection/inflammation, Chronic Dz, Hypothyroidism
```

```
√ Platelet Count                  ─── Renal Dz, Hypothyroidism
Is it high/normal ──yes──         ─── Blackfan-diamond anemia
    │                             ─── Transient erythroblastopenia
    │ no (eg low)                 ─── Congenital dyserthopoietic anemia
    ▼
√ Bone marrow.   ──yes──  Leukemia, Metastatic tumor
Are Blasts present?
    │
    │ no
    ▼
                 ─── Aplastic anemia, Fanconi's anemia
                 ─── Transient erythroblastopenia
                 ─── Lipid storage diseases.
```

Fig 10-1. Anemia

V. Management

A. Children 6 months - 2 years with hypochromic, microcytic anemia most likely have a dietary iron deficiency.

1. Elemental iron 5 mg/kg/po daily given in 3 divided doses (between meals) continue x 2 months.
2. Iron rich foods (meat, eggs, green vegetables, enriched cereals).
3. Limit cow's mild intake to 24 oz/day.
4. Recheck Hb/Hct in 1-2 weeks (it should rise during first week of treatment) and again at 1-2 months (child should no longer be anemic).

Reference

Barkin R and Rosen P, eds. Emergency Pediatrics, 2nd edition. St. Louis: C.V. Mosby Co., 1986.

Stockman JA. Anemia in children. Differential Insight 1(1):13, June 1979.

BITES

I. **Overview:** Children often are bitten by various insects and animals raising concerns about rabies, infection, soft-tissue trauma, permanent disfigurement. Must treat patient and parental anxieties. Main risk of animal bite is wound infection and disfigurement; not rabies (must consider rabies with some animal bites, however).

   A. Etiologic organisms.
      1. Animal bites: staph aureus, strep sp., clostridium sp., pasteurella sp., streptobacillus moniliformis.
      2. Human bites: over 40 species including: staph sp., strep sp., Eikenella sp.
      3. Tick bites: Borrelia burgdorferi (Lyme disease), rickettsial (Rocky Mountain spotted fever).

II. **Evaluation**

   A. History:
      1. Type of animal: suspect rabies if bat, skunk, raccoon, fox, badger, coyote, other large carnivores, or unprovoked attack from dog or cat. Rabies possible but not likely with squirrels (varies with geographical locale--contact health department). Very low likelihood of rabies with mice, rats, gophers, chipmunks, rabbits, domestic cats and dogs.

III. **Management:** If rabies suspected act quickly. Rabies is essentially uniformly fatal. Anti-rabies measures are more effective the earlier they are begun.

   A. General:
      1. Wash wound with lots of soap and water for 15 minutes followed by 70% alcohol wash.
      2. Call police if animal still present. If animal present or dead, avoid further contact. Live animals must be observed 10 days by a veterinarian. Contact local animal shelter or county health department.
      3. Check tetanus status and give booster if > 5 years.
      4. Wound treatment: Irrigate. Consider plastics or ENT referral if facial laceration. In general, human bites

should not be primarily closed because of the high risk of infection. Animal bites may be closed depending upon the condition of the wound.

      5. Antibiotics for human bites: dicloxacillin, amoxicillin/clavulinic acid, or cephalosporin. Antibiotics are not necessary for animal bites unless infection already present.

B. Rabies treatment: (as indicated)

1. Rabies immune globulin. Provides passive immunity. 20 iu/kg x 1.
2. Human diploid cell Rabies Vaccine. Provides active immunity. One cc dose x 5 on days 0, 3, 7, 14, and 28.

IV. Tick Bites

A. Removal: two popular and effective methods for tick removal.

1. Slow constant traction with forceps with slight twisting.
2. Soaking tick with occlusive solution (nail polish, petrolatum). Occlusive solutions may take 30-60 minutes to work.
3. Other measures, such as holding hot match near the tick, are not recommended and have not been shown to be effective.

B. Prevention: wear long clothes in woods, other endemic areas. Wear insect repellant. Daily skin inspection; ticks take several hours to become firmly embedded. Removal is much easier if done before this occurs.

C. Watch for fever, rash, adenopathy in week following bite. If these develop, consider Rocky Mountain spotted fever, tick fever. Lyme disease rash (erythema chronicum migrans) classically has spreading, large erythematous area at site of bite with area of central clearing. Rash may develop 4-6 weeks after bite.

V. Spider bites

A. Of concern in North America are brown recluse spider, black widow spider, and scorpion. Suspect possible arachnid bite if blister forms at site, extreme pain, muscle spasm.

1. Black Widow: shiny, jet black with red markings on dorsal surface, and long legs. Body and legs about 1".
2. Brown Recluse: Brown, long legs. Body and legs about 1 1/2" long. Dark, fiddle-shaped area on head. Causes blister and pain in 4-8 hours after bite.

B. Treatment: venous tourniquet between site and heart. Ice pack at blister/bite site (do not freeze the area). Bring spider in if available.

1. Black widow bite will produce cramping pain at site within an hour which spreads to entire body. Many other systemic symptoms may be present including N/V, headache, pruritis, dyspnea. May be hypertensive. In adults, symptoms begin to abate after a few hours, disappearing in 48-72 hours. In children or adults with underlying medical condition, bite can be fatal.

    a. Symptomatic treatment: hypertensive crisis treated with nitroprusside. Diazepam can relieve muscle spasms. Calcium gluconate 10 ml of 10% solution over several minutes may relieve many of the symptoms. Dantrolene has also been shown to provide relief of muscle spasm. Severe envenomations, children less than 16, pregnant women, elderly adults or adults with significant pre-existing medical condition should receive anitvenin (Merck, Sharp, and Dohme).

2. Brown recluse spider bites may produce mild burning at site initially. This is followed in several hours by pain with area of ischemia at site surrounded by erythematous ring. Center may blister and then necroses. May spread for several hours to days. Systemic symptoms of fever, chills, rash, malaise are common. Many recommend systemic steroids but these have not been shown to be effective. Dapsone may be effective in limiting the extent of local destruction.

3. Other spiders: usually not serious unless allergic response. Treat with ice to area of bite and thorough cleansing.

References

Graef JW and Cone TZ, eds. <u>Manual of Pediatric Therapeutics, 3rd edition</u>. Boston: Little, Brown & Company, 1985.

Mills J, *et al*, eds. <u>Current Emergency Diagnosis and Treatment, 2nd edition</u>. Los Altos: Lange 1985.

Schmitt BD, ed. <u>Pediatric Telephone Advice, 1st edition</u>. Boston: Little, Brown & Company, 1980.

PARASITES

I. **Pinworms** (enterobius vermicularis)
   A. Symptoms: Perianal itching, vulvitis, vaginitis, restlessness.
   B. Examination for pinworms.
      1. Parents inspect perianal area about an hour after the child goes to sleep. Look for white worms, about 1/4 to 1/2 inch long.
      2. Pinworm smear (cellophane tape method) obtained by pressing clear cellophane tape against perianal area (sticky side against the skin) in the morning before bathing. Tape is placed on a microscope slide and examined for evidence of ova.
   C. Treatment: All members of household should be treated simultaneously. Hand washing and fingernail cleanliness may help reduce chance of transmission/ autoinfection.
      1. Mebendazole 100 mg in 1 dose for adults and children older than 2 years. Repeat in 2 weeks.
      2. Pyrantel pamoate 11 mg/kg (up to one gram) in 1 dose. Repeat in 2 weeks.

II. **Pediculosis** (Lice).
   A. Overview: Pediculosis is caused by Pediculus humanus (body louse) and/or Phthirus pubis (Pubic "crab" louse). Symptoms are primarily intense pruritus. Transmission is through contact with combs, hats, brushes, clothing, sexual contact, bedding, towels.
   B. Evaluation.
      1. History of intense itching. Inquire as to possible contact with infected person.
      2. Pediculosis capitus: oval eggs (nits) along hair shafts and stuck to hair shafts. Hair may be matted. Adult lice seen in hair or on comb.
      3. Pediculosis corporis: Excoriations, especially around belt line, mid back, and shoulders. Macular (early) and papular (later) lesion seen. Lice and ova sometimes hard to find, look in seams of clothing.

C. Treatment.
   1. Apply 1% permethrin (NIX) topically. Topical pyrethrins (RID) also very effective. Leave on overnight, then wash off. May repeat in about one week.
   2. Treat all members of household simultaneously.
   3. Wash all clothes, bedding, towels, hats in hot water and dry in hot dryer.
   4. If eyelashes, eyebrows affected, treat by applying petroleum jelly until symptoms clear.

Reference

Graef JW and Cone TZ, eds. Manual of Pediatric Therapeutics, 3rd edition. Boston: Little, Brown & Company, 1985.

11/ GENITOURINARY

John E. Littler, M.D. and Garry R. Weischedel, M.D.

LOWER UTI - FEMALE

I. **Signs and Symptoms**: Dysuria, frequency, tenesmus, nocturia, enuresis, incontinence, urethral pain, suprapubic pain, fever, flank pain, CVA tenderness (50% are cystitis only).

II. **Etiology**: colonization by fecal flora - usually E. coli (75-95%). Other organisms include Klebsiella (5%), Enterobacter, Proteus, Pseudomonas, and others.

III. **Lab Findings**
   A. UA (clean catch mid stream).
      1. Hematuria: from inflamed epithelium, gross or microscopic.
      2. Pyuria: usually > 5 WBC per HPF. May not be present.
      3. Bacteriuria.
      4. Gram stain.
   B. Culture and sensitivity: to determine organism and evaluate effectiveness of treatment.

IV. **Other Conditions**
   A. Urethral syndrome.
      1. UTI symptoms with negative culture or normal UA.
      2. Rule out low colony count infections, chlamydia, trichomonas, or other vaginitis.
      3. Consider yeast, herpes, carcinoma in situ, external irritants, interstitial cystitis, Staphylococcus saprophyticus.
      4. Treatment is empiric, may include antibiotics, estrogens, urinary anesthetics.
      5. Urology referral may be indicated.
   B. Interstitial cystitis.

1. Frequency, urgency, and rarely urge incontinence with periurethral and/or suprapubic pain on bladder filling that is improved by voiding.
2. Etiology unclear.
3. Refer to urology for cystoscopy and possibly biopsy.

V. **Treatment** (for uncomplicated UTI)
   A. Single-Dose Regimens.
      1. Amoxicillin 3 gm.
      2. Sulfisoxazole 2 gm.
      3. Trimethoprim (TMP) 320 mg with sulfamethoxazole (SMZ) 1600 mg.
      4. Nitrofurantoin 100 mg.
   B. Three-day Regimens.
   C. Standard Oral Regimens.
      1. Sulfisoxazole 2 gm then 1 to 2 gm qid for 10 days.
      2. Nitrofurantoin 50 mg qid for 7 to 10 days.
      3. Cephalexin 500 mg qid for 7 to 10 days.
      4. TMP 160 mg SMZ 800 mg bid for 7 to 10 days.
      5. Ampicillin 500 mg qid for 7-10 days.
      6. Amoxicillin 500 mg tid for 7-10 days.
      7. Norfloxacin and ciprofloxacin are both very effective (and very expensive). Indicated for resistant organisms.
   D. Consider phenazopyridine hydrochloride, 200 mg tid times 2 days for topical urinary tract relief if indicated. Be sure to inform patient that this will produce an orange/red tinge to the urine.

LOWER URINARY TRACT INFECTIONS IN MALES

I. **Etiology:** Ascending infection from the urethra most common, hematogenous, lymphangitic spread or extension from adjacent organ possible. Pathogens - E-coli (80%) Proteus, Enterobacter, Pseudomonas, Serratia, Streptococcus faecalis, and Staphylococcus species are the most common.

II. **Localization of Lower UTI**
   A. Divided urine collection may help localize infection.
      1. First voided 10 ml represent urethral.
      2. Mid-stream collection represents bladder.
      3. Prostate represented by prostatic secretions from massage and first voided 10 ml post massage.

III. **Bacterial Cystitis**
   A. Signs/Symptoms: frequency, urgency, dysuria, nocturia, suprapubic discomfort, hematuria, low back pain. Systemic symptoms are absent.
   B. Lab: UA shows pyuria, bacteriuria, no casts. C&S reveals > 105 colonies/ml.
   C. Treatment: depends on C & S. Usually ampicillin 500 mg qid, nitrofurantoin 100 mg qid, or TMP 160 mg/SMZ 800 mg bid for 7-10 days are effective. Intravenous urography/cystoscopy (once urine is sterile) may be indicated.

IV. **Acute Bacterial Prostatitis** (see Fig 11-1)
   A. Signs/symptoms: both systemic (fever, chills, malaise, low back pain) and urinary (frequency, pain, urgency, varying degrees of retention). Prostate is very tender, boggy, and perhaps hot to touch (do NOT massage; risk of bacteremia).
   B. Lab: Leukocytosis, bacteriuria, hematuria, pyuria. C&S required.
   C. Therapy
      1. Hospitalization is often necessary for IV antibiotics (aminoglycoside pending culture results).
      2. Avoid urethral catheterization.

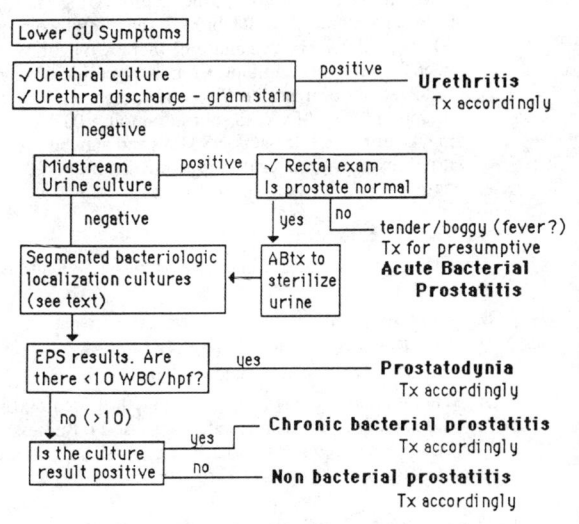

```
┌─────────────────────────┐
│ Lower GU Symptoms       │
├─────────────────────────┤
│ ✓Urethral culture       │  positive
│ ✓Urethral discharge –   │──────────── **Urethritis**
│   gram stain            │             Tx accordingly
└─────────────────────────┘
         │ negative
         ▼
┌──────────────┐  positive  ┌─────────────────┐
│ Midstream    │──────────▶│ ✓ Rectal exam   │
│ Urine culture│           │ Is prostate     │
└──────────────┘           │ normal          │
         │ negative        └─────────────────┘
         ▼                   yes │    │ no
┌─────────────────────────┐      │    └── tender/boggy (fever?)
│ Segmented bacteriologic │   ┌──▼──┐     Tx for presumptive
│ localization cultures   │◀──│ABtx │     **Acute Bacterial**
│ (see text)              │   │to   │     **Prostatitis**
└─────────────────────────┘   │steri│
         │                    │lize │
         ▼                    │urine│
┌─────────────────┐           └─────┘
│ EPS results. Are│  yes
│ there <10 WBC/  │────────── **Prostatodynia**
│ hpf?            │           Tx accordingly
└─────────────────┘
         │ no (>10)
         ▼
┌─────────────────┐ yes
│ Is the culture  │────────── **Chronic bacterial prostatitis**
│ result positive │           Tx accordingly
└─────────────────┘ no
                  ──────────  **Non bacterial prostatitis**
                              Tx accordingly
```

Fig 11-1. Management of Prostatitis

3. If hospitalization is unnecessary TMP/SMX, carbenicillin or minocycline may be used.
4. 3 weeks is minimum treatment.

V. Chronic Bacterial Prostatitis

A. Sign/symptoms: low back and perineal discomfort, voiding symptoms similar to acute bacterial prostatitis but with a more insidious onset, no systemic signs, rarely painful ejaculation. Prostate exam is normal.

B. Lab: Localizing cultures. Needle biopsy of prostate is useless. EPS reveals inflammatory cells. UA will show WBC and bacteriuria if secondary cystitis is present

C. Therapy: unfortunately few antimicrobial agents achieve therapeutic levels in prostatic secretions in setting of no acute inflammation. Possible regimens include TMP/SMX bid x 12 weeks, Carbenicillin 500 mg 2 tab qid x 4 weeks, minocycline 100 bid x 4 weeks, erythromycin 500 mg qid x 4 weeks. Failure of therapy may indicate need for parenteral antibiotics (aminoglycoside x 3 days) followed by oral antibiotics. Low dose prophylactic therapy (TMP-SMX qHS, nitrofurantoin 100 mg qid) may offer relief. Sitz baths, NSAID's and anticholinergic drugs (exybutynin chloride, propantheline bromide) may help. TURP offers cure in 30% of cases.

VI. Nonbacterial Prostatitis

A. Etiology: unknown. Chlamydia is suspected but not proven.

B. Signs/Symptoms: as for chronic bacterial prostatitis.

C. Lab: EPS reveals inflammatory cells but no bacteria. No causative agent is found in any cultures.

D. Therapy: minocycline 100 mg bid or erythromycin 500 mg qid x 4 weeks is recommended but often unsuccessful. Other measures include sitz baths, NSAID's, prostatic massage (controversial) and reassurance.

VII. Prostatodynia; Prostate pain without prostatic infection or inflammation; formerly called prostatosis.

A. Signs/Symptoms: as for chronic bacterial prostatitis.

B. Lab: absence of inflammatory cells or bacteria.

C. Therapy: reassurance. Consider alpha adrenergic blockers (Prazosin) if symptoms include hesitancy and slow stream. Consider psychiatric consult.

VIII. Epididymitis

A. Etiology.

1. Sexually transmitted form associated with urethritis, commonly caused by Chlamydia and/or N. gonorrheae.

2. Non-sexually transmitted form associated with UTI or prostatitis, commonly caused by Enterobacter, or Pseudomonas.
3. Causes such as trauma, tuberculosis, reflux, or as a complication of TURP or systemic infection are less common.

B. Sign/Symptoms:--similar to urethritis/prostatitis/cystitis. Epididymis is painful and swelling/tenderness may extend to groin, lower abdomen, and/or flank. Fever, urethral discharge, and reactive hydrocele are common.

C. Lab: white count is elevated with left shift. UA may show pyuria/bacteriuria. C & S is indicated.

D. Differential Diagnosis: mumps orchitis, tumor, testicular abscess, torsion, and trauma must be considered.

E. Therapy.
   1. General measures: bed rest, scrotal elevation and support, analgesics, ice (early), heat (late), and spermatic cord block with lidocaine may be used.
   2. Antibiotics: Chlamydia - tetracycline 500 mg qid or doxycycline 100 mg bid x 21 days. Gonococcal - ampicillin 500 mg qid x 21 days, ceftriaxone 125-250 mg IM once. Other regimens are acceptable. If not sexually transmitted, TMP-SMX DS bid pending C&S results.

IX. Urethritis

A. Gonococcal Urethritis.
   1. Sign/symptoms: urethral discharge (yellow-brown), dysuria, pruritus, possibly meatal erythema.
   2. Lab: calginate swab of the urethra (at least one hour after last voiding) inserted 2-3 cm for gram stain should show 4 WBC per HPF. Gram negative intracellular diplococci is evidence of N. gonorrheae. Growth on Thayer-Martin media is proof of infection.
   3. Therapy: Amoxicillin 3 gm plus probenicid 1 gm po once, or ceftriaxone 125-250 mg IM once. Treat sexual partner(s).

B. Nongonococcal Urethritis.
   1. Etiology: Most commonly (80%) due to chlamydia trachomatis or Ureaplasma urealyticum. Other causes include Candida, Herpes, and trichamonas.
   2. Sign/symptoms similar to gonococcal urethritis although discharge (if present) is often clear or whitish. Asymptomatic infection is common.
   3. Lab: gram stain of urethral swabbing reveals > 4 WBC per HPF but lacks gram negative intracellular diplococci. C&S is necessary although often negative in the improperly collected specimen.
   4. Therapy: tetracycline 500 mg po qid or doxycycline 100 mg po bid x 7 days, or erythromycin 500 mg qid x 7 days. Treat partner(s).
C. Postgonococcal urethritis: occurs in patients treated for gonococcal urethritis but remain symptomatic. This is usually due to concurrent chlamydia infection and responds to appropriate treatment.
D. Reiter's syndrome consists of urethritis, conjunctivitis, arthritis, and characteristic mucocutaneous lesions, and has been associated with Chlamydia infection.

ACUTE PYELONEPHRITIS

I. **Definition.** Infection of upper urinary tract (kidney and renal pelvis).

II. **Etiology.** Ascending fecal flora, most commonly E. coli. Other agents include proteins, Pseudomonas, Klebsiella, Enterobacter, Staphylococcus, and Enterococcus. Note: Proteus species (and some Klebsiella species) produce urease which causes alkaline urine and favors struvite and apatite (calcium phosphate) stones.

III. **Clinical Presentation**
   A. Symptoms of cystitis (frequency, dysuria, nocturia, hematuria, urgency), flank pain, fever, chills, often nausea, and vomiting with diarrhea.
   B. Signs include fever, CVA tenderness.
   C. Lab: Leukocytosis with left shift, elevated ESR, U/A reveals pyuria, white cell casts, hematuria, bacteriuria, mild proteinuria. C&S of blood and urine are mandatory. BUN/Cr are usually normal in uncomplicated acute pyelonephritis.
   D. Other studies: Abdominal plain films may reveal stones which may indicate special management. IVP, although usually normal, is indicated to screen for possible complicating factors, such as stones or obstructive uropathy. Renal biopsy is not indicated. Radionuclide imaging with gallium may be indicated to determine the site of infection and distinguish acute pyelonephritis from renal or perinephric abscess. VCUG, to document the presence of vesicoureteral reflux, is best delayed until several weeks after clearing.

IV. **Treatment**
   A. Generally will require hospitalization for IV hydration and antibiotics. An aminoglycoside and a penicillin, or a second or third generation cephalosporin. Norfloxacin and ciprofloxacin are very effective against the vast majority of organisms causing infections of the urinary tract. Two weeks of oral antibiotics following IV antibiotics are commonly used.

B. Infected stones or obstruction must be recognized early and dealt with effectively in order to avoid complications.

V. **Chronic Pyelonephritis.** Results from repeated acute attacks and results in renal scarring which in turn leads to renal insufficiency and frequently HTN. Such patients need a full evaluation to search for predisposing risk factors (such as obstructive uropathy). Surgical measures are often necessary to correct anatomic defects or cure (by nephrectomy) renin-mediated hypertension associated with unilateral atrophic pyelonephritis. Prophylactic antibiotic therapy to avoid recurrence of acute pyelonephritis is frequently indicated.

SEXUALLY TRANSMITTED DISEASES

I. **Syphilis**: caused by spirochete Treponema pallidum.
   A. Primary.
      1. Sign/symptoms: hallmark sign is the chancre, a painless sore that usually presents 2-4 weeks after exposure. These are 1-2 cm in diameter, may be multiple and appear as shallow ulcerations with noninflamed margins and occur most commonly on mucous membranes abraded during sexual contact. Chancres heal spontaneously and slowly without scarring in 2-12 weeks. Unilateral or bilateral inguinal lymphadenopathy may be present.
      2. Lab: dark field exam of scraping of suspicious lesions will reveal spirochetes. VDRL or RPR are positive in 50% and may remain negative for up to 3 weeks after the appearance of the chancre. FTA-ABS is the quickest, least expensive and most specific and sensitive examination.
      3. Therapy: see table 11-1. Patients may experience fever, chills, arthralgias, myalgias, and nausea several hours after treatment (the Jarisch-Herxheimer reaction) which usually subsides within 24 hours. VDRL titers usually return to nonreactive within one year of treatment.
   B. Secondary.
      1. Signs/symptoms: Hallmark sign is a widespread, symmetric rash, often involving palms or soles (80%). Rash is usually erythematous but otherwise variable in appearance and normally occurs 4-8 weeks after chancre. Condyloma lata, oral or genital mucous patches, systemic symptoms (50%), and symmetric adenopathy also occur. These lesion of secondary syphilis resolve with or without treatment in 2-10 weeks.
      2. Lab: dark field exam of condyloma lata of genital mucous patches is often positive. VDRL is highly reactive in 90% but should be confirmed with FTA-ABS.
      3. Therapy - see table 11-1.

II. **Gonorrhea**: caused by gram negative diplococcus Neisseria gonorrheae. (For discussion of gonococcal disease in the male, see section on urethritis).
   A. Signs/symptoms: the primary site of infection is the endocervix with secondary infection of the rectum or urethra. Yellow-white discharge may be present but the infection is frequently asymptomatic. Other infections include proctitis, pharyngitis, salpingitis, and disseminated disease (pustulovesicular lesions with arthralgias/arthritis).
   B. Lab: gram stain of smear reveals gram negative intracellular diplococci. Culture on Thayer-Martin (chocolate agar) media.
   C. Therapy: see table 11-1. Repeat cultures should be obtained 3-7 days after treatment to assure adequate treatment.

III. **Chancroid**: caused by gram-negative rod Hemophilus ducreyi.
   A. Sign/symptoms: a papule which becomes a pustule that ulcerates. Lesions are deep with flat, ragged erythematous borders that may extend into subcutaneous tissue. Adenopathy is common, systemic signs of fever, headache, and malaise occur in 50%.
   B. Lab: smear reveals gram-negative rods in chains ('school of fish'). Culture on enriched chocolate agar with vancomycin may be positive, biopsy is diagnostic.
   C. Therapy: see table 11-1.

IV. **Lymphogranuloma Venereum**: caused by Chlamydia trachomatis Types I, II, and III.
   A. Signs/symptoms: a papule or pustule that appears 5-21 days after exposure. This lesion often goes unnoticed. Adenopathy (usually unilateral) occurs 1-2 weeks later. These painful nodes may become fluctuant and form bubos or chronic draining sinuses. Rectal strictures from anorectal node involvement can be seen. Systemic symptoms, including rashes, are common.

- B. Lab: complement fixation titers should show a four fold increase after 4 weeks. Culture of aspirate for C. trachomatis is diagnostic.
- C. Therapy: see table 11-1. I&D of nodes is rarely indicated.

V. **Granuloma Inguinale**: caused by gram-negative bacterium Calymatobacterium granulomatosis.
- A. Signs/symptoms: a papule that erodes, producing a velvety red granulomatous plaque that gradually extends. Inguinal swelling (pseudobubos) is a subcutaneous granulomatous process rather than a true adenopathy. These may erode through the skin.
- B. Lab: intracytoplasmic inclusion bodies (Donovan bodies) in monocytes on Wright's or Giemsa's stain of smears is characteristic. No reliable culture is available. Biopsy may be necessary.
- C. Therapy: see table 11-1.

VI. **Herpes Simplex Genitalis**: caused by herpes simplex virus type II (occassionally type I).
- A. Signs/symptoms: often asymptomatic. Incubation is 2-10 days. Primary lesion is manifest by grouped painful vesicles on an erythematous base which ulcerate and heal without scarring. Fever and adenopathy are common. Secondary lesions are similar to primary except duration and severity are less and accompanying fever and adenopathy are rare.
- B. Lab: Tzanck smear of base of a fresh vesicle (Giemsa stain) reveals multinucleated giant cells. Culture requires 48-72 hours.
- C. Therapy: see table 11-1.

VII. **Condyloma Acuminata**: caused by human papilloma virus.
- A. Signs/symptoms: soft, flesh colored verrucous papules in genital areas.
- B. Lab: serology may be necessary to rule out condyloma lata of secondary syphilis. Biopsy (rarely necessary) is diagnostic.
- C. Therapy: Podophyllin (10-20%) in tincture of benzoin is applied then thoroughly washed off in 1-4 hours. Warts

484   Genitourinary

are treated weekly. Alternative therapies include cryotherapy, electrosurgery, or excision.

VIII. **Pediculosis Pubis**: caused by Phthirus pubis, the 'crab' louse.
   A. Signs/symptoms: yellow-gray dots clinging to skin. Red specks on the skin may represent excrement. Nits are seen as white dots attached to hairs. Pruritus is major symptom.
   B. Lab: Lice are easily recognized either grossly or under magnification.
   C. Therapy: Lindane 1% lotion applied to involved areas, leave on 8-12 hours, one application only.

IX. **Scabies**: caused by mite Sarcoptes scabiei.
   A. Signs/symptoms: Pruritic papules, crusted lesions, and burrows or linear channels beneath the skin with a grey speck at one end are commonly seen. Most commonly seen between fingers, and on extremities, and trunk, not on face.
   B. Lab: low power microscope of scraping reveals the mite (characterized by four pairs of legs).
   C. Therapy: Lindane 1% lotion is applied neck down, left on for 12 hours, and showered off. Application may be repeated in 7 days. Crotamiton 10% may also be used, especially for infants, q Hs x 2. Clothing and bed linen must be laundered at the same time. Family contacts should be treated.

X. **Molluscum Contagiosum**: caused by pox virus.
   A. Signs/symptoms: dome shaped papules, 2-6 mm with central umbilication.
   B. Lab: incision of papule reveals white waxy core. Smear of contents reveals swollen epithelial cells. Biopsy is diagnostic.
   C. Therapy: Curettage, cryosurgery, or electrodessication.

XI. **Candidiasis**: caused by yeast Candida albicans.
   A. Signs/symptoms: in the male, red erythematous pruritic skin with peripheral pustules. In the female, pruritic vaginal mucosa and profuse creamy white discharge.

Sexually Transmitted Diseases 485

More common in diabetics or patients on long term antibiotics.

B. Lab: smear or culture reveals C. albicans.

C. Therapy: on skin, good hygiene and bid topical antifungal cream such as clotrimazole, miconazole, or nystatin. Antifungal vaginal suppositories.

XII. **Trichomoniasis**: caused by protozoa trichomonas vaginalis.

A. Signs/symptoms: often asymptomatic. Vaginal/urethral discharge or pruritus are the most common complaints.

B. Lab: T. vaginalis is motile and best seen under low power.

C. Therapy: see Table 11-1. Be sure to treat partner(s).

Table 11-1. Treatment of Sexually Transmitted Diseases

Type or State	Drug of Choice	Dosage	Alternatives
GONORRHEA			
Urethritis or Cervicitis	Ceftriaxone	125-250 mg IM once	Amoxicillin 3 g. p.o. plus probenecid 1 g. p.o. times one. Spectinomycin 2 g. IM once
CHLAMYDIA TRACHOMATIS			
Lymphogranuloma venereum	Doxycycline	100 mg bid x 21 days	
	Erythromycin	500 mg p.o. qid x 21 days	
VAGINAL INFECTIONS			
Trichomoniasis	Metronidazole	2 g. p.o. once or 250 mg tid x 7	
in pregnancy	Clotrimazole	100 mg vaginally at h.s. x 7 days	
SYPHILIS			
Primary, secondary, or latent less than one year	Penicillin G benzathine	2.4 million U IM once	Tetracycline 500 mg p.o. qid x 15 days. Erythro-

Genitourinary

Table 11-1 (continued)

Type or State	Drug of Choice	Dosage	Alternative
			mycin 500 mg p.o. qid x 15 days
CHANCROID	Ceftriaxone	250 mg IM once	Trimethoprim-sulfamethox-azol 2 tablets p.o. bid x 7 days
	Erythromycin	500 mg p.o. qid x 7 days	
GRANULOMA INGUINALE	Tetracycline	500 mg qid x 2-4 weeks	Streptomycin 1 gram qid x 7 days
	TMP/SMX/DS	1 bid x 2-4 weeks	
HERPES SIMPLEX	Acyclovir	200 mg 5/ x 10 (primary). 200 mg 5/ x 5 (recurrent)	

BENIGN PROSTATIC HYPERTROPHY (BPH)

I. **Etiology.** Exact cause unknown. Associated with dihydrotestosterone (DHT) levels, possibly also estrogen. Two factors are necessary; time and functioning testis.

II. **Clinical Presentation**

   A. Enlargement occurs silently, only when bladder outlet obstruction occurs do symptoms present. These include decreased force and caliber of urinary stream, hesitancy, retention, post-micturition dribbling, double voiding (patient voids and is able to void again in 5-10 minutes), and overflow urinary incontinence (on straining or coughing). Irritative symptoms such as dysuria, frequency, nocturia, urgency, hematuria, and incontinence occur frequently. Flank pain during micturition, suprapubic pain, and azotemic symptoms occur less commonly.

   B. On exam, bladder may be distended, and prostate is enlarged, smooth, and symmetric. The gland may be soft or firm and possibly nodular. However the nodules lack the stony hard consistency associated with carcinoma.

   C. Lab: U/A may reveal signs of infection. If the obstruction has been severe enough to impair renal function, BUN and creatinine may be elevated.

   D. X-ray findings: Plain film may reveal prostatic calculi. IVP may show upper tract or bladder changes secondary to obstruction (hydroureteronephrosis, bladder trabeculation and thickening, bladder diverticula or calculi). VCUG may be indicated. Post void catheterization will reveal residual urine.

III. **Treatment**

   A. Cystoscopy with biopsy evaluates the degree of obstruction and the pathology of the disease.

   B. A temporary indwelling Foley catheter may help acute episodes but is only a stopgap measure.

   C. Surgical measures, most commonly transurethral prostatectomy (TURP), are the preferred and definitive therapy.

- D. Antibiotics should be used to control infection when indicated. Alpha blocking agents, such as phenoxybenzamine, may offer symptomatic relief.
- E. If exam reveals nodularity of the gland, referral to a urologist is indicated.

HEMATURIA

I. **Etiology.** There are many possible causes of hematuria. Few will produce hematuria of hemodynamic significance--urgent surgical consult is required if this occurs. Possible causes include trauma, tumor, kidney stones, infection of bladder, prostate, or kidney, glomerulonephritis, urethral structure/foreign body, use of anticoagulants, and systemic disorders that produce vasculitis.

II. **Evaluation** (for trauma-related hematuria, see section on Trauma)

   A. History: will often provide evidence for etiology with symptoms of infection (fever, dysuria), urolithiasis (pain), use of anticoagulants.

   B. Physical exam: may provide evidence to indicate etiology. Prostate may be tender, suprapubic region tender, CVA tenderness, trauma to perineum/urethra.

   C. Laboratory:

   1. Urine analysis: document hematuria, assess for possible infection as indicated by WBCs, possible WBC casts, bacteria. Presence of red cell casts suggests glomerulonephritis.

   2. Serum creatinine indicated if glomerulonephritis suspected. PT/PTT, bleeding time as indicated.

   3. Painless hematuria should prompt suspicion of tumor. IVP and cystoscopy are indicated even if hematuria resolves.

   4. If other complaints or findings are present suggesting systemic disorder, obtain CBC, sed rate, possibly ANA.

III. **Treatment**

   A. Infectious: Treat infection as indicated for cystitis, prostatitis, pyelonephritis. Urine analysis should be repeated to assure that infection was not incidental and hematuria has resolved.

   B. Urolithiasis: see section on urolithiasis.

C. Other disorders: as indicated. Glomerulonephritis should prompt a consultation with a nephrologist.

UROLITHIASIS

I. **Overview.** Urinary tract stones are a common cause of both hematuria and abdominal/flank/groin pain. Development of stones is related to factors that increase the concentration of the stone components in the urine: decreased urine volume and/or increased excretion of stone components. Stones are composed of calcium, oxalate, urate, cystine, xanthine, and phosphate, and form in the renal pelvis. Size ranges from microscopic to the size of the entire renal pelvis.

II.

  A. Clinical presentation

    1. History commonly includes past history of stones. Pain is usually severe, radiating from back, down flank and into groin. Intermittent, not improved by position change. Hematuria may be noted. Nausea and vomiting are common. Predisposing factors may be present: recent reduction in fluid intake, medications that predispose to hyperuricemia, history of gout.

    2. Physical examination generally will reveal costovertebral angle tenderness. Tachycardia may be present, or bradycardia from vasovagal reaction. Vitals are usually stable.

    3. Laboratory: urine analysis will demonstrate gross or microscopic hematuria in most cases. Urine culture should be obtained. BUN and creatinine should be obtained. Most stones can be seen on KUB. In a patient with past history of documented kidney stones and typical findings on history, physical, and laboratory (hematuria, normal BUN/Cr), excretory urogram is not necessary. In all other cases, IVP should be obtained to evaluate renal function, rule out obstruction, and to document stones in urinary tract.

  B. Initial treatment: consists of analgesia, adequate hydration, and straining urine to obtain specimen for analysis. Potent analgesics (narcotics) are usually required. Admission to hospital is required if parenteral analgesics required, persistent vomiting prevents adequate oral hydration, suspected pyelonephritis, elevated BUN/Cr, oliguria/anuria. Obstructing stones that do not pass will require removal (surgical or endoscopic). Glucagon and nifedipine have been reported to relieve pain and aid in passing of stones by virtue of their affect on smooth muscle. A recent study has not shown that to be the case with nifedipine.

C. Continuing care: all patients with kidney stones should increase their daily fluid intake regardless of the composition of the stones. Analysis of the stones may identify specific preventive measures.

1. Uric acid stones: should evaluate for hyperuricosuria. Allopurinol inhibits uric acid synthesis and may be helpful. Alkalinization of urine will also be of some benefit.

2. Calcium stones: hypercalciuria may occur in hyperparathyroidism, sarcoidosis, but is often idiopathic. Thiazide diuretics may decrease calcium excretion. Dietary intake may need to be reduced.

3. Triple phosophate stones: occur in the setting of high urinary pH seen in chronic urinary infections with urease-producing organisms. Antibiotics and acidification of the urine are indicated.

ACUTE SCROTAL PAIN AND SCROTAL MASSES

I. **Acute Scrotal Pain**
   A. Etiology: multiple causes, generally history will indicate likely cause. Differential diagnosis includes trauma, orchitis, epididymitis, hernia, urolithiasis, torsion of the testicle.
   B. Evaluation (Figure 11-2).
      1. History: trauma, nature/location/duration of pain, associated symptoms, recent infection of urethra/bladder/prostate.
      2. Examination: localization of painful structure is important for diagnosis. Assess for inguinal hernia, urethritis, possible parotitis.
      3. Laboratory: will be directed by findings on history and physical. Urine analysis should be obtained to assess for hematuria, evidence of infection.
   C. Causes:
      1. Trauma: may be difficult to get accurate history if unusual sexual practices involved. Persistence necessary. Ultrasound of scrotum and testicles can be quite useful in assessing trauma.
      2. Urolithiasis: indicated by hematuria, often there is or has been associated flank pain. Examination will reveal normal scrotal contents.
      3. Hernia: incarcerated hernia may cause only scrotal pain. Examination may reveal the presence of bowel sounds in the scrotum. Signs of intestinal obstruction should be present. Ultrasound is diagnostic.
      4. Epididymitis: often a history of prior urethral symptoms. Commonly occurs in sexually active men. Culture urethral discharge and urine. Pain of epididymitis is often lessened by elevating the scrotum.
      5. Torsion of the testicle: urologic emergency, torsion present for longer than 4 to 6 hours will result in loss of the testicle. Exam may provide diagnosis with localized tenderness of the testicle, elevation of the testicle. If torsion has been present for some time, epididymis will also be swollen and tender, preventing differentiation. Cremasteric reflex will be absent on

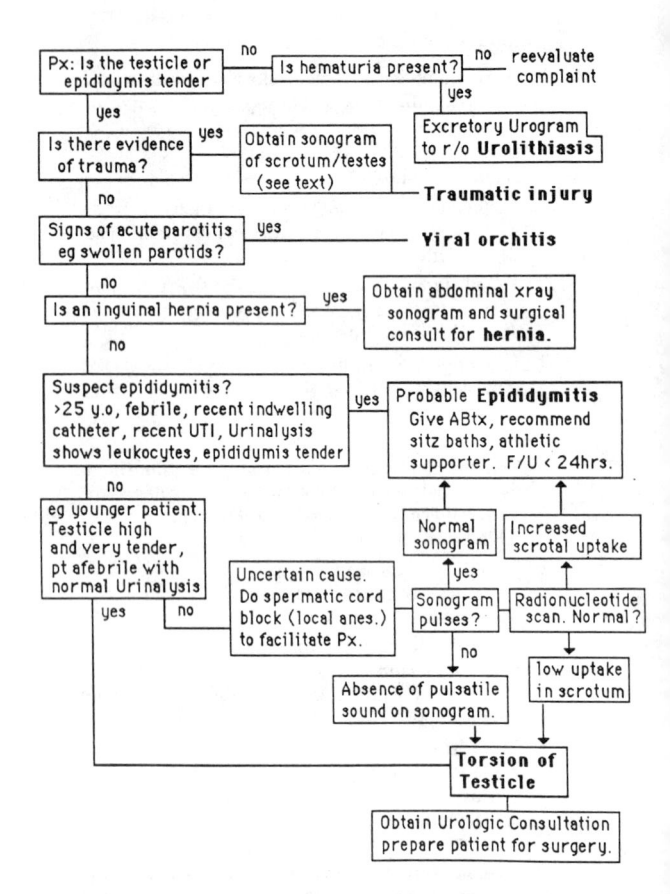

Fig 11-2. Acute Scrotal Pain

the affected side. Doppler may be used to assess for presence of testicular artery pulses. Ultrasound may also be useful. In no case should urgent consultation with a urologist be delayed if torsion is clinically suspected. Manual detorsion may be attempted (if immediate surgical evaluation is not possible) by infiltrating the spermatic cord near the external inguinal ring with 5ml of 2% lidocaine and counter-rotating the affected testicle. Standing below the patient's scrotum, the right testicle would be detorsed by counterclockwise rotation, the left by clockwise rotation.

II. **Painless Scrotal Masses**. Etiology: possible causes include tumors of the testicle or spermatic cord, spermatoceles, hydroceles, varicoceles, hernias, lipomas. Most are painless or associated with only mild pain. Acute, severe pain should prompt evaluation as discussed above. Occasionally tumors will have acute pain, possibly due to hemorrhage.

- A. Varicocele: very common. Usual clinical presentation is adolescent or young adult male with incidentally noted swelling in left scrotum. Physical examination is generally diagnostic with varicosities palpated above and separate from testicle. Enlarges with Valsalva maneuver. Treatment consists of firm scrotal support if symptomatic. Further evaluation/referral indicated for the following:
    1. Large or bilateral varicocele in young adolescent. May result in inhibited growth of left or both testicles, possibly resulting in decreased function (testosterone production, spermatogeneis).
    2. Adult male that is a member of infertile couple.
    3. New-onset varicocele in male older than 30.
    4. Right-sided varicocele without concomitant left-sided varicocele.
- B. Hydrocele: typically presents as gradually enlarging painless cystic structure. Will trans-illuminate. Ultrasound may be advisable as hydrocele can be secondary to tumor.
- C. Spermatocele: usually asymptomatic. Firm but somewhat compressible mass located superior to and separate from the testicle in the spermatic cord. Ultrasound can aid in diagnosis. Requires no treatment.

D. Testicular tumor: usually young adult. Usually painless. Firm, nontender mass will be found on testicle. Will not trans-illuminate. Ultrasound will confirm location of mass. Urological consult required for evaluation.

RENAL FAILURE

I. **Acute Renal Failure.** Sudden loss of renal function as evidenced by oliguria/anuria, increase in BUN and/or serum creatinine.

   A. Etiology.

   1. Renal: glomerular (rapidly progressive glomerulonephritis), vascular (renal artery or vein thrombosis, vasculitis), and tubulointerstitial (ATN; most common, see below).

   2. Prerenal: diminished renal perfusion due to volume depletion, inadequate cardiac output, volume redistribution ("third spacing" from cirrhosis, burns, nephrotic syndrome, etc.).

   3. Postrenal: obstruction of the urinary tract from prostate disease, retroperitoneal disease.

   B. Diagnosis: urine output less than 400ml/24 hr, elevated BUN and creatinine.

II. **Acute Tubular Necrosis.**

   A. Acute renal failure resulting from renal ischemia or renal damage from toxic insults. Renal function generally returns to adequate level if patient survives acute phase, which usually lasts 1-2 weeks.

   B. Causes:

   1. Ischemic: shock, sepsis, hypoxia.

   2. Toxic: radiologic contrast media, heavy metals, aminoglycosides, myoglobinuria from burns, trauma, polymyositis, etc.

   C. Evaluation: diagnosis often apparent because of clinical history. Rule out obstructive process (ultrasound of kidneys, ureters helpful).

   a. Differentiate from postrenal and prerenal causes by low urine osmolality and elevated urine sodium concentration. Fractional excretion of sodium can differentiate between ATN and prerenal azotemia:

   $$\frac{(Urine\ Na/plasma\ Na)}{(Urine\ Cr/plasma\ Cr)} \times 100 \quad \begin{array}{l} ATN > 1\% \\ Prerenal < 1\% \end{array}$$

b. Urine analysis may reveal renal epithelial cells, cellular casts.

III. Prerenal Azotemia

A. Commonly caused by dehydration (often due to excessive diuretic therapy). Indicated by signs of decreased renal function with BUN elevated out of proportion to serum creatinine, often greater than 15-20:1.

B. Treatment:
1. Adequate intravascular volume will prevent progression to oliguric/anuric failure.
2. Treatment is as below if renal failure results.

IV. Treatment of Acute Renal Failure

A. Careful monitoring of fluid and electrolyte status. Fluids should be restricted to replacement of losses. Dietary intake of K^+ and phosphates should be severely restricted. Hyperphosphatemia may be prevented by use of oral aluminum hydroxide to absorb dietary phosphates. Calcium should be monitored, will tend to fall if phosphorus rises. Hyperkalemia should be treated as indicated. Fluid overload may require dialysis.

B. Monitor acidosis. Mild to moderate metabolic acidosis should be anticipated and may be well-tolerated. Severe acidosis may require oral bicarbonate solutions. These contain significant quantities of Na^+.

C. Monitor carefully for signs of infection (a common cause of mortality during acute renal failure).

D. Dialysis indicated for symptomatic pericarditis, severe hyperkalemia or hyperkalemia that does not respond to Kayexalate, severe acidosis, significant fluid overload, uremic symptoms (especially neurological).

V. Chronic Renal Failure (CRF)

A. Clinical syndrome of chronic compromise of renal function that can be categorized into three major groups:
1. Inadequate renal reserve, characterized by inability to compensate for extreme water/solute loading or deprivation.

2. Renal insufficiency, characterized by elevated BUN and markedly diminished capacity for dealing with water/solute fluctuations, but otherwise can maintain homeostasis.

3. Renal failure, characterized by progressive increase in BUN to the point of causing uremia, fluid and electrolyte imbalance.

B. Etiology: common causes include diabetes, hypertension, glomerulonephritis, polycystic kidney disease, obstructive uropathy. Many other causes exist.

C. Clinical Manifestation: early manifestations may include only nocturia due to inability to concentrate urine. Fatigue, altered mental status, peripheral neuropathy, anorexia, N/V, pruritus indicate uremia. HTN is common. Fluid and electrolyte imbalances result in varying signs and symptoms. Loss of erythropoietin and vitamin-D function result in anemia and osteodystrophy.

D. Treatment:

1. Dietary restrictions are required to maintain appropriate fluid and electrolyte balance. Protein restriction can reduce acidosis and symptoms from elevated BUN. Dietary K^+ intake will generally require restriction only late in the course. Phosphate intake should be limited. Calcium and Vit-D will need to be supplemented later in the course.

2. Fluid and sodium should be restricted only as indicated (generally required late in the course, but not early).

3. Dialysis: hemodialysis and chronic ambulatory peritoneal dialysis. Absolutely indicated for uremic pericarditis, progressive motor impairment, fluid overload not responsive to other interventions or producing CHF, severe acidosis and hyperkalemia. Otherwise is reserved for those symptoms of CRF that will respond to dialysis and have become bothersome enough to require this intervention.

4. Transplant: an alternative to dialysis. Decision to proceed with dialysis and/or transplant requires the assistance of nephrologist.

References

Driscoll CE, *et al*, eds. <u>Handbook of Family Practice</u>. Chicago: Year Book Medical Publishers, 1986.

Hanno PM and Wein AJ, eds. <u>A Clinical Manual of Urology</u>. Connecticut: Appleton-Century-Crofts, 1987.

Rakel RE and Conn HF, eds. <u>Textbook of Family Practice, Third edition</u>. Philadelphia: W.B. Saunders Company, 1984.

Tanagho EA and McAninch JW, eds. <u>Smith's General Urology, 12th edition</u>. Connecticut: Appleton & Lange, 1988.

12/ EYES, EARS, NOSE AND THROAT

J. Matthew Johnson, M.D. and John E. Littler, M.D.

RED EYE

I. **Differential Diagnosis.** (Table 12-1)

II. **Evaluation**
   A. History. Duration, rapidity of onset, activity at time of onset, visual changes, pain, itching, discharge or mattering, tearing, photophobia, foreign body sensation.
   B. Exam.
      1. Visual acuity. If not normal, rule out refractive error using pinhole test. Deficit in visual acuity that cannot be accounted for warrants consultation with an ophthalmologist.
      2. Palpate for pre-auricular nodes, tenderness or induration of the lids and periorbital tissues.
      3. Inspect for discharge, mattering, tearing.
      4. Pupils. Pupil may be constricted in corneal injury and iritis, mid-dilated and fixed with glaucoma.
      5. Conjunctiva. Inspect for distribution of redness, ciliary flush. Examine palpebral conjunctiva for cobble-stoning seen in allergic conjunctivitis.
      6. Lids. Evert upper and lower lids to rule out foreign body.
      7. Shine flashlight parallel to iris from the temporal side to assess the depth of the anterior chamber.
      8. Determine intraocular pressure (Schiotz or applanation tonometer) if glaucoma is suspected.
      9. Stain cornea with fluorescein to rule out corneal abrasion or infection. Corneal abrasion will appear as discrete areas which take up the stain. Herpes keratitis will show up as a dendritic staining.

Table 12-1. The Red Eye

	Conjunctivitis			Corneal Injury or Infection	Iritis	Acute Glaucoma
	Bacterial	Viral	Allergic			
Vision	-	-	-	↓ or ↓↓	↓	↓↓
Pain	-	-	-	+	+	+++
Photophobia	-	+/-	-	+	++	-
Foreign body sensation	-	+/-	+/-	+	-	-
Itch	+/-	+/-	++	-	-	-
Tearing	+	++	+	++	+	-
Discharge	Mucopurulent	Mucoid	-	-	-	-
Preauricular adenopathy	-	+	-	-	-	-
Pupils	-	-	-	NL or small	Small	Mid-dilated and fixed
Conjunctival hyperemia	Diffuse	Diffuse	Diffuse	Diffuse and ciliary flush	Ciliary flush	Diffuse and ciliary flush
Cornea	Clear	Sometimes faint punctate staining or infiltrates	Clear	Depends on disorder	Clear or lightly cloudy	Cloudy
Intraocular pressure	NL	NL	NL	NL	↓, NL or ↑	↑↑

C. Lab:
 1. Conjunctival smears are time consuming and usually not necessary. PMN's on gram stain suggest bacterial conjunctivitis, lymphocytes suggest viral conjunctivitis, and eosinophils suggest allergic.
 2. Purulent discharge should be cultured.

III. Management

A. Red eye associated with decreased visual acuity, eye pain, or corneal damage, or acute glaucoma should be referred immediately to an ophthalmologist.

B. Conjunctivitis:(See section on treatment of conjunctivitis).

C. Corneal lesions.
 1. Ulcer: refer to an ophthalmologist.
 2. Herpes simplex keratitis: Start patient on idorcuidine vidarabine ointment five times daily and erythromycin ointment bid, followup with an ophthalmologist within 24 hours.
 3. Corneal abrasion: Traditionally antibiotics are instilled along with a cycloplegic to prevent spasm of iris/ciliary body, and tight sterile patch applied. Recheck in 24 hours. No contact lenses for 2 weeks.
 4. Foreign Body: (See Procedures)

D. Iritis.
 1. Primary iritis should be seen by an ophthalmologist within 24-48 hours.
 2. Measure intraocular pressure as a baseline, begin topical steroids (dexamethasone) and cycloplegic to prevent formation of synechiae.

E. Acute Glaucoma.
 1. Initiate treatment with acetazolamide 500 mg IV.
 2. Pilocarpine 2% up to q 15 minutes to break the attack.
 3. Refer to an ophthalmologist.

References

Crumley RL, ed. <u>Common Problems of the Head and Neck Region</u>. Philadelphia: W.B. Saunders Company, 1986.

Driscoll CE, *et al*, eds. <u>Handbook of Family Practice</u>. Chicago: Year Book Medical Publishers, 1986.

CONJUNCTIVITIS

I. **Definition:** Inflammation of the conjunctiva leading to vascular dilation, cellular infiltration, and irritation.

II. **Differential Diagnosis** (Table 12-2)

Table 12-2.

Sign	Bacterial	Viral	Allergic	Toxic	TRIC
Injection	Marked	Mod	Mild-Mod	Mild-Mod	Mod
Hemmorhage	+	+	--	--	--
Exudate	Purulent	Scant/Watery	Stringy/White	--	Scant
Chemosis	++	+/-	++	+/-	+/-
Pseudomembrane	+/-	+/-	-	-	-
Papillae	+/-	-	+	-	+/-
Follicles	-	+	-	+	+
PAN	+	++	-	-	-
Pannus	-	-	-	-	+

III. **Bacterial Conjunctivitis**

  A. Acute: Etiology.

   1. Staph aureus is most common.
   2. Staph epidermidis.
   3. Strep pneumoniae, common in children.
   4. Strep pyogenes, forms pseudomembranes.
   5. H. influenza, common in children.
   6. Moraxella lacunata, can become a chronic infection.
   7. Neisseria gonorrhea, infection can produce bilateral conjunctivitis. Occurs in newborns from maternal genital tract. Usually apparent by days 2-4.

  B. Chronic Conjunctivitis. Staph. aureus is most common, associated with a concomitant blepharitis. Other agents include Proteus, Klebsiella, Serratia, E. coli. Moraxella lacunata can produce a blepharoconjunctivitis.

  C. Diagnosis.

   1. Conjunctival cultures.

C. Diagnosis.
   1. Conjunctival cultures.
      a. Should be obtained prior to use of topical anesthetics which reduce the yield of the culture.
      b. Moisten a sterile tip applicator and wipe the lid margins and conjunctival cul-de-sac. Plate on blood and chocolate agar and obtain gram stain.
      c. Cytologic features of conjunctivitis (Table 12-3).

Table 12-3.

Cell	bacterial	viral	allergic	toxic	TRIC
PMN	+	+	-	+	+
Lymphs	-	-	-	+	-
Plasma cells	-	-	-	-	+
Multi-nucleated cells	-	+	-	-	-

D. Treatment.
A. Clinical diagnosis alone. 10% sulfacetamide every 3-4 hours. Chloramphenicol or tobramycin drops are an alternative if H. influenza and Moraxella are suspected.
B. Local measures:
   a. Warm compresses.
   b. If blepharitis is involved, dandruff shampoo to scalp and eyelids.
   c. Steroid ointment to lid margins for 10-14 days decreases lid inflammation.
C. Suspected Neisseria infections.
   a. Topical tetracycline or bacitracin ointment qid in neonates and every 2 hours for two days followed by five times a day in adults.
   b. If smears or cultures confirm Neisseria, patient requires systemic antibiotics.

References

Crumley RL, ed. Common Problems of the Head and Neck Region. Philadelphia: W.B. Saunders Company, 1986.

Driscoll CE, et al, eds. Handbook of Family Practice. Chicago: Year Book Medical Publishers, 1986.

GLAUCOMA

I. **Definition**. An elevation in intraocular pressure significant enough to cause a loss of vision.

II. **Prevalence**. Two percent of Americans older than 35.

III. **Pathophysiology**
   A. Open angle glaucoma: results from resistance to flow through the trabecular meshwork.
   B. Closed angle glaucoma: peripheral iris covers the trabecular meshwork, preventing flow of aqueous humor.

IV. **Screening Methods**
   A. Tonometry: pressures greater than 21 mm Hg suggest glaucoma.
      1. Schiotz. Most practical for primary care physicians. Not as accurate as applanation tonometry.
      2. Applanation. More accurate. Requires more training. Hand held applanation devices may be available.
   B. Ophthalmoscopy.
      1. First change is vertical elongation of the cup, usually inferiorly.
      2. Later changes include increase in depth and width of the physiologic cup, nasal displacement of central retinal vessels, and progressive pallor of the optic nerve head.
      3. Asymmetry of the appearance of the right and left optic discs and cups may be a sign of early glaucoma.
   C. Visual fields.
      1. Visual field loss is silent and occurs first in the periphery.
      2. Automated perimetry is an effective screening method and is available to primary care physicians.

V. **Clinical Presentation**
   A. Open angle glaucoma. Asymptomatic until loss of vision has advanced significantly.
   B. Closed angle glaucoma. See Evaluation of the Red Eye.

VI. Management

A. Open angle:
  1. Management is primarily carried out by an ophthalmologist.
  2. Beta-blockers (Timolol): decrease aqueous humor production. Can have systemic side effects including heart block, heart failure.
  3. Epinephrine: decreased production of aqueous humor, may increase outflow. Usually no systemic side effects.
  4. Pilocarpine: contracts ciliary body, facilitates outflow.
  5. Laser trabeculoplasty and other surgical intervention used with medical management as necessary.

B. Acute angle closure glaucoma.
  1. Pilocarpine 2% drops. Use two drops every 15 min.
  2. Acetazolamide 500 mg IV to initiate therapy.
  3. Immediate consultation with ophthalmologist.

References

Crumley RL, ed. Common Problems of the Head and Neck Region. Philadelphia: W.B. Saunders Company, 1986.

Driscoll CE, et al, eds. Handbook of Family Practice. Chicago: Year Book Medical Publishers, 1986.

VERTIGO

I. Overview

A. "Dizziness" is a common symptom. Evaluation depends upon careful history. If patient describes sensation of moving/spinning/falling, then vertigo is present and evaluation must proceed for evidence of vestibular pathology. Main differential is between central and peripheral origin.

B. Differential diagnosis:
   1. Central:
      a. vertebral basilar insufficiency.
      b. multiple sclerosis.
      c. post-traumatic vertigo.
      d. seizure.
      e. migraine.
   2. Peripheral.
      a. motion sickness.
      b. Meniere's disease (labyrinthine hydrops).
      c. benign paroxysmal positional vertigo.
      d. labyrinthitis.
      e. acoustic neuroma.
      f. cervical vertigo.

C. Evaluation: peripheral vestibular disorders are characterized by severe spinning sensation, nausea with vomiting, and nystagmus. Nystagmus is either horizontal or rotatory. Peripheral disorders usually also exhibit tinnitus, change in hearing acuity. Central vertigo generally has less intense symptoms. Nystagmus may be present and may be horizontal, rotatory, or vertical. Vertical nystagmus indicates central lesion as does nystagmus that changes direction with position changes. Position testing (placing patient supine with left ear down, right ear down, and head hanging over end of table) can help differentiate peripheral from central. Peripheral disease is characterized by long latency period between attaining a position and the onset of symptoms (15-20 seconds), fatigability. Central lesions demonstrate a short latency period (or none), nonfatiguing.

II. Specific Disorders

A. Meniere's disease:

1. characterized by intermittent episodes of vertigo (usually severe enough to cause nausea, vomiting, diaphoresis), tinnitus, and decreased hearing acuity. Spells last from 20 minutes to 24 hours.
2. Treatment is with salt-restriction and thiazide diuretics. This will improve symptoms in about 75% of patients. Surgical options are available for treatment failures.

B. Benign paroxysmal positional vertigo.

1. Characterized by brief episodes (10-20 seconds) of vertigo in response to position changes. Generally there is no associated tinnitus or hearing loss. The vertigo does not recur until there is another change in position.
2. Treatment is with labyrinthine exercises--patients are instructed to assume the position that produces the vertigo as frequently as possible, which eventually results in central suppression.

C. Viral labyrinthitis.

1. Characterized by severe vertigo with nausea and vomiting following an upper respiratory infection. Nystagmus is present. Hearing acuity is not affected. Symptoms last for several days with gradual improvement. Generally there are no sequela.
2. Treatment is symptomatic with antiemetics, rehydration (sometimes hospitalization is required), and medications to suppress vertigo. These include meclizine 12.5 - 25 mg p.o. q 6 hr, or diazepam 2-4 mg p.o. t.i.d.

D. Acoustic neuroma.

1. Characterized by unilateral tinnitus and hearing loss, and vertigo. Unilateral neurosensory hearing loss will be present on exam. Audiometric brain stem evoked response will be delayed. CT scan should be obtained.

2. If acoustic neuroma is suspected, referral to otolaryngologist is indicated.

References

Crumley RL, ed. Common Problems of the Head and Neck Region. Philadelphia: W.B. Saunders Co., 1986.

Driscoll CE, *et al*, eds. Handbook of Family Practice. Chicago: Year Book Medical Publishers, 1986.

OTITIS MEDIA

I. **Pediatric Otitis**

   A. Children from birth to about age 5 are subject to middle ear infection by organisms different from those that affect older children and adults (see below). Children also have a higher frequency of ear infections (as many as 75% of children will have at least one ear infection by age 3). Organisms commonly involved include:

   - Hemophilus influenzae (usually type A or untypable; not type B).
   - Strep. pneumoniae.
   - Strep, group A.
   - Branhamella catarrhalis.
   - none (probably viral).
   - (in children 6 weeks of age or less there is an increased incidence of Staph aureus, E. coli, and Klebsiella).

   B. Clinical course: symptoms of irritability, otalgia (which may be suggested in young children by tugging at ears), fever will commonly present after a viral URI, during which congestion of the mucosal membranes results in dysfunction of the eustachian tube and development of inadequately aerated middle ear, which in turn provides a culture media adequate for the development of acute suppurative otitis media. After treatment, most children will have persistent middle ear effusions which will gradually resolve over the following weeks. Some recommend two weeks of prophylactic antibiotics for persistent middle ear effusion in children under two years of age because of the higher incidence of re-infection. The effusion will not respond with more rapid resolution to decongestants.

   C. Diagnosis; history will usually provide some of the features described above. Physical examination will demonstrate some or all of the following findings:

   - decreased mobility of the tympanic membrane (felt by many to be the most reliable indicator of otitis media)
   - hyperemia of the TM.

- bulging of the TM, usually from purulent exudate, with loss of landmarks--light reflex, umbo and short process of the malleus.
- perforation of the TM with purulent exudate in the external canal
- fever

It is absolutely essential to perform a thorough examination to rule out a concurrent infectious process (pneumonia, meningitis).

D. Treatment: standard treatment includes analgesics and antipyretics (acetaminophen, 10-15 mg/kg/dose), adequate hydration, and antibiotics for 10-14 days, directed at the common organisms.

1. Amoxicillin 40 mg/kg/day, divided t.i.d. This will cover the commonly involved organisms with the exception of beta-lactamase producing Hemophilus and Branhamella species. Well-tolerated, available in 125 mg/5ml and 250 mg/5ml oral suspensions, 250 mg chewable tablets, and capsules.

2. Trimethoprim-sulfamethoxazole oral suspension is dosed 1 ml/kg/day, divided b.i.d. (8 mg/kg of T and 40 mg/kg of S per day). Generally effective against the commonly involved organisms with the exception of some group A strep.

3. Erythromycin-sulfisoxazole oral suspension is dosed 50 mg/kg/day of erythromycin divided t.i.d. or q.i.d. Suspension has 200 mg/5ml of erythromycin. Effective against all of the commonly involved bacteria.

4. Cefaclor oral suspension dosed 40 mg/kg/day divided t.i.d. or b.i.d. Available in 125 mg/5ml, 250 mg/5ml, and 187/5 ml and 385/5 ml. Generally effective against all the commonly involved bacteria.

5. Amoxicillin/clavulanic acid, dosed the same as amoxicillin. Clavulanic acid inhibits beta-lactamase, thereby restoring amoxicillin's activity against otherwise resistant strains of Hemophilus and Branhamella.

E. Follow-up: ears should be rechecked at the end of the course of antibiotics to ensure resolution. Middle ear effusion can be expected. For unresolved otitis, consider switching to an antibiotic with coverage of resistant organisms (cefaclor, amoxicillin/clavulanic acid). Prophylaxis may be of some benefit in children with frequent episodes (>3 in 6 months). Trimethoprim/sulfa, amoxicillin, and sulfamethoxazole are commonly used at about half the recommended dose for acute otitis, given once daily for 1-3 months. Effectiveness of this is not clearly established. For multiple episodes or otitis that does not clear with adequate antibiotic therapy, consider referral to an otolaryngologist for possible myringotomy and ventilation tubes.

II. **Acute Otitis Media:** adult and older children

   A. Commonly involved organisms are group A Strep and Pneumococcus.

   B. Diagnosis: history will usually include otalgia, sensation of fullness or impaired hearing. Examination will reveal similar findings as in children.

   C. Treatment: since resistant organisms are much less likely, treatment with penicillin V or erythromycin is generally effective (250 mg q.i.d.).

III. **Serous Otitis**

   A. Characterized by the presence of mildly retracted TM with decreased mobility, clear middle ear effusion. History commonly includes recent URI or allergic/seasonal rhinitis, with sensation of ear fullness, occasionally tinnitus or hearing loss. Otalgia is usually not present.

   B. Diagnosis is based upon history as above, physical findings of dull, immobile eardrum with possible fluid level, abnormal Rinne and Weber testing indicating conductive hearing loss on affected side.

   C. Treatment: in children with definite bilateral hearing loss, should consider referral to otolaryngologist for myringotomy and tubes as prolonged hearing loss may have adverse affect on school performance. In adults or children without significant hearing loss, decongestants may be of some benefit if the serous otitis is due to viral URI. Antihistamines or nasal steroids may help if allergic rhinitis is underlying cause. Valsalva maneuvers (to "pop ears") known as the Toynbee maneuver, may re-establish proper eustachian tube function. If no improvement in about 2 months, consider referral to otolaryngologist.

References

Crumley RL, ed. <u>Common Problems of the Head and Neck Region</u>. Philadelphia: W.B. Saunders Co., 1986.

Driscoll CE, *et al*, eds. <u>Handbook of Family Practice</u>. Chicago: Year Book Medical Publishers, 1986.

PHARYNGITIS

I. **Etiology**

   A. Common organisms include "cold viruses" (adenovirus, rhinovirus), Epstein-Barr virus, Group A strep. Other organisms that have been identified as causing pharyngitis are Corynebacterium hemolyticum (most commonly seen in teenagers and young adults, may have associated scarlatiniform rash), Mycoplasma, Branhamella catarrhalis (55% of adults with laryngitis will have Branhamella involved), Neiserria gonorrhea and Chlamydia. Other causes to consider include sinusitis or rhinitis with posterior nasal drainage causing irritation of the pharynx.

   B. Evaluation.

   1. History should reveal associated viral URI symptoms of congestion, cough, headache/body ache, low-grade fever, or high fever, headache, abdominal pain as may be seen with strep pharyngitis. If not acute (symptoms longer than 10-14 days), evaluate for allergic rhinitis or sinusitis as cause.

   2. Physical exam should include evaluation for other causes of fever (pneumonia, meningitis). Tender anterior cervical adenopathy is asssociated with strep pharyngitis, although not reliably so. Posterior adenopathy suggests mononeucleosis. Lymphoid hyperplasia of the posterior pharynx is consistent with allergic disorders and viral pharyngitis. Exudate on the tonsils or pharynx can be associated with either bacterial or viral cause.

   3. Lab should include rapid test for Strep group A antigen unless there is another reason to treat with antibiotics (concurrent otitis, sinusitis, bronchitis). Even in this setting rapid strep test can be useful in choosing an antibiotic and for families with other children at home.

   C. Treatment for group A strep pharyngitis is with PCN-V, 50 mg/kg/day divided q.i.d., up to 250 mg q.i.d. Benzathine penicillin G can be used if compliance is of concern or for convenience, dosed 600,000 units IM for children less than 27 kgs, 1,200,000 units IM for all others. Erythromycin is an alterntive to penicillin, same dose. Oral treatment must be for 10 days. If Corynebacterium, Mycoplasma, or Branhamella are suspected because of associated clinical features, erythromycin should be used.

II. **Complications**

A. Recurrent tonsillitis (>3/yr) is a relative indication for tonsillectomy. Pharyngeal or peritonsillar abscess is an indication for tonsillectomy.

B. Patients with documented recurrent strep infections should be tested post treatment for possible carrier state. If present, this can be eliminated by use of penicillin (as for acute treatment) and rifampin, dosed 20 mg/kg (not to exceed 600 mg/day), given once daily for four days.

References

Crumley RL, ed. Common Problems of the Head and Neck Region. Philadelphia: W.B. Saunders Co., 1986.

Driscoll CE, et al, eds. Handbook of Family Practice. Chicago: Year Book Medical Publishers, 1986.

SINUSITIS

I. Acute Sinusitis
   A. Paranasal sinuses are the maxillary, sphenoid, ethmoid, and frontal sinuses. Each is a paired set with ostia providing communication with the nasal cavity. Acute infection of a sinus generally occurs as a complication of a viral URI. The inflammation of the respiratory mucosa in response to a viral infection can result in obstruction of the sinus ostia, allowing build up of mucosal secretions and overgrowth by bacteria. Commonly involved organisms are:
      - Pneumococcus.
      - Hemophilus.
      - Staph aureus.
      - Anaerobic streptococci.
      - Branhamella catarrhalis.
   B. Diagnosis:
      1. History will generally reveal recent URI, sensation of pressure or pain in the face over the sinus, pain radiating into teeth (with maxillary sinusitis), purulent nasal discharge or postnasal drainage, headache, fever. Patient may relate that symptoms worsen with placing head in dependent position.
      2. Physical examination may reveal a purulent discharge from the area of the sinus ostia or in the nasopharynx. There may be tenderness over the affected sinus. Transillumination of the sinuses can be useful but care must be taken in interpretation of findings.
      3. X-ray findings include mucosal thickening, air-fluid levels, and opacification of the sinus. In general, x-rays are indicated if complications are already present or if symptoms/signs fail to improve with treatment. Usually history and physical examination are adequate for diagnosis.
   C. Treatment:
      1. Antibiotics: should be used 14-21 days.
         a. amoxicillin, 50-100 mg/kg/day divided t.i.d., not to exceed 500 mg/dose.

Sinusitis

      b. erythromycin, 250-500 mg q.i.d.

      c. trimethoprim/sulfamethoxazole, double strength tablets, one b.i.d.

      d. cefaclor, 50-100 mg/kg/day, divided t.i.d., not to exceed 500 mg/dose.

    2. Topical decongestants:

      a. Afrin nasal spray t.i.d. for up to three days.

      b. Otrivin nasal spray t.i.d. for up to three days.

      c. hot water vapor inhalation as often as possible.

D. Management and complications: failure of the acute sinusitis to resolve with oral antibiotics and topical decongestants is indication for x-ray evaluation and lavage of the affected sinuses. If this does not produce improvement, surgical drainage is indicated. Extension of the infectious process may result in facial cellulitis, orbital cellulitis, osteomyelitis, intracranial infection. If these occur, hospitalization for intravenous antibiotics and surgical drainage is indicated.

II. **Chronic Sinusitis**

A. Distinct clinical entity characterized by chronic obstruction of sinus drainage with edema and thickening of the sinus mucosa, resulting in chronic congestion, headache or facial pain present for weeks to months.

B. Diagnosis: x-rays are quite useful in this setting to rule out acute sinusitis and evaluate for potential causes such as neoplasm or abscess.

C. Treatment is based upon the underlying pathology; allergic rhinitis, neoplasm, etc.

References

Crumley RL, ed. <u>Common Problems of the Head and Neck Region</u>. Philadelphia: W.B. Saunders Co., 1986.

Driscoll CE, *et al,* eds. <u>Handbook of Family Practice</u>. Chicago: Year Book Medical Publishers, 1986.

RHINITIS

I. **Allergic**

   A. Characterized by nasal congestion, clear discharge, sneezing in response to exposure to specific allergen. Commonly is seasonal due to pollens, spores, but may also be perennial due to house dust, danders. May have associated symptoms of allergic conjunctivitis or asthma. Allergic rhinitis may precipitate episodes of asthma. Relatively strong familial tendency.

   B. Diagnosis:
   1. History will generally reveal the symptoms as above. Care should be taken to elicit history of possible allergens.
   2. Examination may reveal boggy, pale nasal mucosa. Wright's (or other) stain of nasal smear will frequently show eosinophils. Skin testing may be done although will generally not be necessary for obvious seasonal allergy.

   C. Treatment:
   1. Avoidance of allergens as possible, especially house dust and animal danders.
   2. Topical steroids--treatment of choice for allergic rhinitis without other allergic symptoms. Beclomethasone (Vancenase/Beconase) and flunisolide (Nasalide) are available as metered dose nasal inhalers. Typical regimen is burst and taper to maintenance with one puff each nostril four times daily times three days, then one puff each nostril three times daily times three days, then one puff each nostril twice daily. Some individuals may be able to reduce dose to one puff each nostril once daily. The aqueous spray preparations may be better tolerated.
   3. Antihistamines--mainstay of treatment. Can be inexpensive, and generally quite effective. Sedation is main problem. Less sedating antihistamines such as Seldane are somewhat less effective. Chlorpheniramine remains as effective as any other antihistamine and is the least expensive. Generally, patients can gradually increase dose to that necessary to con-

Rhinitis

trol symptoms without inhibitory adverse effects. Higher doses of chlorpheniramine can be given twice daily--sustained release preparations are not required.

4. Immunotherapy for desensitization is an alternative, especially for those with serious allergic asthma.

II. Vasomotor

A. Characterized by exaggerated response of nasal mucosa to normal irritants such as weather change (cold, moisture), irritants (smoke). Symptoms are similar to those of allergic rhinitis, although congestion tends to be most prominent and sneezing or itching less common.

B. Diagnosis is generally indicated by the history, with lack of physical findings to suggest allergic rhinitis. Patient is likely to have secondary chronic rhinitis medicamentosa.

C. Treatment:
1. Education regarding the nature of the disorder and the importance of not using topical decongestant and/or antihistamine sprays.
2. If symptoms are severe enough to warrant treatment, systemic decongestants and/or antihistamines may be tried. Efficacy is not high. Topical nasal steroids can also be used--these do not cause rhinitis medicamentosa.

III. Chronic Rhinitis Medicamentosa

A. Rhinitis caused by medications, usually topical decongestants which produce a rebound vasodilatation after a few days use. Several systemic medications can also cause nasal congestion, including several antihypertensives, some major tranquilizers, estrogens.

B. Diagnosis is by history. Patient may have vasomotor rhinitis underlying the rhinitis medicamentosa.

C. Treatment: discontinue use of topical nasal spray decongestants.

References

Crumley RL, ed. <u>Common Problems of the Head and Neck Region</u>. Philadelphia: W.B. Saunders Co., 1986.

Driscoll CE, *et al*, eds. <u>Handbook of Family Practice</u>. Chicago: Year Book Medical Publishers, 1986.

13/ DERMATOLOGY

John E. Littler, M.D.

ACNE

I. **Etiology:** Believed due to excess sebum secretion with occluded follicular orifices and accumulation of anaerobic bacteria, primarily Propionibacterium acnes. Commonly begins in adolescence with stimulation of the sebaceous glands by sex hormones. May occur later in life due to cosmetic use or from systemic steroids. Males affected more frequently than females.

II. **Types of Acne and Their Treatment**

   A. Comedonal.
   1. Characterized by whiteheads and blackheads (closed and open comedones) with minimal inflammatory component. May have small cysts and pustules.
   2. Treatment is topical and takes a minimum of two weeks to show improvement. Essential to educate patient regarding the expected time course for treatment results and the importance of avoiding attempts to extrude blackheads or superficial pustules which may result in deeper, potentially scarring lesions:
      a. Benzoyl peroxide, available in various strengths and lotions or gels. Should be applied as frequently as required to just produce some drying or even scaling, but not irritation.
      b. Vitamin A (Retin-A gel or lotion), again applied often enough to produce dryness and scaling, but a minimum of irritation. Quite effective for acne without a significant inflammatory component.

   B. Papulopustular.
   1. Characterized by a significant inflammatory component with inflamed papules and pustules present in addition to the comedones.
   2. Treatment is with the above listed topical agents and antibiotics. As the inflammatory component

decreases with treatment, antibiotics are tapered and discontinued.

    a. For less severe cases, topical erythromycin, clindamycin or tetracycline may be used.

    b. Systemic antibiotics may be required with more severe cases. Tetracycline or erythromycin are used, 500 to 1,000 mg daily initially. This is continued for at least 6 weeks before treatment failure can be determined. With significant improvement, the dose can be gradually tapered and eventually discontinued.

C. Nodulocystic acne.
   1. Characterized by comedones, inflammatory papules/pustules, and deep, inflamed, nodules and cysts. Often results in scarring.
   2. Treatment:
      a. Topical drying agents (benzoyl peroxide, vitamin A) as above.
      b. Antibiotics (systemic) as above.
      c. Intralesional corticosteroids, triamcinolone 5 mg/ml, for cysts. Inject enough to cause the cyst to blanch. Some recommend needle drainage of the cyst first, although this is probably not necessary.
      d. Oral isotretinoin (Accutane) is effective but many feel this is most appropriately supervised by physicians with experience in its use.

Reference

Rakel RE and Conn HF, eds. Textbook of Family Practice, Third edition. Philadelphia: W.B. Saunders Company, 1984.

URTICARIA

I. **Acute**
   A. Characterized by white or red wheals which are transient, pruritic. May be associated with angioedema--swelling of the subcutaneous or submucosal tissue. Either of these may be the first sign of anaphylaxis.
   B. Causes include drug allergy (especially penicillins), foods (shellfish, nuts, citrus fruits), pollens, infections, physical agents (pressure, heat, cold).
   C. Treatment:
      1. Emergent treatment of anaphylaxis or airway obstruction (see chapter 1).
      2. Subcutaneous epinephrine may be used for initial treatment of severe urticaria or angioedema. Effect, although dramatic, is of short duration.
      3. Antihistamines: diphenhydramine or hydroxyzine hydrochloride. Both available for IM injection, as capsules, and as elixirs. Hydroxyzine is probably somewhat more effective, dosed 25 to 50 mg q 6 hours.
      4. H2 blockers may be used in addition to the above listed H1 blockers for severe or refractory cases, for example, cimetidine 300 mg q 6 hours.
      5. Do not use systemic steroids.

II. **Chronic**
   A. Urticaria/angioedema that persists beyond 6 weeks or recurs multiple times. Often times this is not IgE mediated and usual medications are not as helpful.
   B. Etiologies include idiopathic (common), food/drug/physical agents as above, infections, collagen-vascular disease, hereditary disorder, thyroid disorder.
   C. Evaluation is not likely to reveal a cause unless history, including family history, and physical have suggested a specific cause. Screening labs should include CBC, sed rate, screening chemistries to include liver and thyroid function, and UA. Other more specific tests are obtained as indicated from the history and physical.

D. Treatment:
    1. Avoidance of any identified inciting agent.
    2. Antihistamines as above. Other options for H1 blockers include cyproheptadine 4-8 mg tid, Terfenidine, and astimazole.
    3. H2 blockers may be of some benefit as additional measures.
    4. Tricyclic antidepressants, especially amitriptyline, are potent antihistamines and may be used if the above measures fail.

ECZEMA

I. **Definition**: a superficial inflammatory condition of the skin. Severe acute cases may include vesiculation. Otherwise characterized by erythema, pruritis, crusting or scaling. Chronic cases may become lichenified.

II. **Types**: may be caused by contact with irritants of many different types (producing damage either directly or by delayed hypersensitivity reaction), or by "endogenous" factors.

   A. Endogenous:
   1. Seborrheic: affects scalp, face (especially eyebrows, nasolabial folds). Characterized by scaling, sometimes pruritis.
   2. Nummular: generally seen on extremities, characterized by raised, round, erythematous lesions that are usually scaly, sometimes pruritic.
   3. Atopic: seen in young children, usually with personal or family history of allergies/asthma. Often improves after age 4. Tends to affect the face, extremities (especially antecubital and popliteal fossae). Characterized by erythema and lichenification.
   4. Dyshidrotic: characterized by small vesicles on the palms or soles and between digits.

   B. Contact: many different types of compounds can cause eczematous reactions, including soaps, cosmetics, topical medications, chemicals used in manufacturing clothing/gloves/shoes, metal compounds. Distribution of lesions and careful history may identify the source. Patch testing with common contact allergens may be helpful if source cannot be identified.

III. **Basic Principles of Treatment**

   A. Avoidance of causative or contributing agents.
   B. Drying agents, such as Burow's solution of dilute acetic acid, for oozing or heavily vesiculated lesions.
   C. Topical corticosteroids. On face or intertriginous areas avoid fluorinated steroids.
   D. Anti-pruritics as needed.

CONTACT DERMATITIS

I. **Contact Dermatitis**: An inflammatory process of the skin characterized by erythema, vesicles, edema, crusting and scaling. Often quite pruritic. Initiated by contact of the skin with particular substances.

   A. Poison ivy/oak/sumac:

   1. Very common cause of contact dermatitis. Oleoresin from the plants is precipitating agent. Primary exposure results in characteristic rash after several days. Subsequent exposures will take 12-48 hours to produce the rash. Characteristic is linear groupings of vesicles on exposed areas. More severe reactions may include puffiness of the eyes and face, and genitalia. New lesions may appear throughout the course and are not due to scratching the initial lesions but rather to systemic sensitization.

   2. Treatment: topical treatment is indicated for less severe cases.

      a. Wet to dry soaks of astringent solutions (such as Burow's solution, dilute acetic acid which can be prepared 1 part white vinegar to 10 parts water) for weeping areas.

      b. Potent topical steroids such as 0.1-0.5% triamcinolone, 0.25% dexamethasone.

      c. Antipruritics may be of some benefit (diphenhydramine, hydroxyzine).

      d. For severe cases with involvement of a significant portion of the skin, large areas of bullae, or swelling of the face or genitalia, oral corticosteroids are very effective. Course should be at least 2 weeks (shorter course of steroid may result in rebound flare), with initial dose of prednisone 60 mg q day, then tapered over 2-3 weeks.(Example; 60 mg qd x 1 week; then 30 mg qd x 1 week, then 20 mg qd x 1 week.)

   B. Other causes of contact dermatitis may include rubber, perfumes, nickel, some textiles. History is essential in determining the precipitating agent as primary treatment is avoidance. Patch testing with suspected materials may confirm offending agent. Topical steroids and drying solutions as above are generally adequate for treatment.

DECUBITUS ULCERS

I. **Overview**

Decubitus ulcers result from pressure on soft tissues, usually overlying bony prominences, because of prolonged immobility. The pressure results in ischemic necrosis of the soft tissues with ulceration. Most common sites are over the sacrum, malleoli, greater trochanters and ischia.

II. **Clinical Presentation**
   A. Predisposing factors:
      1. Immobility due to some type of physical (cast, splint,) or physiologic (paralysis) restraint.
      2. Diminished sensation.
      3. Poor peripheral circulation.
      4. Poor nutritional status.
   B. Stages in development:
      1. Erythema of skin without loss of integrity of cutaneous structures or underlying tissues.
      2. Erythema of skin with blistering and desquamation, edema, occasionally induration.
      3. Necrotic skin with exposure of underlying tissues.
      4. Necrosis through cutaneous structures and involving fat or muscle. May eventually extend to bone.
      5. Secondary infection may occur with extension of the destructive process to deeper and surrounding tissues.

III. **Treatment**
   A. Prevention by maintaining adequate nutrition, cleanliness and dryness, frequent repositioning of patients at risk, and frequent skin inspection.
   B. Early lesions: removal of pressure by use of padding and appropriate positioning, careful attention to skin care with gentle massage to stimulate circulation. Do not use heating pads.
   C. Ulcerations: necrotic tissue may require careful debridement, either surgically or with hydrophilic beads or cleansing solutions. Wet to dry dressings q 6 to 8 hours. If

evidence of cellulitis is present, systemic antibiotics will be required. If wound fails to show signs of granulating in, split-thickness grafting may be required.

D. Deep ulcers with involvement of fat or muscle: surgical debridement is required. Closure with a full thickness skin or skin-muscle flap may be required.

Reference

Holvey DN and Talbott JH, eds. <u>The Merck Manual of Diagnosis & Therapy, 12th edition</u>. New Jersey: Merck & Company, 1972.

SKIN CANCERS AND PRE-CANCERS

I. **Pigmented Lesions:**

   A. Congenital nevi: present at birth or within first few days of life. Evidence suggests that there may be increased risk for malignant degeneration. These nevi may be sensitive to sex hormones and change in size or character at time of puberty. Removal before that time may be advisable.

   B. Common nevi: classified as lentigo (flat, uniformly pigmented), junctional (flat to slightly elevated, brown to black), compound (dark, slight to greatly elevated), intradermal, and halo. Generally appear during childhood and adolescence. Most malignant melanomas do not arise from pre-existing nevi. Removal for histological examination is indicated for:
   - sudden enlargement.
   - irregular color change, especially blue, red or white.
   - bleeding, ulceration, inflammation, pain or itching.

   Should be removed by simple excision, unless too large. Then biopsy is indicated.

   C. Malignant melanoma: malignancy of melanocyte origin; may arise anywhere in the body that melanocytes exist. Lesions that should be biopsied (by simple excision) include those that demonstrate the characteristics listed above, any pigmented lesion with variegated colors, irregular surface, or irregular borders. For adequate histological diagnosis, biopsy should be full thickness with a small border of normal appearing surrounding skin. Depth of invasion is the primary determinant of prognosis.

II. **Lesions Related to Sun Exposure**

   A. Actinic keratoses: slightly erythematous, scaly, sometimes tender papules with irregular borders occurring on sun exposed areas--forehead, cheeks, backs of hands. Essentially a squamous carcinoma in situ, with progression occurring only very slowly (unless on lip or mouth). Treatment is cryotherapy. Recurrences and new lesions are common as they are the result of years of sun damage and indefinite follow-up is indicated. Patients should be instructed to use sun screen.

B. Squamous cell carcinoma: erythematous, indurated, scaly or crusted, nodule or papule. May ulcerate. Very slow to progress unless on lip or mouth. Treatment consists of biopsy for diagnosis, then wide excision or excision by Moh's procedure. Careful, indefinite follow-up required.

C. Basal cell carcinoma: usually small, shiny firm nodules. Sometimes ulcerated, commonly with waxy appearance, central umbilication, and telangiectasias. Treatment consists of biopsy of suspicious lesions, then local excision/electrodessication/curettage or Moh's procedure. Follow-up required indefinitely.

Reference

Holvey DN and Talbott JH, eds. The Merck Manual of Diagnosis & Therapy, 12th edition. New Jersey: Merck & Company, 1972.

14/ NEUROLOGY

Mark J. Mabee, M.D.

HEADACHE

Headache is a common presenting complaint which need not be a diagnostic dilemma. Thorough history is the key to making the appropriate diagnosis.

I. **Etiologies.**

   Trauma, infection, vasospasm, increased intracranial pressure, tumor, subarachnoid hemorrhage, glaucoma, muscle contraction, inflammatory, hypertension, sinusitis, drugs, temporomandibular joint syndrome, depression, psychogenic.

II. **Clinical Features** (Table 14-1)

III. **Treatment**
   A. Muscle Contraction.
      1. Aspirin, acetaminophen in adequate doses.
      2. Nonsteroidal anti-inflammatories (NSAIDS) for pain relief and anti-inflammatory effect on muscles.
      3. Neck massage and local heat.
      4. Biofeedback and relaxation techniques.
      5. Avoid narcotics.
   B. Migraine.
      1. Acute.
         a. Aspirin or acetaminophen.
         b. Ergot derivatives (effective also in aborting and prevention).
      - Ergotamine: 2 mg SL at start of attack, then 2 mg q 30 min., up to 6 mg in 24 hrs and 12 mg in 1 week.
      - Cafergot: 1-2 mg po at start, 1-2 mg po q 30 min. Max 6 mg per 24 hr. and 12 mg per week.
      - Dihydroergotamine: 1 mg IM at start, then 1 mg q hr up to total of 3 mg. If IV give 1 mg initially, then 1 mg

in one hour. Prochlorperazine may be given 5 mg IV immediately prior to DHE.

- Midrin: 2 capsules initially, then 1 capsule q 1 hr up to 5 in 12 hours.

    c. Narcotics (The cautious use of IM narcotic with an adjunctive agent for nausea/anxiety may be required. Essential to monitor the frequency with which this modality is used.)

- Meperidine 50-100 mg IM with
- Promethazine 25-50 mg IM or
- Hydroxyzine 25-50 mg IM or
- Chlorpramazine 25-50 mg IM. (Thorazine has been used as a single agent for acute treatment, dose of 1 mg/kg IM, or 0.4 mg/kg IV.)

2. Prophylaxis.

    a. Propranolol: 20-60 mg po qid.

    b. Verapamil: 240 mg po q day.

    c. Amitriptyline: 50-100 mg q hs or divided bid.

    d. NSAIDS.

    e. Methysergide: 2 mg po q day divided qid, retroperitoneal fibrosis may occur with chronic treatment. Must not be used longer than 6 months without a 2-3 week drug holiday.

    f. Life Style - foods, chemicals, relaxation techniques.

3. Status Migraine - migraine continues > 24 hours. There is quite often a sterile inflammation around the affected vessel. The use of steroids may hasten the resolution of prolonged migraine.

    a. Dexamethasone (Decadron-LA) 16mg IM.

Table 14-1. Clinical Features of Headaches

Type	Location	Age and Sex	Clinical Characteristics	Interval	Aggravating Factors	Associated Features
Common migraine	Frontotemporal, unilateral, sometimes bilateral	Children, young to middle-aged adults, both sexes, female > male	Throbbing and/or dull ache; worse behind one eye or ear, nausea or vomiting. Becomes generalized	Irregular interval, weeks to months. Tends to disappear in middle age and during pregnancy	Bright light, noise, tension, alcohol. Dark room and sleep Scalp sensitive, pressure helps relieve	Nausea in some cases
Classic migraine	Same as above	Same as above	Same as above; visual prodrome common.	Same as above	Same as above	Blindness and scintillating lights, unilateral numbness, disturbed speech, vertigo, confusion
Cluster	Orbital, temporal, unilateral	Adolescent and adult males (80-90%)	Intense, nonthrobbing pain, usually nocturnal	Nightly for several weeks to months; recurrence: years later	Alcohol in some	Lacrimation, congested eye
Tension headaches	Generalized	Children, adolescents, and adults, both sexes	Pressure (nonthrobbing); tightness, aching	One or more periods of months to years	Fatigue and strain	Depression, nervousness, anxiety, insomnia

Adapted from Petersdorf RG, et al, eds. Harrison's Principles of Internal Medicine, 10th edition. New York: McGraw Hill, 1983.

DEMENTIA

Dementia is a loss of intellectual abilities sufficiently severe to interfere with social or occupational functioning. Impairment in memory, abstract thinking, judgment, personality change with clear consciousness are characteristic. A combination of the preceding impairments occur with insidious onset and a uniformly progressive deteriorating course.

I. Etiologies

   A. Treatable Causes: tumor, normal pressure hydrocephalus, subdural hematoma, vitamin B12 deficiency, liver disease, depression, syphilis, fungal meningitis, toxins (bromide), uremia, myxedema, Cushing's disease, thiamine deficiency, CO poisoning, congestive heart failure, medications (commonly implicated drugs: cimetidine, propranolol, digoxin, theophylline), hypoxia, hypertension, hypercalcemia, lung cancer, subacute bacterial endocarditis.

   B. Nontreatable Causes: Alzheimer's disease, arteriosclerotic (multi-infarct), Jakob-Creutzfeldt disease, Huntington's chorea, Niemann-Pick disease.

   E. Differential Diagnosis Mnemonic.
   - Depression.
   - Endocrine (T3, T4, TSH).
   - Metabolic (electrolytes, calcium, PO4, Mg, BUN, Creatinine, SGOT, Alk Phos, LDH, or Panel).
   - ETOH (+ meds and other drugs).
   - Nutritional (B12, Folate).
   - Trauma, tumor (CT head).
   - Infection (CBC, UA, CXR, VDRL) Inflammation (ESR).
   - Alzheimer's (Psychometric Testing, EEG)

II. Evaluation

   A. History - family members helpful.

   B. Physical Exam - with complete neurological exam.

   C. Mental Status Exam - See Mini Mental Status Exam.

   D. Lab (Table 14-2):

III. **Treatment**

No consistently effective agents available at this time. Treat specific causes if possible.

Table 14-1. Evaluation of Dementia

Initial Studies	Additional studies (as indicated)
Urine drug screen for sedatives	Urinalysis
Complete blood count	Chest x-ray
Psychometrics	Electrocardiogram
SMA-20*	Drug levels (barbiturates, bromides)
Electrolytes (Na, K, CO_2, Cl, Ca, PO_4, Mg)	Heavy metal screens (blood, urine)
Blood area nitrogen/creatinine	Lumbar puncture
Liver function tests	Arteriography
T_3, T_4, TSH**	Serum cortisol
Erythrocyte sedimentation rate	Blood cultures
B_{12}, folate	Arterial blood gases
Serologic test for syphilis	
Electroencephalogram	
Computed tomographic scan	

* Sequential multiple analyses of 20 chemical constituents.

** Serum triiodothyronine, serum thyroxine, serum thyroid-stimulating hormone.

Adapted from Black KS and Hughes PL. Alzheimer's disease: making the diagnosis. American Family Physician 36(5):199, November 1987.

Reference

Weiner HL and Levitt LP, eds. <u>Neurology for the House Officer, 3rd edition</u>. Baltimore/London: Williams and Wilkins, 1983.

MENINGITIS

I. **Acute Bacterial Meningitis**
   A. Etiology: several bacteria can cause meningitis in adults, including meningococcus, pneumococcus, Group A strep., and others. Predisposing factors include compromised immune status or parameningeal focus of infection such as sinusitis, otitis, mastoiditis.
   B. Clinical presentation: ranges from rapidly progressing septic picture with development of seizures and coma over 24 hours or less to more slowly progressing illness over several days.
      1. Fever, headache, neck stiffness, nausea and vomiting are characteristic symptoms.
      2. Mental status changes are usually present and progress from irritability to confusion, stupor, and coma. Physical exam will also reveal evidence of meningeal irritation with stiff neck, Brudzinski's sign (flexion of the neck produces involuntary flexion of knees) and Kernig's sign (resistance to straightening knees from thigh-flexed position).
   C. Evaluation: if history and physical examination suggest the possibility of meningitis, lumbar puncture should be performed. If papilledema or focal neurological signs (other than cranial nerve deficits) are present, CT scan should be obtained. If a clinical diagnosis of meningitis is made, treatment should be started immediately and should not await the results of laboratory exams. Lumbar puncture, CBC with diff, blood cultures, electrolytes if indicated. CSF should be sent for cell count, gram stain, culture, glucose and protein. Latex agglutination for meningococcus, H. influenzae, and pneumococcus can be obtained on CSF, serum, or urine. Organisms on gram stain or CSF white cell count of 100/ml or more with predominant neutrophils indicate acute bacterial meningitis. CSF glucose is commonly decreased and protein elevated.
   D. Treatment: initial recommendations (adjust according to cultures/sensitivities):

1. In an adult without immunocompromise, the most likely organisms are meningococcus, pneumococcus and Group A strep. All of these are generally quite sensitive to penicillin G, 50,000 units/kg q 4 hours.
2. In an immunocompromised or elderly patient, other organisms may be involved and empiric therapy would include 3rd generation cephalosporin with good pseudomonas coverage (ceftazidime) and an antipseudomonal aminoglycoside such as gentamicin or tobramycin.

II. **Aseptic (viral) Meningitis**
   A. Etiology: inflammation of the meninges without evidence of bacterial involvement. Organisms that have been associated with viral meningitis include adenoviruses, CMV, EBV, enteroviruses, herpes simplex viruses, and others. There may be associated encephalitis.
   B. Clinical presentation: essentially the same as with acute bacterial meningitis, but tends to be more slowly progressive over several days. Fever, headache, stiff neck, nausea/vomiting.
   C. Evaluation: is the same as with bacterial meningitis. CSF shows elevated WBC but usually not above a few hundred/ml. Predominantly lymphocytes. Glucose is normal or only slightly decreased.
   D. Treatment:
      1. If uncertain of diagnosis and acute bacterial meningitis suspected, hospitalize and begin antibiotic treatment as above.
      2. Supportive treatment including adequate hydration. If adequately hydrated and capable party available at home to observe, may discharge with appropriate instructions regarding signs of progression or complication.

Reference

Mills J, *et al*, eds. <u>Current Emergency Diagnosis and Treatment, 2nd edition</u>. Los Altos: Lange, 1985.

SEIZURES

Epilepsy is the state of recurrent seizures. A seizure is the outward manifestation of aberrant electrical activity in almost any part of the brain (cerebral, subcortical, cerebellar). Types of seizure activity range from tonic-clonic to absence, and may be simple or complex.

I. **Etiology**
   A. Causes: Trauma (subdural/epidural hematoma, contusion), neoplasm, cerebrovascular accident, congenital, fever, anoxia, hypoxia, epileptic drug withdrawal, infection (meningitis, abscess, granuloma, encephalitis), toxins (drugs, ETOH, CO, lead, mercury), Allergy, Subarachnoid hemorrhage, thrombus, hypertension, metabolic--nutritional (electrolytes, glucose, PKU, B vitamins), A-V malformations, hereditary, degenerative, idiopathic.
   B. Common Causes by Age.
      1. 0-20 - Congenital.
      2. 20-35 - Trauma.
      3. 35-50 - Tumor.
      4. 50 - CVA

II. **Diagnosis**
   A. Based mainly on history. The onset, character, duration, and course are usually characteristic for a particular seizure disorder. Classification and common clinical features as below (Table 14-3).
   B. Ancillary Methods.
      1. EEG.
      2. Lab: Directed by history, but may include CBC, UA, electrolytes, BUN, calcium, glucose, SGOT, alk phos, bilirubin, toxin screen, blood alchol, antiepileptic medication levels.
      3. Consider lumbar puncture.
      4. CT of Head (if indicated).

III. Treatment

A. Directed by Seizure Type (Table 14-4).

Table 14-3. Classification of Epileptic Seizures in Adults

	Type of Seizure	Common Clinical Features
Partial or Focal	Simple partial (consciousness not impaired): Motor signs only, sensory symptoms present, autonomic phenomena present, psychic symptoms present	Focal motor or sensory disturbances (Jacksonian epilepsy)
	Complex partial (consciousness impaired): Simple onset, then impaired consciousness, impaired consciousness at onset, partial seizures evolving to generalized seizures	Automatisms; bizarre behavior; visceral, olfactory, or gustatory auras
Generalized	Absence	Brief loss of awareness; staring; blinking; little or no motor activity
	Myoclonic	Isolated clonic jerks, often evoked by sensory stimulus; common in degenerative and metabolic brain disease
	Clonic Tonic Tonic-clonic	Generalized major motor convulsions; loss of consciousness; postictal depression of cerebral function
	Atonic	Brief loss of consciousness and postural muscle tone
Continual	Status epilepticus	Continual seizures; incomplete recovery between attacks; may be generalized or partial

Adapted from Rubenstein E and Federman DD, eds. Scientific American Medicine, Volume 2. New York: Scientific American Inc., 1989.

Table 14-4. Treatment of Seizures

Type of Seizure	Drug of Choice	Alternative
Primary Generalized Tonic-Clonic (Grand Mal)	Carbamazepine Phenytoin Valproate	Phenobarbital Primidone
Partial, Including Secondarily Generalized	Carbamazepine Phenytoin	Phenobarbital Primidone
Absence (Petit Mal)	Ethosuximide Valproate	Clonazepam

Adapted from Abramowicz M, ed. The Medical Letter on Drugs and Therapeutics. 31(783), January 13, 1989.

IV. **Status Epilepticus**

Status Epilepticus is a true medical emergency. Prompt treatment is essential to prevent brain damage and possible death. Definition: continuous seizures lasting greater than 30 minutes with impaired consciousness; prolonged absence; or consciousness intact, but prolonged partial activity.

A. Treatment Protocol.

1. 0-5 min seizure activity.

- ABCs.
- Oral airway and Oxygen if needed.
- History, neurological and physical exam.
- Draw blood for Antiepileptic drug levels, glucose, BUN, electrolytes, metabolic screen, drug screen, ABGs.

2. 6-9 min seizure activity.

- IV of normal saline.
- Give 25 gm. glucose and B vitamins.

3. 10-30 min seizure activity.

- Phenytoin 20 mg/kg IV at rate not greater than 50 mg/min. (ONLY in normal saline solution).
- Monitor EKG and Blood Pressure.
- Diazepam 10-20 mg IV if convulsions during phenytoin infusion.

4. 31-60 min seizure activity.
- If seizures persist, phenobarbital 10 mg/kg at 100 mg/min IV.
5. 1 hour seizure activity.
- If seizures persist, barbiturate coma, general anesthesia

CEREBROVASCULAR DISEASE

Stroke is the third leading cause of death in the U.S. Fortunately, the overall incidence of stroke is declining with increased attention the risk factors (HTN). Cerebral ischemia may result in a transient or permanent neurological deficit.

I. **Definitions**
   A. Transient Ischemic Attacks (TIAs): Neurologic symptoms or deficits clearing in < 24 hours.
   B. Reversible Ischemic Neurological Deficit (RIND): A neurologic deficit which persists > 24 hours, but < 7 days.
   C. Stroke.
      1. Progressing ("In Evolution"): Progression of increasing neurologic deficits.
      2. Completed: Stable neurologic deficit, which may show some improvement over the next few months without complete resolution.

II. **Etiologies**

   Hypertension, embolus, intracranial hemorrhage, tumor, complicated migraine, sepsis, atherosclerosis (thrombosis), oral contraceptives.

III. **Diagnosis**
   A. History and Physical.
      1. Look at onset, duration, pattern of deficit.
      2. Search for embolic sources (recent MI, Hx of drug abuse, valvular disease, carotid stenosis, atrial fibrillation).
      3. Thorough neurological exam to determine location of lesion.
         a. Carotid circulation lesions: Produce contralateral deficits (hemiparesis, hemisensory loss, homonymous hemianopsia).
         b. Vertebral-basilar circulation lesions: Produce deficits in occipital region and brainstem. "Drop Attacks" common.

- Brainstem symptoms: Vertigo, nystagmus, diplopia, ataxia, sensory loss, hoarseness, dysphagia, hearing loss, weakness.
- Occipital cortical symptoms: Homonymous visual field deficit.

B. Ancillary Studies.

1. CT Scan: Intracerebral hemorrhage seen well immediately, infarction best seen after 36 hours. Useful to exclude tumor, abcess, subdural hematoma, subarachnoid hemorrhage.
2. Lumbar Puncture: Primarily performed to identify infective etiologies (meningitis, endocarditis).
3. Lab: CBC + diff, ESR, glucose, electrolytes.
4. Chest x-ray, ECG. Atrial arrhythmias, including atrial fibrillation, are common in the setting of stroke and may not be cause but rather result of stroke.

IV. Treatment

A. Anticoagulation: Indicated specifically for cardiac thrombus, continue as long as source exists. Should not be used in setting of hemorrhagic stroke or hypertensive crisis. Many recommend anticoagulator of all non-hemorrhagic strokes if not contraindicated.

1. Acutely: Heparin 5,000 to 10,000 units bolus, then 1,000 to 2,000 units/hr IV pump. PTT 1.5 to 2.0 times the control. Check PTT and adjust every 4 hrs until steady state, then daily.
2. Oral Therapy: Warfarin 10 to 15 mg po q day x 3-5 days, then 2-15 mg as daily maintainence dosage. Dosage based on PT at 1.5-2.5 times control depending on exact indication. Check daily until steady state, then every 2 weeks or as indicated. Not of proven benefit for RIND or TIA (except for vertebral basilar TIAs).

B. Antiplatelet Therapy (aspirin): Indicated for TIA and RIND. Shown to reduce incidence of stroke and death. Dosages range from 80 mg to 1300 mg/ day. At 80mg (1 baby aspirin) /day the incidence is decreased to 2% per year.

Reference

Orland M, *et al*, eds. <u>Manual of Medical Therapeutics, 25th edition</u>. Boston: Little, Brown & Company, 1986.

15/ PSYCHIATRY

John E. Littler, M.D.

PRINCIPLES OF COUNSELING

I. **Overview**
   A. Important Basic Principles:
      1. All members of the household should be involved in the counseling process in one way or another as all members are affected by and affect the "patient with the problem."
      2. The family physician providing counseling is not an observer of the family system but a participant in the process.
      3. The physician-patient relationship is never just bilateral; the patient's support system is always involved, even with straightforward medical problems.
   B. Goals of Primary Care Counseling.
      1. Education of the family regarding the nature of medical problems that may be contributing to the family dysfunction, stresses involved in the family life cycle, etc.
      2. Prevention of commonly encountered problems related to family dynamics and the life cycle by anticipatory education and counseling.
      3. Support of the family during periods of stress by providing attentive ear, acceptance of expressed emotions.
      4. Challenge the family to recognize the problems and dysfunctional interactions that have produced or perpetuated the problem.

II. **Counseling Format**
   A. Build therapeutic relationship.
   B. Assess the problem.
   C. Problem solve.
   D. Formulate treatment plan.

E. Summarize the session.

III. Counseling Techniques

1. Engage the family by talking to all members of the family, each individually, starting with one other than "the patient."(Starting with an adult member may be most effective). Adapt to the family's style of conversation to provide the most "at ease" atmosphere possible.

2. Initiate discussion of the problem by asking a family member (other than the patient) to tell about the problem. Further define the problem by having each family member discuss what changes they would like to see. In addition establish the history of the problem by tracing the start of the problem and previous efforts at dealing with it.

3. Structure the session by establishing certain rules, either explicitly or by practice. This alone helps structure the relationship by demonstrating the leadership role of the physician. Rules include:

    a. each person may speak without being interrupted.

    b. announced plans will not be waylaid by interruptions.

    c. guide the discussion back to the issues when necessary.

    d. do not respond to premature requests for solutions.

    e. establish the physical arrangements of the session by arranging seating, observing the choice of seats, moving individuals as needed.

    f. insist upon proper attendance of all involved individuals at the sessions.

4. Demonstrate neutrality: paraphrase each person's major complaint/proposal, articulate both (or more) sides of the conflict.

5. Encourage a collaborative set by communicating the expectation that the family will work together to solve the problem.

6. Facilitate discussion by inducing the members to speak directly with one another.//
7. Deal directly with resistance as demonstrated by absenteeism/tardiness, but do not allow argument with assessments of the problem--ask the family to think about the observation.
8. Once the problem is better understood, members should contract to make changes. Changes should be specific, concrete.
9. Follow up on assignments/contracts.

References

Driscoll CE, *et al*, eds. Handbook of Family Practice. Chicago: Year Book Medical Publishers, 1986.

Rakel RE and Conn HF, eds. Textbook of Family Practice, Third edition. Philadelphia: W.B. Saunders Company, 1984.

AFFECTIVE DISORDERS

I. **Depression**

A. Symptoms can be divided into emotional (dysphoria, irritability, anhedonia, withdrawal), cognitive (self-criticism, sense of worthlessness or guilt, hopelessness, poor concentration, memory impairment, delusions or hallucinations), and vegetative features (fatigue, decreased energy, insomnia, hypersomnia, anorexia, psychomotor retardation or agitation, impaired libido).

B. Diagnosis: DSM-III-R criteria for major depressive syndrome are at least five of the following symptoms present for at least two weeks, representing a change from previous level of functioning. Must include either dysphoria or anhedonia:

- depressed/irritable mood (most of day, almost daily).
- diminished interest/pleasure in all or most activities.
- significant change in appetite or weight in absence of intentional efforts to alter weight.
- insomnia or hypersomnia.
- psychomotor agitation or retardation.
- fatigue or decreased level of energy.
- feeling of worthlessness or inappropriate guilt.
- poor concentration/indecisiveness.
- recurrent thoughts of death/suicidal ideation.

These should be present in the absence of initiating organic factors and without preceding significant emotional loss. There should also be no evidence for previously existing psychotic disorder.

C. Evaluation:

1. History: Several inventories are available to aid in evaluating depression (e.g., the Beck inventory) and may help in following progress during treatment. Many patients will have a positive family history for depression or alcoholism.

2. Examination: Patient should undergo thorough physical examination to evaluate for possible causative or otherwise related medical condition (such as anemia, hypothyroidism, chronic infection, side effect of medications including oral contraceptives and an-

tihypertensives, drug abuse, dependence, withdrawal).

3. Laboratory: Consider screening for above mentioned medical conditions with CBC with differential, general chemistry screen to include electrolytes, renal and liver function, thyroid studies.

D. Treatment:

1. Hospitalization: indicated if definite suicidal ideation (with a plan and access to the means), occasional suicidal thoughts and history of impulsive acts, complicating medical condition, unsatisfactory home environment (lack of appropriate support).

2. Psychotherapy: supportive therapy is always part of the treatment for depression. Other types of psychotherapy may or may not be helpful depending upon the particular circumstances.

3. Medications: indicated for almost all major depressive episodes. Tricyclic antidepressants are most commonly used, although lithium alone is an effective antidepressant and should be used in depressed bipolar. Tricyclics should be started at a relatively low dose (25 to 50 mg/day) and increased as rapidly as side effects allow (increments of 25 to 50 mg about every third day) to a dose of 150 mg/day. Must be continued for at least 3 to 4 weeks before treatment failure can be declared. If no improvement, the dose may be increased further as side effects allow to 300 mg/day maximum.

4. Electroconvulsive therapy: remains the most effective and rapid means of treating major depressive episodes. Indicated for episodes not responding to medications, patients unable to tolerate side effects of antidepressant medications, actively suicidal patients, depressed patients with severe vegetative symptoms. Decision to administer ECT should be by a psychiatrist.

E. Table: Antidepressants (Table 15-1).

Table 15-1. Antidepressants

Drug	Sedation	Anti-cholinergic*	Orthostatic Hypotension
Amitriptyline	+++	++++	++
Desipramine	+	+	+
Imipramine	++	++	+++
Nortriptyline	++	++	+
Fluoxetine	+	+	+
Trazodone	++	+	++

* blurred vision, constipation, dry mouth, urinary retention

Adapted from Katzung BG, ed. Clinical Pharmacology 88/89. Norwalk: Appleton and Lange, 1988.

II. Bipolar Affective Disorder

A. Most patients that have recurrent manic episodes will also have one or more depressive episodes.

B. Mania is characterized by a distinct period of persistently and abnormally euphoric, irritable or expansive mood. During the period of disturbance the patient must exhibit at least three of the following symptoms (four if the mood is only abnormally irritable):

- grandiosity.
- decreased need for sleep.
- pressured speech or unusually talkative.
- racing thoughts or flight of ideas.
- distractability.
- psychomotor agitation or increased goal-directed activity.
- excessive indiscretions without regard for expected painful consequences.

These symptoms should be present without evidence of pre-existing psychotic disorder or possible inciting organic factor.

C. Evaluation.

1. History: necessary to document definite change in level of function, presence of diagnostic criteria. Interview of family or other household members is probably essential. There is a significant genetic component with increased incidence of other affective disorders and alcoholism in first degree relatives.

2. Examination: most important is to evaluate for evidence of inciting organic cause, especially drug abuse or intoxication.

D. Treatment:
1. Hospitalization: indicated for full manic syndrome because the patient's well-being is at risk due to poor judgement.
2. Antipsychotics (such as Haloperidol) generally required for sedation and control of behavior. Lithium is the drug of choice and should be started immediately as the effect is delayed in onset (in part due to the time needed to attain adequate blood levels). Levels must be closely monitored as well as clinical signs of toxicity. Control of acute mania will require serum levels of 0.9 to 1.4 mEq/L. Slightly lower levels are required for prophylaxis. (Prophylaxis is indicated only for those patients that suffer recurrent episodes; many do not).
   a. dose: 600-2400 mg/day. Administered once daily if < 1200 mg/day, twice daily if 1200-2400 mg/day. During acute episodes, where dose is being adjusted rapidly, levels should be checked once or twice weekly.
   b. adverse effects: polyuria/polydypsia occur with predictable frequency. GI irritation and tremor also occur with significant frequency in the short term. Hypothyroidism with goiter may occur.

References

Diagnostic and Statistical Manual of Mental Disorders, 3rd edition - revised. Washington D.C.: American Psychiatric Association, 1987.

Rakel RE and Conn HF, eds. Textbook of Family Practice, Revised edition. Philadelphia: W.B. Saunders Company, 1984.

ANXIETY DISORDERS

I. **Overview**

   A. Anxiety disorders include generalized anxiety disorder, panic attacks, agoraphobia, social phobias, simple phobias, obsessive compulsive disorder and post-traumatic stress disorder. Anxiety is an unpleasant and unwarranted feeling of apprehension, sometimes accompanied by physiological symptoms. An anxiety disorder indicates dysfunction due to anxiety.

   B. Differential diagnosis of anxiety disorders includes anxious depression, drug abuse/withdrawal (alcohol, hypnotic-sedative withdrawal, stimulant use including amphetamines and caffeine), certain personality disorders, and hyperventilation syndrome. Medical conditions that should be considered include benign palpitations, palpitations due to angina or mitral valve prolapse, other cardiac arrhythmias such as supraventricular tachycardias, asthma or COPD, acute intermittent porphyria, hypoglycemia, hyperthyroidism, and pheochromocytoma.

   C. Treatment: for all anxiety conditions will include supportive counseling. For many of these disorders behavior therapy can be helpful, including systematic desensitization. Benzodiazepines are generally effective at symptomatic relief but do not cure the disorder and can easily result in addiction. Beta-blockers can also provide symptomatic relief (especially if there is associated mitral valve prolapse) for those symptoms that are adrenergic. Tricyclic antidepressants (imipramine) are specific for certain of these disorders. Buspirone is a non-benzodiazepine anxiolytic that may be effective for many of the disorders characteized by anxiety.

II. **Generalized Anxiety Disorder**

   A. Characterized by unrealistic or excessive anxiety about two or more life circumstances for a period of at least 6 months with symptoms most days. Symptoms are not related to other anxiety disorder, do not occur during the course of depression, mania, or psychotic disorder, and no organic factor accounts for the symptoms (stimulants, hyperthyroidism). While anxiety is present the patient should demonstrate evidence of motor tension (trembling, tremor, restlessness), autonomic hyperactivity (dyspnea, tachycardia or palpitations), and hypervigilance (exaggerated startle, irritability, insomnia).

B. Treatment includes psychotherapy, training in relaxation techniques, and education. Benzodiazepines should be used sparingly and for brief periods only. Buspirone is considered by many to be the treatment of choice as it is nonsedating and has little potential for abuse. Onset of action is up to 2 weeks. Dose is started at 5 mg t.i.d., increased by 5 mg/day every 2-3 days. Typical dose is in the range of 20-30 mg/day, maximum is 60 mg/day. About half of these patients will become asymptomatic with time.

III. **Panic Attacks**

A. Characterized by discrete episodes of unexpected intense fear, at least four attacks in one month or one or more attacks followed by at least a month of persistent fear of another attack. No organic factor is found to account for the symptoms (mitral valve prolapse does not preclude the diagnosis of panic attack). During the attacks at least four of the symptoms listed below occur:

- dyspnea.
- dizziness, faintness.
- palpitations or tachycardia.
- trembling.
- sweating.
- choking.
- nausea or abdominal discomfort.
- depersonalization.
- paresthesias.
- flushing or chilling.
- chest discomfort.
- fear of dying.
- fear of insanity or uncontrolled behavior.

B. Treatment includes supportive counseling. Tricyclics are specific therapy, generally effective more quickly than for depression and at lower doses. Imipramine is commonly used at dose up to 75-100 mg/day. Benzodiazepines are

IV. Agoraphobia

A. Characterized by a fear of being in situations from which escape might be difficult in the event of suddenly developing symptoms that may be embarrassing or incapacitating (such as panic attack, dizziness, loss of bowel or bladder control, vomiting). The fear results in the patient restricting travel or requiring a companion during trips away from home.

B. Treatment may include behavior therapy with systematic desensitization, benzodiazepines for acute episodes, and tricyclics if panic attacks are part of the disorder. Buspirone may be effective.

V. Simple and Social Phobias

A. Characterized by persistent fear of humiliation or embarrassment in a certain social situation (social phobia) or other circumscribed stimulus (simple phobia). Exposure to the particular stimulus provokes immediate anxiety and the fear results in avoidance that disrupts the patient's social environment or produces significant distress. The patient will generally realize that the fear is excessive.

B. Treatment includes supportive and behavior therapy with desensitization.

VI. Obsessive Compulsive Disorder

A. Characterized by obsessions or compulsions that significantly interfere with the patient's daily functioning because of distress or time consumption. Obsessions are recurrent and persistent thoughts that are experienced as intrusive and which the patient attempts to ignore or neutralize. These thoughts are recognized as not being imposed from without. Compulsions are repetitive, purposeful behaviors that are performed in response to an obsession or according to certain rules, designed to neutralize or prevent discomfort. In general these are recognized as unreasonable.

(of some use in the short term and beta blockers may provide relief from some symptoms.)

B. Treatment is not curative. Behavior therapy techniques may help limit the amount of dysfunction that results from the obsessions/compulsions. Tricyclics occasionally help.

VII. Post-Traumatic Stress Disorder

A. Occurs in individuals that have experienced an extraordinarily distressing event and is characterized by persistent re-experiences of the event in at least one of the following ways:

- intrusive, recurrent recollections of the event.
- recurrent distressing dreams of the event.
- sudden sense of reliving the experience (flashbacks, hallucinations).
- intense distress with exposure to symbols or representations of the event such as anniversaries.

Results in avoidant behavior or decreased general responsiveness and symptoms of increased arousal (difficulty with insomnia, irritability and anger, poor concentration, hypervigilance, exaggerated startle).

B. Treatment should include the supportive therapy appropriate for grief reaction. Prominent features in individual cases may suggest other medical treatments (ex., depressive symptoms may respond to tricyclics, anxiety to buspirone or benzodiazepines).

References

Diagnostic and Statistical Manual of Mental Disorders, 3rd edition - revised. Washington D.C.: American Psychiatric Association, 1987.

Rakel RE and Conn HF, eds. Textbook of Family Practice, Third edition. Philadelphia: W.B. Saunders Company, 1984.

SUBSTANCE ABUSE

I. Overview

A. Psychoactive substance dependence is indicated by at least three of the following:
- substance taken in larger amounts/over longer period than intended.
- persistent desire or unsuccessful attempts to cut down use.
- significant amount of time spent in obtaining, consuming, or recovering from the substance.
- frequent intoxication or withdrawal symptoms at times patient is expected to fulfill major role obligations at school, work, home.
- important social or occupational activities reduced because of substance use.
- persistent use despite knowledge of social, psychological or physical problems caused by its use.
- tolerance.
- withdrawal.
- substance taken to avoid withdrawal symptoms.

II. Alcohol

A. Most commonly abused drug. Contributes significantly to morbidity and mortality in this country. Alcohol abuse is diagnosed if there is impairment of social or occupational functioning due to alcohol use. Dependence is diagnosed if there is evidence of tolerance (increased amounts required to produce effect--blood alcohol level of 150 mg/dl without evidence of intoxication indicates tolerance) or withdrawal. Strong familial component.

B. Diagnosis: suspect alcohol abuse if any of the following complaints are present.
- chronic anxiety/tension.
- insomnia.
- chronic depression.
- headaches, blackouts.
- vague GI problems.
- frequent falls or minor injuries.
- seizures.
- legal or marital problems.

Laboratory evaluation should include CBC, liver enzymes, PT/PTT, and serum protein level. Anticipated complications include gastritis/PUD, nutritional deficiencies, hypertension, pancreatitis, liver disease, insomnia, depression, impotence, myopathy and cardiomyopathy.

C. Management:
1. Must maintain focus on drinking as the primary problem; do not allow the patient to focus your attention on the social/family/work problems that "cause" the drinking problem.
2. If tolerance/ withdrawal are present, the patient will require detoxification. Thiamine, 50-100 mg IM, should be given to prevent Wernicke-Korsakoff syndrome. Any benzodiazepine may be used to decrease the symptoms of withdrawal and as prophylaxis against the development of delirium tremens. Diazepam and chlordiazepoxide are commonly used (ex: chlordiazepoxide given 50 mg po q4 hr x 24 hours, then 50 mg q6 hr x 24 hours, then 25 mg q4 hr x 24 hours, then 25 mg q 6 hr x 24 hours). Some recommend phenytoin for anyone with a history of withdrawal seizures, although even with a loading dose therapeutic levels will not be attained quickly.
3. Most effective counseling approach is group therapy with multidisciplinary treatment team. Involvement in AA should be encouraged. Antabuse can be helpful although it depends upon a patient already motivated to address the drinking problem.

III. **Clinical Presentations of Abused Substances Tables** (15-2 and 15-3)

Table 15-2. Clinical Manifestations of Acute Drug Reactions, By Class of Drug

Signs and Symptoms	Withdrawal Opioids	Depressants	Stimulants
Anxiety	X	X	
Convulsions			X
Delirium		X	X
Fatigue			X
Hallucinations		X	
Headaches		X	

Table 15-2 (continued)

Signs and Symptoms	Withdrawal Opioids	Depressants	Stimulants
Hypertension	X		
Hypotension (orthostatic)		X	
Nausea	X	X	
Pupils, dilated	X		
Reflexes, hyperactive		X	
Tachycardia	X	X	

Adapted from Rakel RE and Conn HF, eds. Textbook of Family Practice, Revised edition. Philadelphia: W.B. Saunders Co., 1984.

Table 15-3. Clinical Manifestations of Acute Drug Reactions, By Class of Drug

Intoxication/Overdose

Signs and Symptoms	Opioids	Depressants	Stimulants	Hallucinogens	Phencyclidine
Anxiety	X	X	X	X	X
Arrhythmia			X		
Coma	X			X	
Convulsions		X	X		X
Delirium	X	X	X	X	X
Euphoria	X	X	X	X	
Fatigue		X			
Hallucinations			X	X	X
Headaches			X		
Hypertension			X	X	X
Hypotension (orthostatic)	X	X			
Hyperthermia			X	X	
Nausea			X	X	X
Nystagmus		X			X
Pupils, dilated			X	X	
Pupils, pinpoint	X				
Reflexes, hyperactive			X	X	X
Respiration, slow and shallow	X	X	X	X	X
Speech, slurred		X			X
Tachycardia			X	X	X
Tremor			X	X	
Violent behavior		X			X

Adapted from Rakel RE and Conn HF, eds. Textbook of Family Practice, Third edition. Philadelphia: W.B. Saunders Company, 1984.

References

Diagnostic and Statistical Manual of Mental Disorders, 3rd edition - revised. Washington D.C.: American Psychiatric Association, 1987.

Rakel RE and Conn HF, eds. Textbook of Family Practice, Third edition. Philadelphia: W.B. Saunders Company, 1984.

ACUTE PSYCHOSIS

I. Overview

A. Characterized by marked impairment of sense of reality (incoherence, loosening of associations, delusions, hallucinations, catatonic or disorganized behavior), generally resulting in impairment of ability to communicate, emotional turmoil, impaired cognitive abilities.

B. Differential diagnosis includes drug-induced (either intoxication or withdrawal), acute exacerbation or presenting episode of chronic psychotic disorder (schizophrenia), episode of major affective syndrome (mania or depression), fever. Organic etiology should be suspected if there is some degree of delirium (clouding of sensorium), no personal or family history of psychotic disorders, patient is older than age 35 and has no prior episodes, condition developed rapidly in patient that was previously functioning well.

C. Treatment initially is with antipsychotics to control behavior (such as haloperidol or chlorpromazine). Longer-term treatment will depend upon the etiology, which may not be apparent until further history is obtained from family/friends or from the patient after symptoms have improved.

II. Antipsychotics (Table 15-4)

Table 15-4. Antipsychotics

Drug	Sedation	EPS*	Anticholinergic**	Orthostasis
Chlorpromazine	+++	++	++	+++
Fluphenazine	+	+++	+	+
Haloperidol	+	+++	+	+
Thioridazine	+++	+	+++	+++
Thiothixene	+	+++	+	+

* dystoria, akathisia, tardive dyskinesia

** dry mouth, constipation, blurred vision, urinary retention

Adapted from Katzung BG, ed. Clinical Pharmacology 88/89. Norwalk: Appleton and Lange, 1988.

References

<u>Diagnostic and Statistical Manual of Mental Disorders, 3rd edition - revised</u>. Washington D.C.: American Psychiatric Association, 1987.

Rakel RE and Conn HF, eds. <u>Textbook of Family Practice, Third edition</u>. Philadelphia: W.B. Saunders Company, 1984.

SCHIZOPHRENIC AND SCHIZOPHRENIC-LIKE DISORDERS

I. **Schizophrenia**
   A. Most common psychotic disorder--affects 1% of the population. Strong familial tendency. Chronic disorder characterized by:
      1. Active episodes with psychotic features of bizarre delusions, hallucinations, incoherence or loosening of associations and marked decrease in level of social functioning.
      2. Signs of the disorder must be present for 6 months with at least one active psychotic episode lasting one week or more.
      3. Prodromal phase (showing a clear deterioration in functioning before the active episode) and residual phase involve at least two of the following symptoms:
      - marked social isolation/withdrawal.
      - marked decrease in level of functioning in social roles.
      - peculiar behavior.
      - impaired personal hygiene.
      - blunted, inappropriate affect.
      - vague, impoverished, or impoverished content of speech.
      - magical thinking (not consistent with cultural norms).
      - unusual perceptual experiences.
   B. Subtypes:
      1. Catatonic: clinical picture dominated by stupor, negativism, rigidity, purposeless excitement, posturing.
      2. Disorganized: characterized by marked incoherence, loosening of associations, disorganized behavior, flat or grossly inappropriate behavior. Worst prognosis.
      3. Paranoid: preoccupation with systematized delusions or hallucinations (auditory) without incoherence, loosening of associations, catatonic or disorganized behavior. Best prognosis.

C. Differential diagnosis includes any condition that may produce active psychotic episodes (see section on acute psychosis).

D. Treatment: acute psychosis is treated with antipsychotic medications. For patients with relapses long-term treatment with antipsychotics is indicated for controlling psychotic symptoms. Dose should be kept at minimum so as to not contribute to impaired level of functioning. Psychotherapy (of various types) may help maintain level of functioning.

II. Brief Reactive Psychosis

A. Clinically similar to schizophrenia with similar psychotic symptoms. However, symptoms appear after stressful event and prodromal symptoms are absent. Duration is less than one month with return to premorbid level of functioning.

B. Differential diagnosis includes those disorders that can produce acute psychosis (which should be looked for carefully in this clinical situation).

C. Treatment includes supportive environment and antipsychotic medications as needed. Patient will have full recovery but will be at risk for future episodes.

III. Schizophreniform Disorder

A. Characterized by the same symptoms as schizophrenia (psychotic, prodromal and residual) but episodes last less than 6 months. Good prognostic signs are early onset of psychotic feature after first noticeable change in behavior, confusion or disorientation at peak of episode, good premorbid function, absence of blunted or flat affect.

B. Treatment is similar to that for acute schizophrenic episodes.

References

Diagnostic and Statistical Manual of Mental Disorders, 3rd edition - revised. Washington D.C.: American Psychiatric Association, 1987.

Rakel RE and Conn HF, eds. Textbook of Family Practice, Third edition. Philadelphia: W.B. Saunders Company, 1984.

EATING DISORDERS

I. **Anorexia Nervosa**

   A. Disorder affecting females 10:1 over males, characterized by onset in adolescence of abnormal body image ("feeling fat" in spite of dramatic evidence to the contrary) and preoccupation with losing weight. Abuse of exercise, diuretics, laxatives is common. Many will also have periods of binge eating. Anorexia nervosa is a life-threatening disorder, with mortality as high as 10%.

   B. Diagnosis: early signs may be withdrawal from family and friends, increased sensitivity to criticism, sudden increased interest in physical activity, anxiety or depressive symptoms. Later signs include those of starvation with amenorrhea. DSM-III-R criteria for diagnosis are:
   - refusal to maintain body weight over a minimal normal weight for age and height.
   - intense fear of becoming fat.
   - disturbed body image.
   - in females, absence of at least three consecutive periods.

   C. Treatment: for the emaciated patient, hospitalization is indicated for nutritional support. Inpatient behavior modification programs are effective while the patient is hospitalized but long-term family and individual therapy is indicated as the strict manipulation of the environment during in-hospital therapy cannot be maintained at home. Spontaneous remission commonly occurs in mid to late 20's.

II. **Bulimia Nervosa**

   A. Eating disorder also much more prevalent in females, with onset generally in adolescence or early 20's. Bulimics tend to be normal or slightly above normal weight. Binge eating, often followed by purging to prevent weight gain, is characteristic. Associated dysphoria or depression is common.

   B. Diagnosis: DSM-III-R criteria are:
   - recurrent episodes of binge eating.
   - feeling of lack of control over eating behavior.

- regular use of self-induced vomiting, laxatives, diuretics, fasting or excessive exercise to prevent weight gain.
- minimum average of 2 binge episodes/week for at least 3 months.
- persistent overconcern with body shape and weight.

C. Treatment should include supportive therapy, behavior therapy, and treatment of depression if present.

References

Diagnostic and Statistical Manual of Mental Disorders, 3rd edition - revised. Washington D.C.: American Psychiatric Association, 1987.

Rakel RE and Conn HF, eds. Textbook of Family Practice, Third edition. Philadelphia: W.B. Saunders Company, 1984.

16/ EMERGENCY PROCEDURES

Tom Francis, M.D.

DEFIBRILLATION/CARDIOVERSION

I. **Indications**
   A. Defibrillation.
      1. Conversion of ventricular fibrillation (V-fib) and pulseless ventricular tachycardia (VT).
   B. Cardioversion.
      1. Conversion of unstable VT with a pulse, stable VT not responsive to antiarrythmics, unstable supraventricular tachycardia (SVT), atrial fibrillation or flutter with cardiovascular compromise.

II. **Contraindications**
   A. Atrial fibrillation with slow ventricular response, digitalis toxicity, sick sinus syndrome, long-standing atrial fibrillation (without prior anticoagulation), atrial fibrillation secondary to hypothyroidism are all relative contraindications.

III. **Materials**
   - defibrillator with monitor.
   - conduction jelly or pads.
   - sedative (diazepam or midazolam are commonly used).
   - materials for support of airway, including oral and nasopharyngeal airways, bag-mask for ventilation, suction.

IV. **Technique**
   A. Defibrillation.
      1. Charge paddles to appropriate energy (see ACLS protocols, Chapter 1). Make sure defibrillator is in unsynchronized mode. Apply conducting jelly to paddles or conductive pads to chest.

2. Place one paddle on right upper chest, below the clavicle, and the other paddle to the left lower chest. Proper paddle placement is essential. Apply approximately 25 pounds of pressure with the paddles.

3. Recheck rhythm and make sure that no one is in contact with the bed or patient. Simultaneously depress paddle buttons to deliver the countershock.

4. Evaluate patient by checking pulse and monitor.

B. Cardioversion.

1. Establish IV access as clinical situation allows. Sedation is preferred if possible (1-5 mg of midazolam IV, or 5-10 mg of diazepam IV). Set defibrillator/monitor unit on synchronized mode and make sure that monitor is marking all QRS complexes.

2. Charge paddles to appropriate energy (see table 16-1). Apply conducting jelly to paddles or conduction pads to patient's chest as above. Apply approximately 25 pounds of pressure to paddles.

3. Check rhythm on monitor and make sure that no one is in contact with the bed or patient. Simultaneously depress the buttons on the paddles and hold in until countershock is delivered.

4. Evaluate patient by checking pulse and rhythm.

Table 16-1.

Rhythm	Recommend energy (adult)
atrial fibrillation	100 Joules, then 200 J, followed by 360 J.
SVT	75-100 J initially.
atrial flutter	25 J initially.
VT with pulse	50 J initially, then 100 J, 200 J, 360 J.

Adapted from Driscoll CE, et al, eds. Handbook of Family Practice. Chicago: Year Book Medical Publishers, 1986.

V. **Complications**

A. Potential complications include skin burns, arcing of the delivered shock, and failure to deliver the countershock.

Reference

Driscoll CE, et al, eds. Handbook of Family Practice. Chicago: Year Book Medical Publishers, 1986.

TUBE THORACOSTOMY

I. **Indications**
   A. Pneumothorax.
   B. Hemothorax.
   C. Drainage of pleural effusion.

II. **Contraindications**
   A. There are no contraindications to chest tube placement in patients symptomatic from the above listed indications.

III. **Materials**
   A. Materials needed are:
   - Iodine and alcohol swabs for preparing skin.
   - Sterile drapes and gloves.
   - #11 scalpel blade and handle.
   - Mayo clamp.
   - Kelly clamp.
   - Silk suture(size 0).
   - Needle holder.
   - Petrolatum-impregnated gauze.
   - Sterile gauze.
   - Tape.
   - Suction apparatus.
   - Chest tube (size 32-40 French depending upon clinical setting).
   - 1% lidocaine, 10 cc syringe with 25 and 22 gauge needle.

IV. **Technique**
   A. Position patient with affected side up. Identify the insertion site, which is generally at the anterior axillary line at the level of the nipple. Prepare the skin with the iodine and alcohol swabs. Insertion site should be anesthetized with 1% lidocaine subcutaneously and along the insertion tract to the pleura. Appropriate position can be checked by aspirating through the needle used for instilling the local anesthetic.
   B. Sterile gloves should be donned and the area draped. The skin should be incised directly over the body of the rib,

the incision length being 1-1/2 times the diameter of the chest tube to be used. The Kelly or Mayo clamp is then used to bluntly dissect superiorly over the superior margin of the next higher rib. The Mayo clamp is then pushed through the parietal pleura with tips closed and with slow steady pressure. Once the pleura has been penetrated the clamps are opened wide to enlarge the insertion tract and removed. Operator's index finger can also be inserted along the tract to further enlarge the opening if needed.

C. The chest tube is grasped near the end to be inserted with the Mayo clamp (jaws of the clamp parallel to the length of the tube), and advanced into the pleural space. Once the tube is inserted so that all drainage ports are inside the thoracic cavity, the tube is connected to suction and sutured in place with silk suture by closing the skin edges of the incision around the tube and tying the suture ends up around the tube. The area should be dressed with petrolatum-impregnated gauze and sterile gauze sponges. Chest x-ray should be obtained.

V. **Complications**

A. Potential complications include:
- hemorrhage at the site of insertion.
- infection.
- hematoma.
- lung laceration.
- laceration of intra-abdominal organs if tube is inadvertently inserted in to the abdominal cavity.

Reference

Mills J, *et al*, eds. <u>Current Emergency Diagnosis and Treatment, Second edition</u>. Los Altos: Lange Medical Publishers, 1985.

VENOUS CUTDOWN

I. Indications

Emergency venous access when other sites are not available, or when multiple sites of access are indicated.

II. Contraindications

- previous use of the intended vein (previous cutdown site, venous stripping, donor site for bypass grafting).
- phlebitis.
- cellulitis over insertion site.
- trauma at the proposed insertion site.
- venous obstructive disease.

III. Materials

- Iodine and alcohol swabs for preparing skin.
- 1% lidocaine without epinephrine for local anesthetic.
- 10 cc syringe and 25 gauge needle.
- gauze and tape.
- sterile gloves and drapes.
- #11 and #15 scalpel blades and handle.
- silk ligatures, size 3-0.
- nylon suture, 5-0.
- needle holder.
- Kelly clamp.
- Mosquito clamp.
- Tissue scissors.
- Forceps.
- IV tubing and IV fluid.
- 2 inch or longer 18 gauge IV catheter.

IV. Technique (Fig 16-1)

A. Identify saphenous vein just anterior to the medial malleolus, or the cephalic vein 1 cm proximal to Lister's tubercle on the distal radius. Prepare the skin with iodine and alcohol. Don gloves and drape the area. Anesthetize the area with 1% lidocaine. A 1-1/2 to 2 cm incision is made transversely across the site. The incision is carried down to the vein by blunt dissection until the vein is completely exposed and the mosquito clamp can be passed under the vein.

B. The distal portion of the exposed vein is ligated with a silk ligature. Pass the second silk ligature beneath the vein and slide it to the proximal portion of the exposed vein, but do not tie it.

C. Support the vein with an open Kelly clamp and perform a venotomy with the #11 scalpel. (In the alternative, a "mini-venous cutdown" may be done with an over-the-needle venous catheter inserted under direct visualization into the vein at this point.) Only the superior surface of the vein is incised leaving the posterior and side walls intact. Insert the IV catheter. IV tubing is connected after blood return is demonstrated. The proximal ligature is tied around the vein and catheter. The skin is closed with nylon suture and the catheter is secured to the skin. Dress the area with gauze and tape.

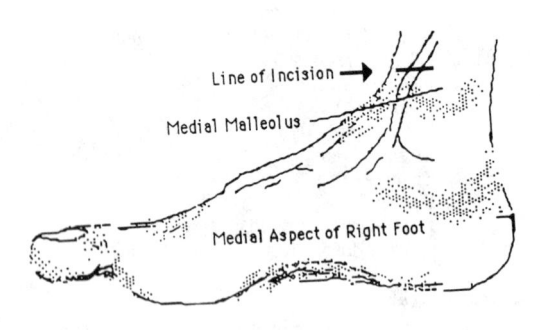

Fig 16-1. Venous Cutdown
* Saphenous Vein

V. **Complications**
- bleeding.
- infection.
- thrombosis.

- phlebitis.
- transection of the vein.
- hematoma.

Reference

Mills J, *et al*, eds. <u>Current Emergency Diagnosis and Treatment, 2nd edition</u>. Los Altos: Lange Medical Publications, 1985.

INTRAOSSEOUS INFUSION

Intraosseous infusion can provide a very rapid and dependable route of vascular access in children age 3 or less (where vascular access is likely to be difficult in settings where it is most urgent). Via this route almost any infusate can be instilled at a rapid rate, including blood and blood products, Plasmanate, glucose, crystalloids, pressor agents including epinephrine, dopamine and dobutamine, and atropine.

I. **Indications**
- emergency fluid infusion, especially in setting of circulatory collapse where rapid IV access is essential.
- difficult IV access.
- burn or other injury preventing access to the venous system at other sites.

II. **Contraindications**
- overlying cellulitis.
- bony lesion at site.
- osteomyelitis.

III. **Materials**
A. Material for preparing the area (alcohol and iodine prep solutions).
B. 1% lidocaine if local anesthesia is appropriate.
C. 3 cc syringe with 25 gauge needle for infiltration of local anesthetic.
D. Sterile gloves and drape.
E. IV infusion set.
F. 18 or 20 gauge short spinal needle or bone marrow needle.

IV. **Technique**
A. Identify landmarks and prepare the insertion site with iodine or alcohol solution. Sites for insertion:
- proximal tibia 2 cm below the tibial tuberosity in the midline.
- distal femur 3 cm above superior aspect of the lateral condyle in the midline.

Intraosseous Infusion 577

B. Infiltrate the overlying skin to the periosteum if the situation indicates.
C. For insertion in the proximal tibia, the spinal needle is directed inferiorly at a 45° angle from the perpendicular. If the insertion site is the distal femur, the needle should angle 45° superiorly. In both instances the goal is to angle away from the region of the growth plate (see Fig 16-2).
D. Advance needle (with stylet in place) through skin, subcutaneous tissue and cortex of bone into the marrow space.

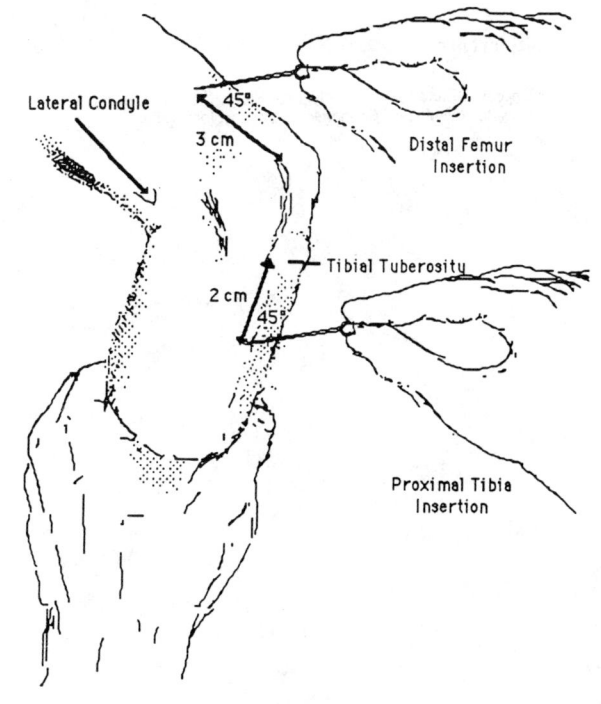

Fig 16-2. Intraosseous Infusion

578 Emergency Procedures

  E. Remove stylet and confirm placement by infusing 5 cc of saline with a syringe.
  F. Detach syringe and connect IV tubing to begin infusion. Secure in position with tape.

V. **Complications**

  A. Potential complications include:
    - local abscess or cellulitis.
    - osteomyelitis.

  (Injury to growth plate has not been identified as a complication that occurs with any significant frequency.)

Reference

Driscoll CE and Rakel RE, eds. <u>Procedures for Your Practice</u>. Oradell, New Jersey: Medical Economics Company, Inc., 1988.

CULDOCENTESIS

Culdocentesis is the transvaginal puncture of the pouch of Douglas to aspirate peritoneal fluid for diagnostic purposes.

I. **Indications**

   A. Early diagnosis of hemoperitoneum.

   B. Preoperative evaluation of patients with suspected ectopic pregnancy.

   C. Obtaining peritoneal fluid for further evaluation in both pathologic and physiologic conditions.

II. **Contraindications**

   A. Patient in whom the cul-de-sac appears obliterated by adhesions or by a palpable mass of unknown nature.

   B. Patient with a uterus fixed in retroversion, thereby obliterating the culd-de-sac.

III. **Procedure** (Fig 16-3)

   A. Materials.

   1. 10 ml syringe with at least a 4 inch, 18 gauge or larger spinal needle.

   2. Povidone-iodine soaked gauze.

   3. Ring forceps.

   4. Tenaculum.

   5. Culture tubes.

   6. Bivalve vaginal speculum.

   B. Technique.

   1. Bimanual exam to rule out obliterated cul-de-sac or mass and to assess position of uterus.

   2. Position patient as for routine pelvic exam. Introduce the vaginal speculum so that good view of the cervix is obtained and swab the vagina with povidone-iodine, focusing on the posterior fornix.

   3. Grasp the posterior lip of the cervix with the tenaculum and gently pull anteriorly and forward to expose the posterior fornix.

4. The spinal needle on a 10 ml syringe containing 2-3 ml of air is rapidly thrust through the posterior fornix and into the cul-de-sac about 3 cm along an axis parallel to the posterior wall of the uterus.
5. The air in the syringe is injected. If resistance is felt, the tip of the needle is in a solid organ and should be repositioned until the air injects without resistance.
6. Suction is applied, and if fluid is present it will flow freely into the syringe. If no fluid is obtained a second or third attempt may be made at a different angle or puncture site.

IV. Complications

A. Introduction of bacteria into the peritoneal cavity.
B. Rupture of adnexal structures.
C. Puncture or laceration of bowel.

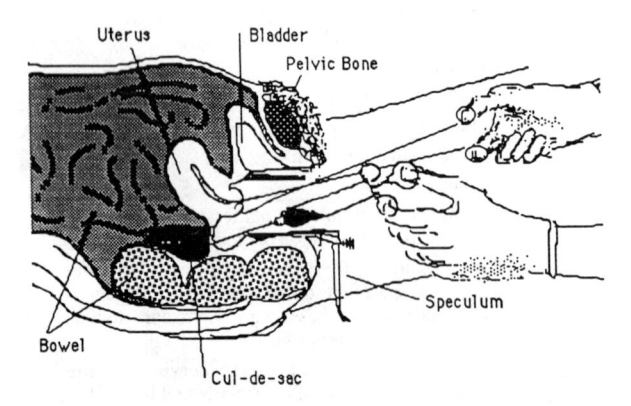

Fig 16-3. Culdocentesis: Left hander's approach.

V. **Results:** see Table 16-2.

Table 16-2.

Fluid retrieved	Interpretation	Further test/Rx
Blood that does not clot after 10 min.	+ culdocentesis	Check Hct of fluid, if > 15% indicates probable ectopic pregnancy. Obtain ultrasound or laparoscopy.
Pus or cloudy fluid	PID	Gram stain, cultures, antibiotics (see PID).
Chocolate-colored fluid	endometriosis, cyst with old blood, chronic ectopic pregnancy	Consider pelvic ultrasound.
Clear fluid	Ascites, ruptured ovarian cyst or normal peritoneal fluid	As clinically indicated
No fluid	Nondiagnostic	As clinically indicated

PARACENTESIS AND PERITONEAL LAVAGE

I. Indications

A. Nontraumatic.
   1. Evaluation of ascites.
   2. Therapeutic, to relieve discomfort due to chronic ascites.
   3. Assessment for possible pancreatitis/peritonitis.

B. Trauma.
   1. Blunt abdominal trauma with suggestive or equivocal eam in stable patient.
   2. Blunt abdominal trauma with factors that make physical exam inaccurate: spinal cord injury, unconscious or severely intoxicated patient.
   3. Multiple trauma victim requiring urgent surgery for other injury. Note: patient with shock and abdominal trauma requires surgery, not lavage.

II. Contraindications

A. Absolute.
   1. Bleeding disorders.
   2. Coagulopathies.
   3. Cellulitis of anterior abdominal wall.

B. Relative.
   1. Patient with previous laparotomy scars.
   2. Hepatosplenomegaly.
   3. Distended bladder.
   4. Known adhesions.

III. Materials

- Sterile gloves.
- Povidone-iodine solution.
- Sterile drapes.
- 10 cc syringe.
- 2 inch, 21 gauge needle.
- 2% lidocaine with epinephrine.
- 50 cc syringe.

Paracentesis and Peritoneal Lavage

- 2 inch, 14 gauge needle.
- Sterile 16 gauge intraluminal catheter.
- 1 liter normal saline.
- Specimen tubes.
- Gauze sponges.

IV. Technique

A. Empty bladder, catheterization optional. Have patient supine. Prep skin with povidone-iodine and drape.

B. 2% lidocaine local 3 cm below umbilicus in the midline, anesthetize a track down to the peritoneum. Insert 14 gauge needle until it "pops" into the abdominal cavity.

C. Aspirate, if frank blood, stop and proceed with emergency laparotomy. If no return of fluid, disconnect syringe and advance 16 gauge intraluminal catheter through the needle and remove needle. Instill 1 liter of normal saline through the catheter. Once instilled, place bottle on floor, and allow it to refill by gravity

D. Send fluid for analysis, (CBC, amylase, Gram stain, C & S, pH, bile, cytology). Remove catheter and dress wound.

V. Complications

- Bowel perforation.
- Bleeding from puncture site.
- Laceration of an epigastric vessel.

VI. RESULTS (Table 16-3)

Table 16-3. Criteria for evaluation of peritoneal lavage fluid.

Positive	Aspiration of >15 ml of gross blood on catheter placement
	Drainage of lavage fluid from another body cavity
	Grossly bloody lavage fluid
	Evidence of food, foreign particles, or bile
	Erythrocytes > 100,000/mm^3 after blunt trauma
	Erythrocytes > 50,000/mm^3 after penetrating trauma
	Leukocytes > 500/mm^3
	Amylase > 100 units/dl

Table 16-3 (continued)

Indeterminate	Small amount of gross blood on catheter insertion Erythrocytes 50,000-100,000/mm^3 after blunt trauma Erythrocytes 1,000-50,000/mm^3 after penetrating trauma Leukocytes 100-500/mm^3
Negative	Erythrocytes < 50,000/mm^3 after blunt trauma Erythrocytes < 1,000/mm^3 after penetrating trauma Leukocytes < 100/mm^3

References

Driscoll CE, *et al*, eds. Handbook of Family Practice. Chicago: Year Book Medical Publishers, 1986.

17/ HOSPITAL PROCEDURES

Tom Francis, M.D.

FETAL SCALP ELECTRODE

I. **Indications:**

   Variations in fetal heart rate for which immediate delivery is not indicated:
   - Pitocin induction.
   - Meconium stained amniotic fluid.
   - Vaginal delivery after cesarean section.
   - Hypertension.
   - Vaginal bleeding.
   - Pre- and post-term pregnancies.
   - IUGR.
   - Diabetes.
   - H/O prior stillbirth.

II. **Contraindications:**
   - Long, closed cervix.
   - Intact amniotic sac.
   - Placenta previa.

III. **Materials:**
   - Sterile drapes.
   - Sterile gloves.
   - Amniotomy hook - optional.
   - Fetal scalp electrode.
   - Monitor.
   - Sterile lubricant.

IV. **Technique:**

   A. Don gloves and drape. Perform vaginal exam to determine dilation, effacement, position and presenting part(s). Perform amniotomy with amniotomy hook if membranes are intact.

   B. Insert scalp electrode over the intra-vaginal hand, and position it onto the presenting part. Be sure to avoid the fontanelles, suture lines, face and genitalia. With the catheter tip firmly seated on the fetal scalp, twist the driving tube to propel the spiral electrode through the skin.

C. Remove guide tube and attach the wires to an electrode strapped to the mother's leg. Be sure an electrocardiographic signal is picked up.

V. Complications:

- Misplacement of electrode.
- Postpartum infection (endometritis).
- Fetal scalp infection.
- Early amniotomy.

Reference

Pritchard JA, MacDonald PC, and Gant NJ, eds. Williams Obstetrics, 17th edition. Connecticut: Appleton-Century-Crofts, 1985.

FETAL SCALP pH SAMPLING

I. Indications

A. Obtaining blood from the fetal scalp is indicated for the evaluation of possible fetal distress as evidenced by late decelerations, significant bradycardia, or prolonged second stage of labor.

II. Contraindications

- intact amniotic sac.
- long, closed cervix .
- low lying placenta or placenta previa.

III. Materials

- Sterile gloves and drapes.
- Lighted endoscope.
- Cotton swabs.
- Ethyl chloride spray.
- Silicone gel.
- Calibrated scalpel blade on long handle.
- Heparinized glass capillary tubes.
- pH analyzer.

IV. Technique

A. Don gloves and drape the patient. Perform bimanual exam to check fetal position and cervical dilatation and effacement. Insert lighted endoscope through the dilated cervix and press it firmly against the fetal scalp.

B. Cleanse the scalp with cotton swabs. Spray scalp with ethyl chloride and coat it with silicone gel to induce hyperemia. Incise the skin with the calibrated blade. Collect a drop of blood with the capillary tube and send for analysis.

V. Results

A. General guidelines for interpreting the pH results are listed below:

- pH > 7.25 no evidence of fetal distress, observe repeat as indicated.
- pH 7.20 -7.25, resample in 30 minutes.
- pH < 7.20, resample immediately.

- Repeat pH < 7.20, Cesarean section for fetal distress.
- Repeat pH > 7.20, as above.

VI. Complications

A. Potential complications include infection, bleeding, maternal infection, early amniotomy.

Reference

Pritchard JA, MacDonald PC, and Gant NF, eds. *Williams Obstetrics, 17th edition*. Connecticut: Appleton-Century-Crofts, 1985.

CIRCUMCISION

(Gomco Clamp Technique)

I. **Indication:** The American Academy of Pediatrics holds that there is no absolute medical indication for routine circumcision of newborns.

II. **Contraindications:**
- Infants 24 hours of age.
- Premature infants not yet ready for discharge.
- Evidence of infection.
- Presence of penile congenital anomalies, including hypospadias, chordee.
- Family history of hemophilia.

III. **Materials:**
- Adjustable infant restraint board.
- Warming lamp and light.
- Sterile gloves and drapes.
- 4 x 4 gauze sponges.
- 1% lidocaine without epinephrine and 1 cc syringe with 27-gauge needle.
- Povidone-iodine.
- Three mosquito clamps.
- Suture scissors.
- Blunt malleable probe.
- Scalpel handle and blade.
- 1" x 9" petrolatum-impregnated gauze.
- 1.1 and 1.3 Gomco circumcision clamps.
- Sterile safety pin.

IV. **Technique:**

A. Infant should be fasting x 2-3 hours. Restrain infant on board beneath warming light. Prep skin with povidone-iodine. Drape with sterile towels.

B. Draw up .1 cc/kg of 1% lidocaine without epinephrine. Inject 1/2 of the 1% lidocaine on each side of the base of the penile shaft at the 10 o'clock and 2 o'clock position. This should be a subcutaneous injection, avoiding surface veins. Wait 3 minutes for anesthesia to take effect.

Hospital Procedures

C. Identify the lumen of the prepuce, insert a mosquito clamp and clamp the edge of the skin at the 10 o'clock position, repeat with a second mosquito clamp at the 2 o'clock position.

D. Hold 10 o'clock and 2 o'clock clamps with non-dominant hand, and insert a third mosquito clamp (closed) through the preputial space (in the 12 o'clock position) to the dorsal base of the glans at the corona, and open the clamp to dissect the prepuce laterally. Repeat on lateral sides of preputial space.

E. Slide an open clamp over the dorsal midline of the prepuce to a point connecting the distal 2/3 and proximal 1/3 of the prepuce. Be <u>certain</u> that the clamp is not in the urethra. Close the clamp to crush the dorsal prepuce for 5 seconds. Remove clamp.

F. Still holding the 10 and 2 o'clock clamps, insert an opened scissors along the crush line with the blunt side beneath the prepuce. Divide the prepuce down the center of the crush line. Peel back the cut edges of the prepuce with the 10 and 2 o'clock clamps. If the initial blunt probing did not fully dissect the glans-prepuce plane, use a blunt probe and/or 4" x 4" gauze until the coronal sulcus is fully exposed.

G. After full dissection, bring the prepuce back up over the glans. Select a 1.1 or 1.3 Gomco bell, and insert it into the plane just dissected. Bring the two edges of the dorsal slit up around the bell and fasten them together with a sterile safety pin. Remove the 10 o'clock and 2 o'clock clamps.

H. Place the open ring of the Gomco circumcision clamp plate over the shaft of the bell and bring the prepuce and safety pin through. Loosen the thumb screw knob to allow the crossbar of the shaft to fall into the grooves of the clamp arm. Hold the plate horizontally, and pull the prepuce through the ring, down to, and including the proximal edge of the dorsal incision. Make sure an equal amount of tissue is pulled through on all sides.

I. Tighten the thumbscrew of the Gomco clamp to produce a symmetric ring crush through the foreskin. Leave clamped for 5 minutes. With the Gomco clamp in place, trim the prepuce with the scalpel blade at the upper plate edge against the bell. Loosen the thumbscrew, remove the clamp, and loosen the bell from the glans with a 4 x 4 gauze sponge. Wrap a petrolatum-impregnated gauze dressing around the raw skin edge.

V. **Follow-Up:**
- Observe for 24 hours for infection or bleeding.
- Keep incised edges clean and dry.
- Apply petroleum jelly to cut edges with each diaper change x 1 week.
- Instruct parents on signs of infection.

VI. **Complications:**
- Hemorrhage at incision site, controlled with pressure, and/or topical epinephrine.
- Infection: topical antibiotics.
- Surgical trauma (careless dissection or excessive denudation of the shaft), inadequate prepuce removal, urethral fistulas, bivalving of the glans, scrotal lacerations.

Reference

Driscoll CE and Rakel RE, eds. Procedures for Your Practice. Oradell, New Jersey: Medical Economics Co., Inc., 1988.

LOCAL AND REGIONAL BLOCKS

I. **Indications:**
   A. Anesthesia for suturing lacerations.
   B. Anesthesia for biopsies.
   C. Anesthesia for deliveries.
   D. Local - when a small area is to be anesthetized.
   E. Regional - if local anesthesia would distort the anatomy, when a particular procedure calls for a great amount of anesthesia to effectively prevent pain.

II. **Contraindications:**
   A. Allergy to local anesthetic (unusual).
   B. The use of epinephrine with an anesthetic in fingers, toes, nose, ears or penis.
   C. The use of epinephrine in patients with hypertension, cardiac rhythm disturbance or other heart disease.
   D. Injection through an area of cellulitis.

III. **Materials:**
   - 1% lidocaine with or without epinephrine.
   - 20 gauge needle, 1 1/2 inch needle.
   - 25-30 gauge needle (5/8 in. - 1 1/2 in.).
   - Syringe.
   - Povidone - iodine skin prep.

IV. **Technique:** for local infiltration
   A. Prep injection site with povidone-iodine. Draw up anesthetic with 20 gauge needle.
   B. Use 25-30 gauge needle, then raise wheal at injection site. Slowly inject the surrounding area of skin. Wait 2-3 minutes, then proceed with procedure.
   C. For wound closure, drip 1% lidocaine into wound and wait 2-3 minutes prior to infiltration of wound edges.

V. Regional Blocks

A. Prep skin and draw up anesthetic. Always raise skin wheal before advancing the needle, and always inject slowly and aspirate to avoid intravascular administration.

B. Digital Blocks: for complete finger anesthesia.
   1. Raise skin wheal at base of finger at the level of the interphalangeal skin creases.
   2. Angle 5/8 in. 25 gauge needle 45° from finger in the horizontal and vertical planes and advance until the bone is reached, then march the needle tip down to the inferior border of the bone, and inject 1-2 cc of lidocaine without epinephrine.
   3. Repeat on opposite side.

C. Metacarpal Block: for complete finger anesthesia.
   1. Raise skin wheal (lidocaine without epinephrine) on dorsolateral and dorsomedial aspect of the metacarpal, just proximal to the MCP joint.
   2. Advance the needle, continuously injecting anesthetic along the metacarpal until the tip is felt on the volar aspect (inject 2 cc).
   3. Repeat on the other side.

D. Field Block: To avoid several injections for multiple lacerations in a confined area.
   1. With 1 1/2 in. long 25 gauge needle, raise a skin wheal with 1% lidocaine without epinephrine. Advance needle in a horizontal plane and continuously inject the anesthetic as it is withdrawn.
   2. Repeat on all sides to completely encircle the wound.

E. Supraorbital Nerve Block: anesthesia for upper eyelid, forehead and scalp to lambdoid suture.
   1. Palpate supraorbital notch immediately above pupil. Raise skin wheal at this site.
   2. Advance needle superiorly until paresthesias are noted. Apply pressure to the upper lid, and inject 2 cc of 1% lidocaine without epinephrine.

F. Infraorbital Nerve Block: anesthesia of the upper lip, nose, lower eyelid and maxillary portion of the face.

1. Palpate infraorbital foramen immediately below midline pupil. Raise skin wheal at this site.
2. Advance the needle until paresthesias are elicited, and inject 2 cc of 1% lidocaine without epinephrine while applying pressure above the infraorbital rim.

G. Mental Nerve Block: anesthesia of the chin and lower lip.

1. Identify the mental foramen which is palpable subcutaneously halfway between the upper and lower border of the mandible. A line drawn connecting the supra and infraorbital foramina and the corner of the mouth would pass through the mental foramen. Prep the skin with ovidone-iodine. Raise a skin wheal at the injection site
2. Advance the 25 gauge needle to, but not into, the foramen, and inject 3 cc of 1% lidocaine without epinephrine.

H. Intercostal Nerve Block: relieve chest wall pain caused by rib fractures.

1. Have patient sit, leaning forward onto a Mayo tray. Identify affected rib and the angle formed by the rib and paraspinous muscle. Raise skin wheal at this angle, over the inferior border of the rib.
2. Advance the needle to just under the inferior border of the rib, aspirate, and inject 5 cc of 1% lidocaine with epinephrine. Marcaine may also be used for prolonged effect.

I. Paracervical Block: To relieve pain of uterine contractions and anesthesia for D & C's.

1. Materials:
- Sterile speculum.
- Povidone-iodine.
- Iowa trumpet needle guard.
- 20 gauge spinal needle.
- 20 gauge, 6 inch needle.
- 10 cc syringe.
- .5% lidocaine without epinephrine.
- .5% Carbocaine without epinephrine.
- Sterile gloves.

2. Position patient in dorsal lithotomy position.

Local and Regional Blocks 595

3. Anesthesia for Dilation and Curettage.
   a. Insert a sterile speculum and cleanse cervix and vagina with povidone-iodine.
   b. Inject 10 cc of .5% lidocaine at the 3 o'clock and 9 o'clock position and 5 cc at the 7 o'clock and 5 o'clock position with a 22 gauge spinal needle to anesthetize the paracervical and uterosacral ligaments respectively. Advance the needle no more than .5 cm into the submucosa.
4. Anesthesia During Labor.
   a. Using sterile technique place the Iowa trumpet in the non-dominant hand and insert into vagina. Place the guard tip into the lateral vaginal fornix in the 3 o'clock position.
   b. Pass the needle through the director, just into the vaginal mucosa. Be sure not to advance more than 1-2 mm.
   c. Aspirate, then inject 5 to 10 cc of .5% Carbocaine into the fornix. Repeat at the 9 o'clock position. Observe for fetal bradycardia.

J. Pudendal Block: anesthesia for vaginal delivery, episiotomy and repair (Fig 17-1).

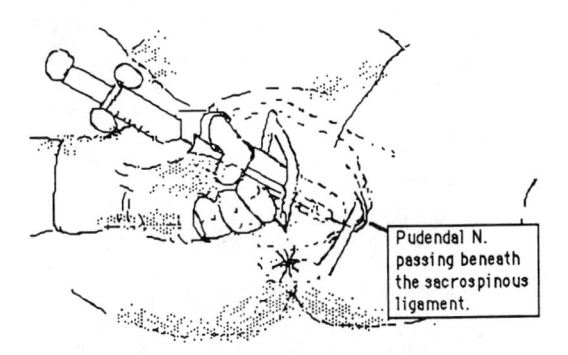

Fig 17-1. Pudendal Block

1. Materials:
- Iowa trumpet.
- .5% Carbocaine.
- 10 cc syringe with 6 inch 20 gauge needle.
- Sterile gloves.
    a. Using sterile technique, place the Iowa trumpet in the non-dominant hand. Insert in the vagina, and position the end of the guard just beneath the tip of the ischial spine.
    b. The needle is inserted, and a submucosal wheal is raised after aspiration. The needle is then advanced and 6 cc of anesthetic is injected.
    c. The needle is then withdrawn back into the needle guard and redirected to a point just above the ischial spine and 2 cc is instilled.
    d. Withdraw the needle and place guard 1cm below ischial spine over the sacrospinous ligament and inject 2 cc into the ligament, withdraw needle and guard.
    e. Repeat process on the opposite side.

ARTERIAL LINE

I. **Indications:**
   - Continuous blood pressure monitoring.
   - When frequent arterial blood gases or other labs are needed, i.e. ventilator patients, diabetic patients.
   - Management of complex MI patients, hypertensive crises.

II. **Contraindications:**
   - Negative Allen's test.
   - Bleeding diathesis.
   - Overlying skin infection.

III. **Materials:**
   - Sterile gloves.
   - Povidone-iodine and alcohol swabs.
   - Rolled towel.
   - Sterile drapes.
   - 20 gauge radial artery catheter.
   - IV tubing.
   - Pressure transducer.
   - 1% lidocaine.
   - 5 cc syringe with 27 gauge 5/8 in. needle.

IV. **Technique:**
   A. Palpate radial pulse and perform Allen's Test. Prep skin with povidone-iodine and alcohol. Place rolled towel under wrist, so wrist lies hyperextended. Drape and don sterile gloves.

   B. Palpate radial artery with non-dominant hand. Raise skin wheal with 1% lidocaine (27 gauge 5/8 in. needle) and instill anesthetic down to the level of the radial artery. Be sure to always aspirate before injecting to avoid intravenous or intra-arterial administration.

   C. Hold 20 gauge radial artery catheter at a 30° angle to the wrist, and advance the catheter towards the pulse until a flashback of blood is noted. Advance another 1-2 mm, then slide the catheter off the needle and into the artery.

D. Hold pressure proximal to the catheter tip to occlude blood flow. Remove the needle, and connect the catheter to the pressure transducer via I.V. tubing flushed with heparinized saline. Tape catheter in place.

V. **Complications:**
- Bleeding.
- Hematoma.
- Thrombotic embolism.
- Infection.
- Catheter tip embolus.
- Arterial spasm.

CENTRAL LINES

I. Indications:
- CVP monitoring.
- Rapid fluid infusion.
- Medication administration.
- Parenteral nutrition.
- Poor peripheral access.
- Conduit for Swan-Ganz catheters, temporary cardiac pacemakers, hemodialysis catheters.

II. Contraindications:
- Bleeding diathesis.
- Overlying skin infection.

III. Materials:
- Sterile gloves and drapes.
- Povidone-iodine and alcohol swabs.
- 16 gauge central venous catheter kit.
- 1% lidocaine without epinephrine.
- Pressure monitor - optional.
- Heparinized saline.
- Sterile gauze.

IV. Technique (Fig 17-2):

A. Position patient supine with slight Trendelenburg. Identify insertion site (infraclavicular or supraclavicular). Supraclavicular approach will be described. Prep skin with povidone-iodine and alcohol. Don gloves and drape patient.

B. Identify landmarks and raise skin wheal at the angle formed by the lateral head of the sternocleidomastoid muscle and the clavicle. Aim needle tip towards contralateral nipple, and inject anesthetic down to the level of the vein, be sure to aspirate before injecting.

C. Attach an 18 gauge long needle to a 10 cc saline filled syringe. Reidentify landmarks, and insert the needle through the skin wheal. Aim towards the contralateral nipple, and advance the needle tip just underneath the clavicle, aspirating while advancing. A flash of blood will indicate successful venipuncture.

600	Hospital Procedures

- D. Advance the needle another 2-3 mm, then remove the syringe. Quickly place finger over hub to avoid air embolism. A free flow of blood confirms placement.
- E. The flexible guide wire is inserted through the needle and into the vein. Do not advance the wire into the right atrium. Remove the needle over the guide wire, making sure the guide wire is securely held throughout removal of the needle. Make a skin incision next to the wire to allow passage of the catheter.
- F. Slide the vein dilator onto the wire, and advance it through the skin and into the vein. Be sure not to advance the guide wire. Remove vein dilator and slide the venous catheter over the wire and into the vein. Be sure to maintain guide wire in position.
- G. Remove guide wire and attach IV tubing to catheter. Suture catheter into position, and dress site with sterile gauze and antibiotic ointment.
- H. Obtain chest x-ray.

V. **Complications:**
- Infection.
- Catheter tip embolus or thrombotic embolus.
- Bleeding.

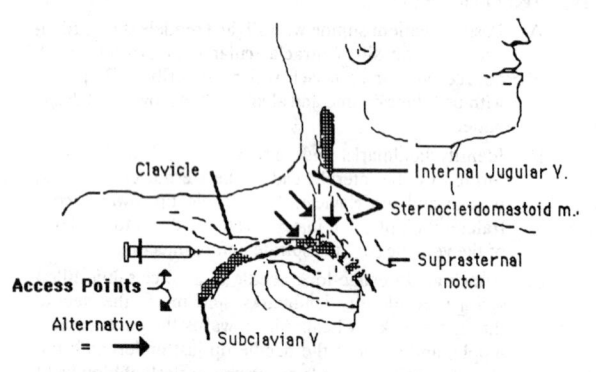

Fig 17-2. Subclavian/Jugular Vein Access

Central Lines

- Hematoma formation.
- Arterial cannulation.
- Pneumothorax.
- Hemothorax.
- Chylothorax.
- Air embolism.
- Arrhythmias.

INTRAUTERINE PRESSURE CATHETER

I. Indications
A. Pitocin induction and augmentation of labor.
B. Evaluation of uterine contractions.
C. Uterine dystocia.
D. Previous C-section.
E. Increased likelihood of fetal compromise or uteroplacental insufficiency.

II. Contraindications
A. Placenta previa or low lying placenta.
B. Long, closed cervix.
C. Intact membranes.
D. Early amniotomy.

III. Materials
- sterile gloves and drapes.
- fluid-filled plastic catheter.
- pressure transducer.
- amniotomy hook.

IV. Technique
A. Don gloves and drape patient in usual fashion. Perform sterile vaginal exam to check position, presentation, dilatation and effacement. Perform amniotomy if indicated.

B. Slide fluid-filled intrauterine catheter over the intravaginal examining hand. Allow catheter tip to slide between the examining hand and the fetal scalp in 6 o'clock position. Slowly advance until the position marker on the catheter is at the introitus. If resistance is met at the 6 o'clock position, try again at the 5 or 7 o'clock positions. DO NOT force the catheter tip against resistance.

C. Connect to pressure transducer and confirm proper functioning.

Intrauterine Pressure Catheter

V. **Complications**
   - early amniotomy, maternal and fetal infection, trauma to fetus, uterine perforation, placental penetration and hemorrhage.

VI. **Interpretations**
   A. Montivedio units: add up millimeters of pressure under each contraction in a 10 minute time span. If 150-250: adequate contractions. If < 150: poor contraction quality. If > 250: hypertonic uterus.

Reference

Pritchard JA, MacDonald PC, and Gant NF, eds. Williams Obstetrics, 17th edition. Connecticut: Appleton-Century-Crofts, 1985.

THORACENTESIS

I. **Indications**: Evaluation of a pulmonary effusion. Provide relief of respiratory distress caused by large effusion.

II. **Contraindications**:
- Severe coagulopathies.
- Small stable effusions.
- Agitated patients.
- Patients responding to medical therapy.

III. **Materials**:
- Povidone-iodine solution and swabs.
- Gauze.
- Alcohol pads.
- Sterile drape and gloves.
- 5/8", 25 gauge needle and 1% Xylocaine.
- 2 inch, 22 gauge needle.
- 3-way stopcock.
- 5 cc syringe.
- 50 cc syringe.
- 3 specimen tubes with stoppers.
- Adhesive tape.
- Optional: vacuum bottle, to bring to 15 gauge needle clamp.

IV. **Technique**

A. Determine puncture site by CXR and percussion. Have patient sit leaning forward. Prep skin with povidone-iodine and alcohol pads. Drape area.

B. Choose entry site below air-fluid interface, above rib. Raise skin wheal with 25 gauge needle and carry anesthesia down through the chest wall. Use 22 gauge 2" needle to anesthetize the pleural surface. "Pop" the needle into the pleural space and confirm location with aspiration of fluid

C. Remove needle, and attach it to the 3 way stopcock and 50 cc syringe. Reinsert and withdraw enough fluid to fill the specimen tubes.

D. To remove a large volume of fluid, fill 50 cc syringe and turn the stopcock to permit emptying. Repeat if necessary. If you will be emptying up to 1 liter of fluid, attach a vacuum bottle by rubber tubing to a 15 gauge needle clamp tubing, and insert needle in clamp and allow vacuum to aspirate the fluid.

E. When finished aspirating, withdraw needle and apply pressure over site for a few minutes and dress with pressure dressing. Observe for dyspnea. Send fluid for cell count and differential, protein, glucose, LDH, culture, gram stain, specific gravity, cytology, AFB, fungal cultures. Obtain post-tap CXR.

V. **Interpretation**: see Chapter 3, Pleural Effusion

VI. **Complications**:
- Pneumothorax.
- Hematoma.
- Hemothorax.
- Infection.

References

Driscoll CE, *et al*, eds. Handbook of Family Practice. Chicago: Year Book Medical Publishers, 1986.

Driscoll CE and Rakel RE, eds. Procedures for Your Practice. Oradell, New Jersey: Medical Economics Co., Inc., 1988.

LUMBAR PUNCTURE - ADULTS

I. Indications:
- New seizure activity.
- Unexplained fever.
- Headache.
- Meningeal signs.
- Confirm leukemia or CNS malignancy.
- Subarachnoid bleeding.
- Dementia evaluation.
- Syncope.
- Asymmetric weakness.
- Hypoesthesia.

II. Contraindications:
- Raised intracranial pressure.
- Patients on anticoagulants.
- Skin infection at puncture site.
- Stiff or unyielding back.

III. Materials:
- Sterile gloves and drapes.
- Povidone-iodine solution.
- 70% alcohol solution.
- 2" x 2" gauze pads.
- 22-25 gauge, 1 1/2 inch spinal needle with stylet.
- Manometer with 3-way stopcock.
- 1% lidocaine without epinephrine in 2 cc syringe with 25 gauge needle.
- Three sterile test tubes.
- Bandaid.

IV. Technique:
A. Have patient lie on side. (With infants and children hold child in either a sitting or left side down position.) Place patient in a knee/chest position with neck flexed.

B. Palpate the L-4 spinous process at the level of the iliac crest and mark the spot with the fingernail. Prep skin starting at the puncture site working outwards in concentric circles. Drape in a sterile fashion

- C. Glove and inject 1-2 cc of local anesthetic into the puncture site. Select the appropriate sized spinal needle (22-25 g) and insert in the midline with the needle parallel to the floor, and the point directed towards the patient's umbilicus.
- D. Advance slowly, and withdraw the stylet every 2-3 mm to see if CSF appears. A "pop" is usually felt upon entering the subdural space, advance the tip another 2-3 mm and check for CSF by withdrawing stylet. If the needle meets bone, withdraw slightly, and redirect needle.
- E. Determine opening pressure with a manometer. Then allow 1 cc of CSF to flow into each of the three sterile vials. Send the first for glucose and protein measurements, second for Gram's stain, C & S, third tube for blood cell count and differential. A fourth tube can be sent for viral titers or cultures, India ink prep, fungal cultures, VDRL, rickettsial titers or cytology. Replace stylet and withdraw the needle.
- F. Dress puncture site with a bandage.

V. Complications:

- Persistent CSF leak.
- Headache (may be avoided if patient remains supine for several hours post lumbar puncture).
- Infection.

URINE COLLECTION

I. **Overview**: Urine collection should first be attempted noninvasively. In the male neonate utilize the Perez reflex.

II. **Technique**: Suspend infant over sterile specimen cup and stroke along the sacral spine, with the thumbnail, beginning at the sacral tip and moving towards the lumbar/dorsal spine region.

Suprapubic Bladder Tap

I. **Indications**: Infant or child under 4 who is not a candidate for urethral catheterization and is unable to void on command. Diagnosis of urinary tract infection. Sepsis workup. FUO workup.

II. **Contraindications**: Empty bladder, bleeding diathesis

III. **Materials**:
- 5-10 cc syringe.
- 23 gauge 1 1/2 inch needle.
- Alcohol or povidone-iodine swabs.
- Adhesive tape.
- Sterile gloves.

IV. **Technique**:
A. Place child supine in "frog leg" position, restrain as needed. Prep skin with alcohol or povidone-iodine.
B. Palpate symphysis pubis with gloved hand (fat crease at symphysis). Attach syringe to needle, and insert it in the midline directly above the symphysis angled toward the infant's coccyx.
C. Aspirate while advancing needle until urine is noted. If needle is advanced 3 cm without return, withdraw and angle needle more caudal and repeat. If no urine is obtained, assume you have a dry tap and withdraw needle.
D. Apply dressing if needed.

V. **Complications:**
- Bleeding
- Hematoma
- Bowel perforation

Reference

Driscoll CE, *et al*, eds. <u>Handbook of Family Practice</u>. Chicago: Year Book Medical Publishers, 1986.

18/ OFFICE PROCEDURES

Tom Francis, M.D.

FOREIGN BODY REMOVAL - EAR

I. **Indications:**
   - Foreign body present in external canal.

II. **Contraindications:**
   - Relative: uncooperative patient.

III. **Materials:**
   - Ear loop or hook.
   - Otoscope.
   - Ear syringe or WaterPik.
   - Mineral oil or viscous lidocaine.
   - Alligator forceps.

IV. **Technique**
   A. Irrigation with a syringe or WaterPik. Be sure TM is intact. Attempt to aim irrigation stream over the foreign body instead of directly at it.
   B. Under direct visualization, place a loop or hook behind the object and remove it.
   C. If a living insect, instill mineral oil or viscous lidocaine and let dwell for several minutes, then irrigate or remove with forceps (under direct visualization).

V. **Complications:**
   - Tympanic membrane ruptured.
   - Trauma to the canal.

Reference

Driscoll CE, *et al*, eds. <u>Handbook of Family Practice</u>. Chicago: Year Book Medical Publishers, 1986.

FOREIGN BODY REMOVAL - EYE

I. Indications:
- Persistent pain.
- Foreign body sensation or history of foreign body.
- Unexplained irritation and erythema.

II. Contraindications:
- Penetrating globe injuries.

III. Materials:
- Topical anesthetic, i.e. Opthaine, Alcaine.
- Cotton-tipped applicators.
- Magnifying loupes.
- Saline for irrigation.
- Eye spud or 25 gauge needle.
- Topical antibiotic.
- Cycloplegic agent (1% Cyclogel, 2% homatropine).
- Eye patches and tape.
- Fluorescent strip.
- Woods lamp.

IV. Technique:
A. Instill topical anesthetic using magnifying loupes.
B. Inspect globe in all gazes, and inspect below lids by pulling down the lower lid, and inverting the upper lid with a cotton tipped applicator.
C. Remove foreign body by:
  1. Pressurized irrigation.
  2. Light touch with a moistened cotton-tipped applicator.
  3. Eye spud or 25 gauge needle
D. If successful, examine eye with fluorescent dye and woods lamp to assess for corneal abrasions. If an abrasion is present instill cycloplegic and topical antibiotic, and patch eye. Recheck abrasions in 24 hours

V. Complications:
- Inability to remove foreign body.

- Inadequate anesthesia.

Reference

Driscoll CE, *et al*, eds. Handbook of Family Practice. Chicago: Year Book Medical Publishers, 1986.

EXCISION OF SKIN LESIONS

There are three techniques to obtain small skin samples: excisional biopsy, punch biopsy, and shave biopsy.

I. **Indications**
   - Whenever a small, full or partial-thickness skin specimen from a lesion is needed for microscopic examination.

II. **Contraindications**
   - Bleeding diathesis (relative).
   - Shave biopsy of melanomas.

III. **Materials**
   A. Skin preparation.
      - Antibacterial soap or alcohol pads.
      - Gloves.
      - 3 cc of 1% lidocaine HCl.
      - 3 cc syringe.
      - 25 gauge needle.
   B. For biopsy.
      - Scalpel with #15 blade.
      - Biopsy punches in various sizes.
      - Iris scissors.
      - Specimen container with 10% formalin.
      - Sterile gauze.
      - Adhesive tape.
      - Silver nitrate sticks or Monsel's solution.
      - Cotton-tipped applicator.
      - Needle holder.
      - Suture materials (4-0 or 5-0 monofilament).

IV. **Technique**

   Cleanse skin with soap or alcohol and infiltrate skin with 1% lidocaine for anesthesia.

   A. Punch Technique.
      1. Select smallest size punch that will yield an adequate specimen. Stretch skin and then twist punch and press

the edge into the tissue, incising into the subcutaneous fat.
2. Elevate the specimen by the edges with forceps and cut the base with scissors or a scalpel. Place specimen in container and send for pathologic examination.

B. Scalpel technique (excision).
1. With a #15 blade make an elliptical incision around site, extending incision into subcutaneous fat. Elevate with forceps and free base with scalpel or scissors. Place specimen in container and send for pathologic examination.

C. Shave.
1. Hold #15 blade scalpel parallel to the skin, pinch the skin, and shave the lesion from the skin. Place in container and send for pathologic examination.
2. Hemostasis is achieved with either pressure, silver nitrate sticks, Monsel's solution, or a suture.

V. **Complications**
A. Bleeding (usually controlled with the above techniques).
B. Infection.
C. Possible blood-borne dissemination of a melanoma.

Reference

Driscoll CE and Rakel RE, eds. Procedures for Your Practice. Oradell, New Jersey: Medical Economics Co., Inc., 1988.

CRYOTHERAPY

I. **Indications**: Destruction of small superficial lesions.
   - Actinic keratosis.
   - Seborrheic keratosis.
   - Hypertrophic sebaceous glands.
   - Molloscum contagiosum
   - Epithelial nevi.
   - Xanthelasma.
   - Venucal.
   - Condylomata.
   - Benign lentigines.
   - Leukoplakia.
   - Cutaneous horns.

II. **Contraindications**
   A. Absolute.
      - Cryoglobulinemia.
      - Cryofibroginemia.
      - Cold anaphylaxis.
   B. Relative.
      - Autoimmune disorders.
      - Raynaud's syndrome.
      - Thin epithelium (eyelids).
      - Damaged skin (irradiated, patients on chronic steroids).

III. **Materials**
   A. Cotton-ball wick method.
      - Cotton-tipped applicator.
      - Cotton balls.
      - Liquid nitrogen in storage unit.
      - #20 surgical blade.
   B. Nitrogen spray method.
      - Liquid nitrogen spray unit.
      - Tips of various sizes.
      - Liquid nitrogen.
      - #20 surgical blade.
   C. Cryoprobe method.

- Cryoprobe with tips of various sizes.
- Nitrous oxide in tank with pressure regulator gauge.
- #20 surgical blade.

IV. Technique

Consider local anesthesia. Pare hyperkeratotic lesions with #20 blade. If malignancy is suspected, always obtain biopsy first.

A. Cotton-ball technique.
  1. Reinforce cotton applicator with more cotton and shape to suit the lesion. Dip applicator in liquid nitrogen and apply to lesion until there is a thin margin of frozen tissue seen around the lesion.

B. Nitrogen spray.
  1. Choose appropriate sized tip. Spray targeted area until freeze zone extends 2-4 mm into normal tissue or 30 sec. thaw time.
  2. Repeat cycle x 1.

C. Cryoprobe.
  1. Choose appropriate tip and attach to probe. Pressurize gun via regulator. Apply small amount of lubricating jelly to lesion.
  2. Place tip on target area and freeze, elevate tip so as to spare underlying tissue. Achieve 30 second thaw time.
  3. Repeat cycle x 1.

V. Complications

- Pain.
- Infection.

VI. Follow-Up

- Inform patient that a blister usually forms and is at times hemorrhagic.
- Provide appropriate wound care instructions.
- Recheck in 3-4 weeks.

Reference

Driscoll CE and Rakel RE, eds. <u>Procedures for Your Practice</u>. Oradell, New Jersey: Medical Economics Co., Inc., 1988.

ELECTRODESICCATION

Destruction of: Verrucae, molluscum contagiosum, seborrheic or actinic keratoses, skin tags, benign nevi, small malignant skin tumors (basal cell), Bowen's disease, small cutaneous vascular lesions.

I. **Indications**
   - Cosmetic.
   - Therapeutic.

II. **Contraindications**
   - Patient with a cardiac pacemaker.

III. **Materials**
   - Antiseptic solution, NO alcohol.
   - 1% lidocaine without epinephrine.
   - 3 cc syringe with 25 g 5/8 in. needle.
   - Hyfrecator with needle electrode.
   - Curette.
   - Sterile forceps.
   - Dressing material.

IV. **Technique**
   A. Prep skin with antiseptic solution. Instill local anesthetic.
   B. Set hyfrecator on low and set dial to 25 (begin with low current and increase as needed). Desiccate lesion until charred and dry.
   C. Scrape with sharp curette. Repeat desiccation x 1 if benign, x 2 if malignant. (Always obtain biopsy specimen if malignancy suspected.)

V. **Complications**
   - Scar formation/keloid formation.
   - Infection.
   - Change in skin pigmentation at site.

Reference

Roberts P, ed. <u>Useful Procedures in Medical Practice.</u>, Philadelphia: Lea & Febiger, 1986.

TYMPANOMETRY

I. Indications:
- Detect negative middle ear pressure.
- Detect tympanic membrane perforation.
- Detect ossicular chain disruption.
- Check patency of ventilation tubes.
- Screening children for audiometry.

II. Contraindications:
Absolute: None.
Relative: Otitis externa.

III. Materials:
- Otoscope and specula.
- Cerumen spoon.
- Automatic tympanometer and recorder.

IV. Technique:
A. Examine ear canal and remove occluding cerumen or exudate. Inspect tympanic membrane. Select appropriate tip for tympanometer.
B. Grasp helix and straighten ear canal. Position probe, when positioned properly the automatic recording device will be triggered.
C. Leave probe in position until the tympanometer signals the conclusion of the test. Repeat in contralateral ear.

V. Interpretation (Fig 18-1):

References

Driscoll CE, *et al*, eds. Handbook of Family Practice. Chicago: Year Book Medical Publishers, 1986.

Driscoll CE and Rakel RE, eds. Procedures for Your Practice. Oradell, New Jersey: Medical Economics Co., Inc., 1988.

Tympanometry

Normal Tympanic Membrane

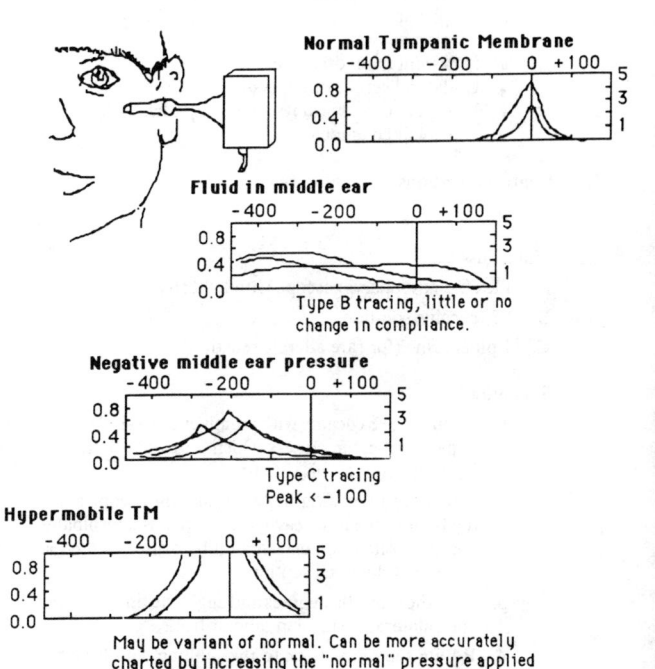

Fluid in middle ear

Type B tracing, little or no change in compliance.

Negative middle ear pressure

Type C tracing
Peak < -100

Hypermobile TM

May be variant of normal. Can be more accurately charted by increasing the "normal" pressure applied to the membrane from 1 to 5 mls.

Fig 18-1. Tympanometry

FLEXIBLE NASOPHARYNGOSCOPY

I. **Indications**
   - Unexplained hoarseness.
   - Stridor and neck/throat pain.
   - Recurrent pneumonia/bronchitis or sinusitis.
   - Dysphagia.
   - Foreign body.
   - Persistent nasal drainage.
   - Unilateral serous otitis media.
   - Unexplained cervical lymphadenopathy.
   - Unexplained earache.

II. **Contraindications**
   - None.

III. **Materials**
   A. Flexible nasopharyngoscope with light source.
   B. 5% cocaine solution.
   C. Epinephrine (for rare allergic reaction).

IV. **Technique**
   1. Instill the 5% cocaine with atomizer or soaked cotton tipped applicator. Assess which nares has better air flow and attempt this side first.
   2. Have the patient mouth breathe and slide scope along the floor of the nasal cavity. Observe nasal turbinates and the ipsilateral eustachian tube orifice located at the end of the nasal septum.
   3. Turn the scope 90 degrees and angle the tip to observe contralateral eustachian tube orifice.
   4. Rotate the scope back to the midline, and have the patient breathe through the nose. Angle the scope 90 degrees downward to advance to the level of the epiglottis to view the larynx. Do not advance past the larynx, as this may cause laryngospasm.
   5. Observe the vocal cords during rest and phonation.

V. **Complications**
- Laryngospasm (as noted above).

VI. **Interpretation**

The following references have illustration of various lesions.

References

Driscoll CE and Rakel RE, eds. <u>Procedures for Your Practice</u>. Oradell, New Jersey: Medical Economics Co., Inc., 1988.

Silberman HD, Wilf H, and Tucker JA. Flexible fiberoptic nasopharyngo-laryngoscopy. <u>Annals of Otology</u>, Rhinology and Laryngology 85(5)5:640, October 1979.

FINE NEEDLE BREAST BIOPSY

I. Indications
- Cytologic evaluation of a breast mass or cyst.
- Distinguish suppurative disease from neoplasm.
- Establish a positive diagnosis of cancer.
- Analyze the estrogen receptor for status of a carcinoma.

II. Contraindications
- Absolute: None.
- Relative: Deep lesions.

III. Materials
- Cameco syringe pistol.
- 20 cc disposable syringe.
- 18, 22 and 25 gauge needles.
- Alcohol pads.
- Microscope slides.
- Spray fixative.
- 1% lidocaine.

IV. Technique

A. Breast exam. Attach syringe to syringe pistol. Prep skin with alcohol pads. 1% lidocaine local anesthesia.

B. Position the mass between the index finger and thumb of your non-dominant hand. Insert the needle quickly through the skin and advance it into the mass. Confirm your location by moving the mass with the needle tip.

C. Apply full suction, and move the needle back and forth within the mass multiple times. Release suction as soon as fluid is retrieved. Discard clear yellow fluid or fluid devoid of particulate matter and reaspirate any remaining mass with a fresh needle.

D. If no specimen is found in the hub, make 10-12 passes for a good sample. Release suction then remove syringe and apply pressure to the puncture site. Disengage the needle from the syringe, fill the syringe with air, reattach to the needle and expel the aspirate onto the slides. Fix the slides immediately and submit it for pathology.

Centrifuge any turbid fluid and prepare a slide from the particulate matter.

V. **Complications**
- Hematoma.
- Infection.
- Pneumothorax.

Reference

Driscoll CE and Rakel RE, eds. <u>Procedures for Your Practice</u>. Oradell, New Jersey: Medical Economics Co., Inc., 1988.

ENDOMETRIAL BIOPSY

I. **Indications**
- Post menopausal bleeding.
- Infertility evaluation.
- Dysfunctional uterine bleeding.
- Patient in need of hormonal therapy (pre and post treatment evaluation).
- Detection of dysplasia in women with a history of pelvic radiation.
- Detection of uterine cancer.
- High risk patients.

II. **Contraindications**
   A. Absolute.
   - Active infection.
   - Pregnancy.

   B. Relative.
   - Inadequate pelvic exam.
   - Cervical stenosis.
   - Uterine flexion.
   - Coagulopathy.
   - Leiomyomata.
   - Severe anemia.
   - Heart disease.
   - Extreme anxiety.

III. **Materials**
- Sterile speculum and gloves.
- Povidone-iodine solution.
- Cotton balls or gauze.
- Graduated dilators.
- Sterile tenaculum.
- 4 mm sterile endometrial suction curette with collecting apparatus and vacuum source.
- Uterine sound.
- Preservative.

IV. **Preparation**
- Premedicate with a non-steroidal anti-inflammatory drug.
- Explain procedure and obtain informed consent.

V. **Technique**

A. Perform bimanual exam to check uterine position and for signs of infection.

B. Insert sterile speculum and inspect cervix. Clean cervix and vagina with povidone-iodine.

C. Grasp the anterior lip of the cervix with a tenaculum, apply gentle traction. Use dilators if the os is stenotic. With post menopausal bleeding, use endocervical curette and collect the sample on filter paper and place in preservative.

D. Sound the uterus. Insert suction curette, apply suction (51-71 mm Hg pressure) and pull the curette out with small sweeping motions. For a diagnostic evaluation curette at all hours of the clock. For a fertility evaluation sample at 3 and 9 o'clock.

E. Aspirate some preservative into the system. Disconnect collecting chamber and fill with preservative, send for evaluation. Remove instruments, and have patient remain recumbent for a few minutes.

VI. **Complications**
- Pain and cramping.
- Bleeding from tenaculum site.
- Uterine perforation.
- Vasovagal syncope.
- Infection.
- Allergic reaction to povidone-iodine.

Reference

Driscoll CE and Rakel RE, eds. <u>Procedures for Your Practice</u>. Oradell, New Jersey: Medical Economics, Co., Inc., 1988.

ARTHROCENTESIS

I. Indications
- Analysis of joint fluid.
- Therapeutic (relief of pain by drainage of tense effusion or instillation of medication).

II. Contraindications
- Infection of nearby skin or soft tissue.

III. Technique
A. General principles of technique.
1. Careful identification of landmarks.
2. Preparation of skin with povidone-iodine and alcohol.
3. Local anesthesia of overlying soft-tissues with 1% lidocaine.
4. Advancement of needle with constant negative pressure.

B. Shoulder (Fig 18-2).
1. Patient should be in a sitting position with arm in lap (this positions the shoulder in mild internal rotation and adduction). Identify insertion site inferior and slightly lateral to tip of coracoid.
2. Prepare site as above.
3. Direct needle dorsally, laterally, and slightly superiorly into joint space.

C. Wrist (Fig 18-3).
1. The wrist should be positioned prone with about $20°$ of flexion. Identify insertion site by marking the distal ends of the ulna and radius. The insertion site is ulnar to the extensor pollicis longus tendon.
2. Prepare the site as above.
3. Direct needle perpendicular to the skin.

D. Elbow (Fig 18-4).
1. Position patient with elbow at $90°$, palm prone. Identify insertion site on the lateral aspect of the elbow in the shallow depression immediately anterior and inferior to the lateral epicondyle of the humerus.

2. Prepare the skin as above.
3. Direct the needle perpendicular to the skin.

E. Knee (Fig 18-5).
   1. Patient should be supine with quadriceps muscle relaxed (patella should be freely moveable). Identify the insertion site immediately beneath the lateral or medial edge of the patella.
   2. Prepare the skin as above.
   3. Direct the needle parallel to the plane of the underside of the patella.

IV. **Intra-Articular Steroids**

A. Large joints such as the knee or shoulder may be injected with the equivalent of 80 mg of methylprednisolone acetate in 1 to 2 ml of 1% lidocaine.

B. Smaller joints such as the wrist, elbow or ankle may be injected with 20 to 40 mg of methylprednisolone acetate in 0.5 to 1 ml of 1% lidocaine.

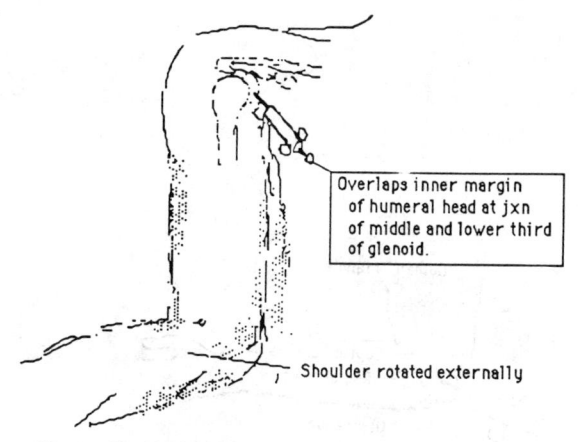

Overlaps inner margin of humeral head at jxn of middle and lower third of glenoid.

Shoulder rotated externally

Fig 18-2. Shoulder Joint Access (Anesthetics or Aspirates)

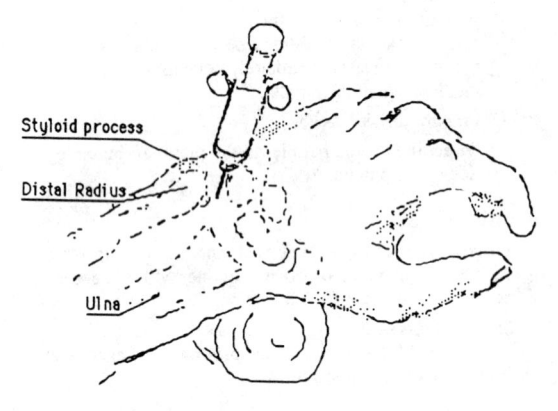

Fig 18-3. Wrist Joint Access

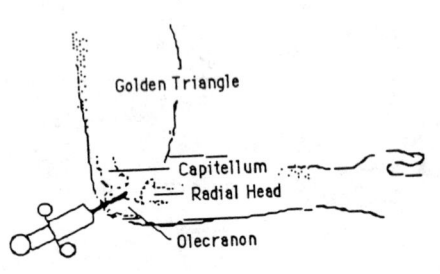

Fig 18-4. Elbow Joint Access

Arthrocentesis

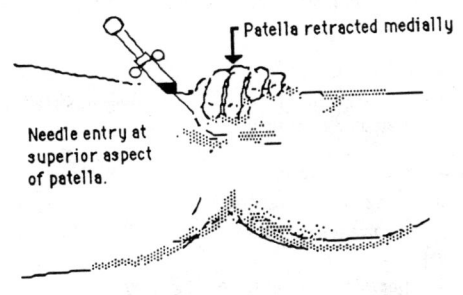

Fig 18-5. Knee Joint Access

INGROWN TOENAILS

I. Overview
- Normally occur on the tibial side of the great toe, but may occur bilaterally. Recurrence is a significant problem.

II. Indications For Treatment
- Unacceptable frequency, pain, swelling, infection, and granulation formation.

III. Contraindications
A. No absolute contraindications.
B. Relative contraindications.
- Diabetes mellitus.
- Peripheral vascular disease.
- Bleeding diathesis.
- Use of phenol with pregnancy.

IV. Materials
- 5 cc 1% lidocaine without epinephrine.
- 5 cc syringe with 25 gauge 5/8 inch needle.
- Betadine and alcohol swabs.
- Sterile cotton.
- Splinter forceps.
- Surgical scissors.
- Silver nitrate sticks.
- Hemostat (small and large).
- Antibiotic ointment.
- Tube gauze.
- Adaptic or other non-stick dressing.
- Tincture of iodine.

V. Technique
A. Initial lesion of < 2 months.
1. Place digital block with 1% lidocaine without epinephrine.
2. Roll lateral edge of nail plate up and away from nail fold with small hemostat. Place rolled cotton between nail plate and nail bed. Apply tincture of iodine.

3. Cauterize with silver nitrate any granulation tissue. Dress with adhesive bandage.

B. Treatment of recurrent lesion.

1. Place digital block and prepare skin with Betadine and alcohol.
2. Fully insert single blade of hemostat between nail plate and bed. Incise nail to the base along the track created by the hemostat.
3. Grasp incised edge and roll it toward affected nail fold and remove. Dry nail bed with cotton applicator and apply phenol to germinal matrix and nail bed. Cauterize granulation tissue with silver nitrate.
4. Dress with antibiotic ointment, non-stick dressing, and tube gauze. Recheck in 2 days.

VI. **Complications**
- Bleeding.
- Infection.
- Recurrence (1%).
- Pain.

Reference

Driscoll CE and Rakel RE, eds. Procedures for Your Practice. Oradell, New Jersey: Medical Economics Co., Inc., 1988.

VASECTOMY

Surgical division of the vas deferens for permanent male sterilization.

I. **Indications**
   - Sterilization.

II. **Contraindications**
   - Bleeding diathesis.
   - Epididymitis/orchitis or other concurrent GU infection.
   - Large varicocele or other anomaly, hindering delineation of normal anatomy.

III. **Materials**
   - Betadine scrub and alcohol pads.
   - Sterile gauze and drapes.
   - #15 scalpel blade.
   - Towel clips (2).
   - 2 hemostats.
   - Iris scissors.
   - Alice clamp (1).
   - 4-0 Dexon suture.
   - Specimen container with 10% formalin (2) L&R.

IV. **Technique**

   (Note: several techniques are described for separating the remaining ends of the vas post-excision. This technique is the one used by the author.)

   A. Before coming to the office, patient should shave all hair from scrotum, then bathe. Prep skin with Betadine and/or alcohol. Isolate area with sterile drapes.

   B. Bring vas deferens to skin surface and hold between first, second and third fingers. Make 1/2 inch incision directly over vas and bluntly dissect down to vas.

   C. Once isolated, place Alice clamp so as not to allow vas to fall back into scrotum.

- D. Carry blunt dissection distal and proximal to expose 2 cm of the vas. Place towel clips around both ends and remove Alice clamp.
- E. Double ligate proximal and distal ends with Dexon suture. Place hemostats partially across the proximal and distal ends of the vas, and excise a 1.5 cm portion between the Dexon sutures. Place specimen in appropriately labeled container and send for pathologic examination.
- F. Fulgurate proximal and distal ends. Oversew proximal end and surrounding tissue so as to place it in a separate, superficial tissue plane.
- G. Remove clamps and close skin incision with Dexon suture. Repeat on opposite side.

V. **Post-Op Instructions**

- Scrotal support x 24-48 hours.
- Rest.
- Analgesics.
- Elevate and ice scrotum.
- Shower after 24 hours.
- 1 week check up.
- Check sperm count after 25-30 ejaculations or 6 weeks post-procedure.
- Continue contraception until azoospermia confirmed.

VI. **Complications**

- Pain.
- Bleeding and bruising.
- Infection.
- Swelling.
- Spermatocele formation.
- Recanalization.
- Psychological sexual dysfunction.

Reference

Driscoll CE and Rakel RE, eds. Procedures for Your Practice. Oradell, New Jersey: Medical Economics Co., Inc., 1988.

FLEXIBLE SIGMOIDOSCOPY

I. Indications

- Screening age 50, 51 (then every 3-5 years if first two negative).
- Melena or hematochezia.
- GI pain or cramping.
- Changes in bowel habits (stool caliber, constipation, diarrhea, differences in frequency).
- Anemia.
- Unexplained weight loss.
- Guaiac (+) stool.
- X-ray evidence of colorectal disease.
- Suspected foreign body.
- Patients with a history of colorectal lesions or inflammatory bowel disease.
- Family history of polyps or colorectal cancer.

II. Contraindications

- Acute diverticulitis with fever.
- Suspected bowel perforation.
- Peritonitis.
- Recent MI or severe cardiovascular disease.
- Ischemic bowel disease.
- Large aortic or iliac aneurysms.
- Patients with history of multiple abdominal surgeries and radiation therapy.
- Suspected complete or GI obstruction.
- Toxic megacolon.
- Patients with prosthetic heart valves without antibiotic prophylaxis one hour prior to procedure.

III. Materials

- Adjustable table.
- Water-soluble lubricant.
- Gloves.
- Occult blood testing cards.
- Anoscope.
- Flexible fiberoptic sigmoidoscope with light source.
- Suction.
- Air and water sources.

Flexible Sigmoidoscopy

- Biopsy forceps and brush.

III. Bowel Preparation

A. Clear liquids for 24 hours before procedure.

B. Biscodyl suppository 24 hours before procedure.

C. 10 oz. of magnesium citrate the afternoon before procedure.

D. Two Fleets enemas at one and two hours before the procedure.

IV. Technique

A. Have patient in left lateral decubitus, Sim's knee-chest position, or supine with the right leg flexed.

B. Perform digital rectal and anoscopic exam and check for occult blood. Lubricate the anus and scope and insert the scope under direct visualization.

C. Insufflate minimal amounts of air to distend the colon and allow visualization. Scope should be advanced only under direct visualization of the lumen.

D. Inspect rectal mucosa. Advance to recto-sigmoid junction and negotiate a 90 degree angle by use of torquing and gentle insertion and partial withdrawal (dithering) techniques. Torque the scope clockwise to help advance it into the sigmoid colon. Advance the scope through the sigmoid colon and into the descending colon if using a long enough scope.

E. Begin systematic examination of the colonic mucosa with gentle, slow scope withdrawal. Use biopsy forceps and brush to perform a biopsy on any suspect regions. Inspect behind folds.

V. Interpretation

A. "Red out" -- pushing scope against bowel wall.

B. Blanching of colonic mucosa -- indicates too much pressure against the bowel wall.

VI. Documentation

- Exam indications.
- Bowel prep type and adequacy.

- Findings of digital and anoscopic exam.
- Insertion technique and ease of insertion.
- Depth of insertion.
- Mucosal findings.
- Anatomic site, depth of appearance of lesions.
- Site of biopsy or photographs.
- Patient's tolerance of procedure.

VII. Complications

- Discomfort.
- Bowel perforation.

Reference

Driscoll CE and Rakel RE, eds. <u>Procedures for Your Practice</u>. Oradell, New Jersey: Medical Economics Co., Inc., 1988.

Reference Data

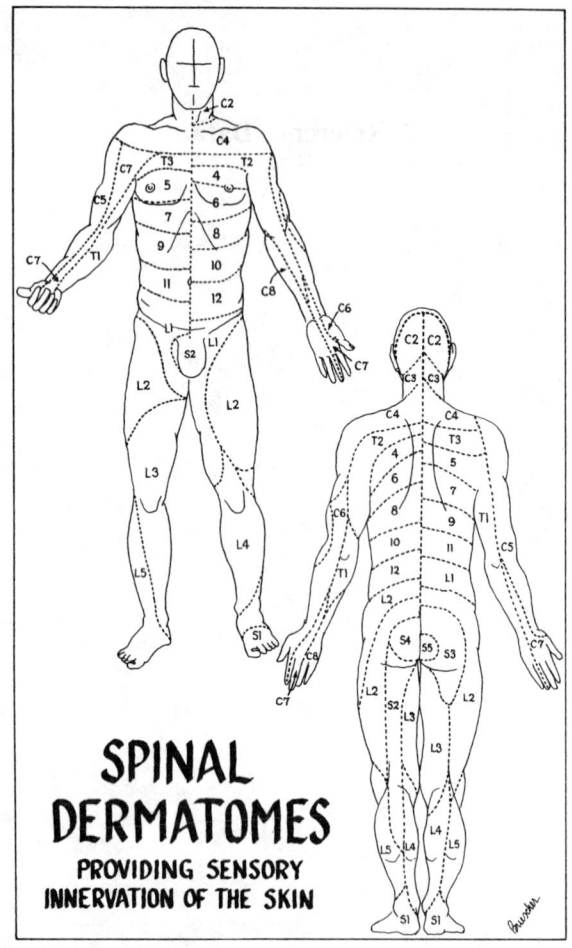

From Rowe PC: *The Harriet Lane Handbook*, ed 11. Chicago, Year Book Medical Publishers, 1987, p. 363. Used with permission.

Reference Data   641

Nomogram for the determination of body surface area of children and adults.
(Reproduced, with permission, from Boothby & Sandiford: Boston M&S J
1921;185:337.) (Revised 1979.)

Nomogram for the determination of body surface area of children. (Reproduced, with permission, from Du Bois: Basal Metabolism in Health and Disease. Lea & Febiger, 1930.)

Nomogram for the determination of body surface area of children and adults.

Nomogram for the determination of body surface area of children.

Ref: Way LW (ed): Current Surgical Diagnosis and Treatment, 7th edition.
Lange Medical Publications, Los Altos, CA, 1985, p. 1188, with permission.

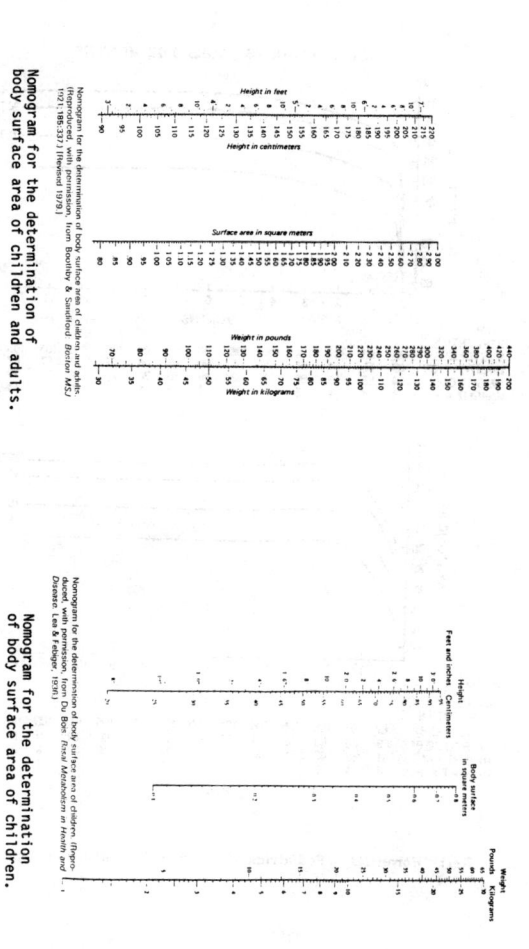

BLOOD PRESSURES, AGES 0-12 MONTHS

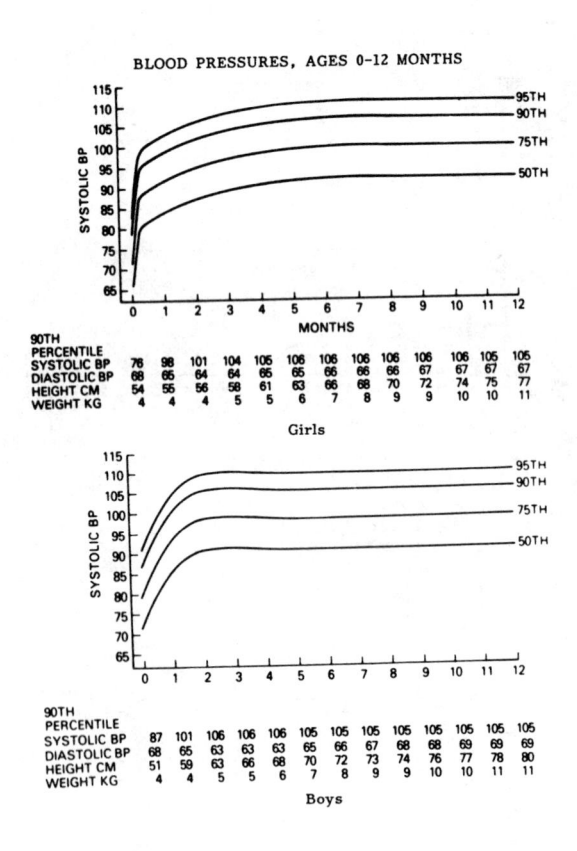

Girls

90TH PERCENTILE													
SYSTOLIC BP	76	98	101	104	105	106	106	106	106	106	106	105	105
DIASTOLIC BP	68	65	64	64	65	65	66	66	66	67	67	67	67
HEIGHT CM	54	55	56	58	61	63	66	68	70	72	74	75	77
WEIGHT KG	4	4	4	5	5	5	6	7	8	9	9	10	11

Boys

90TH PERCENTILE													
SYSTOLIC BP	87	101	106	106	106	105	105	105	105	105	105	105	105
DIASTOLIC BP	68	65	63	63	63	65	66	67	68	68	69	69	69
HEIGHT CM	51	59	63	66	68	70	72	73	74	76	77	78	80
WEIGHT KG	4	4	5	5	6	7	8	9	9	10	10	11	11

Ref: Horan MJ. Pediatrics 1987; 79:1-25. With permission.

Reference Data

BLOOD PRESSURES, AGES, 1-13 YEARS

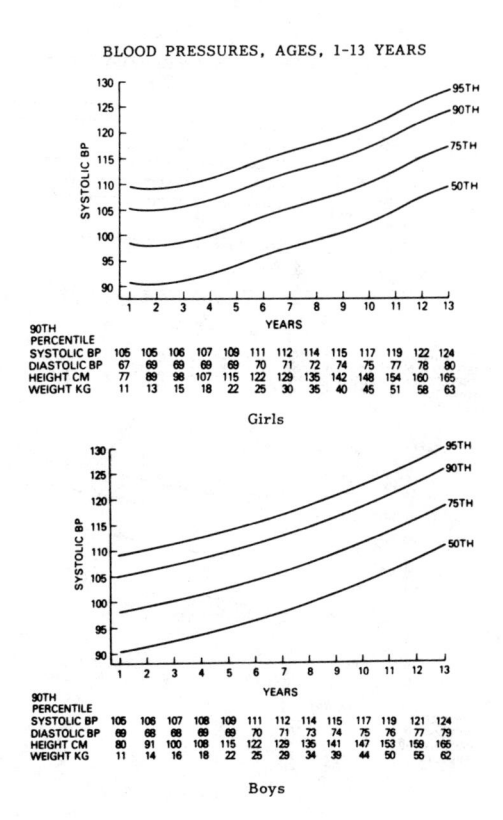

Girls

90TH PERCENTILE													
SYSTOLIC BP	105	105	106	107	109	111	112	114	115	117	119	122	124
DIASTOLIC BP	67	69	69	69	69	70	71	72	74	75	77	78	80
HEIGHT CM	77	89	98	107	115	122	129	135	142	148	154	160	165
WEIGHT KG	11	13	15	18	22	25	30	35	40	45	51	58	63

Boys

90TH PERCENTILE													
SYSTOLIC BP	105	106	107	108	109	111	112	114	115	117	119	121	124
DIASTOLIC BP	69	68	68	69	69	70	71	73	74	75	76	77	79
HEIGHT CM	80	91	100	108	115	122	129	135	141	147	153	159	165
WEIGHT KG	11	14	16	18	22	25	29	34	39	44	50	55	62

Ref: Horan MJ. Pediatrics 1987; 79:1-25. With permission.

BLOOD PRESSURES, AGES, 13-18 YEARS

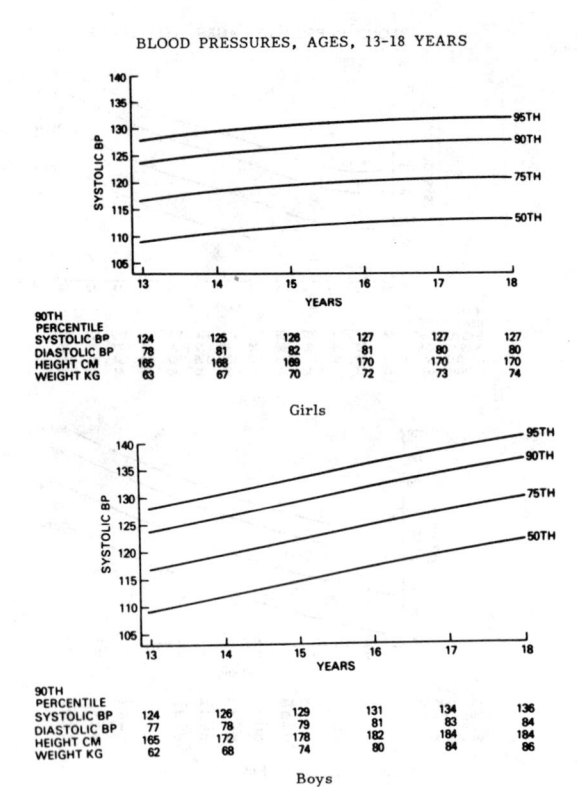

Girls

90TH PERCENTILE						
SYSTOLIC BP	124	125	126	127	127	127
DIASTOLIC BP	78	81	82	81	80	80
HEIGHT CM	165	168	169	170	170	170
WEIGHT KG	63	67	70	72	73	74

Boys

90TH PERCENTILE						
SYSTOLIC BP	124	126	129	131	134	136
DIASTOLIC BP	77	78	79	81	83	84
HEIGHT CM	165	172	178	182	184	184
WEIGHT KG	62	68	74	80	84	86

Ref: Horan MJ. Pediatrics 1987; 79:1-25. With permission.

Normal Values - Hematology

Age	Hgb (gm%) mean (-2SD)	Hct (%) mean (-2SD)	MCV (fl) mean (-2SD)	MCHC (gm/%RBC) (mean (-2SD)	Rectic (%)	WBC/mm³ x 100 mean (-2SD)	Plts (10³/mm³ mean (±2SD)
26-30 wk gestation [1]	13.4 (11)	41.5 (34.9)	118.2 (106.7)	37.9 (30.6)	-	4.4 (2.7)	254 (180-327)
28 wks	14.5	45	120	31	(5-10)	-	275
32 wks	15.0	47	118	32	(3-10)	-	290
Term[2] (cord)	16.5(13.5)	51(42)	108(98)	33(30)	(3-7)	18.1(9-30)[3]	290
1 - 3 days	18.5 (14.5)	56 (45)	108 (95)	33 (30)	(3-7)	18.1 (9-30)[3]	290
2 wk	16.6 (13.4)	53 (41)	105 (88)	31.4 (28.1)		11.4 (5-20)	252
1 month	13.9 (10.7)	44 (33)	101 (91)	31.8 (28.1)	(0.1-1.7)	10.8 (5-19.5)	
2 months	11.2 (9.4)	35 (28)	95 (84)	31.8 (28.3)			
6 months	12.6 (11.1)	36 (31)	76 (68)	35 (32.7)	(0.7-2.3)	11.9 (6-17.5)	
6mon - 2yrs	12 (10.5)	36 (33)	78 (70)	33 (30)		10.6- (6-17)	
2 - 6yrs	12.5 (11.5)	37 (34)	81 (75)	34 (31)	(0.5-1.0)	8.5 (5-15.5)	(150-350)
6 - 12yrs	13.5 (11.5)	40 (35)	86 (77)	34 (31)	(0.5-1.0)	8.1 (4.5-13.5)	
12 - 18 yrs					(0.5-1.0)		
male	14.5 (13)	43 (36)	88 (78)	34 (31)	(0.5-1.0)	7.8 (4.5-13.5)	*
female	14 (12)	41 (37)	90 (78)	34 (31)	(0.5-1.0)	7.8 (4.5-13.5)	*
Adult							
male	15.5 (13.5)	47 (41)	90 (80)	34 (31)	(0.8-2.5)	7.4 (4.5-11)	*
female	14 (12)	41 (36)	90 (80)	34 (31)	(0.8-4.1)	7.4 (4.5-11)	*

[1] Values are from fetal samplings. [2] Under 1 month, capillary Hgb exceeds venous: 1hr-3.6gm difference; 5 days-2.2 gm difference; 3 wks-1.1 gm difference. [3] Mean (95% confidence limits).

Cerebrospinal Fluid

Cell Count		%PMNs
Preterm mean	9.0 (0-25.4 WBC/mm^3)	57%
Term mean	8.2 (0-22.4 WBC/mm^3)	61%
>1 mo	0-7	0

Glucose		
Preterm	24-63 mg/dl	(mean 50)
Term	34-119 mg/dl	(mean 52)
Child	40-80 mg/dl	

CSF Glucose/Blood Glucose (%)
- Preterm 55-105
- Term 44-128
- Child 50%

Lactic Acid Dehydrogenase: Mean 20 U/ml (range 5-30 U/ml)

Myelin Basic Protein: <4 ng/ml

Pressure: Initial L.P. (mm H$_2$O)
- Newborn 80-110 (<110)
- Infant/Child <200 (lateral recumbent position)
- Respiratory movements 5-10

Protein		
Preterm	(mean 115)	65-150 mg/dl
Term	(mean 90)	20-170 mg/dl
Children	Ventricular	5-15 mg/dl
	Cisternal	5-25 mg/dl
	Lumbar	5-40 mg/dl

Biophysical Profile Scoring: Technique

Biophysical variable	Score = 2	Score = 0
1. Fetal breathing movements	>1 episode of >30 s in 30 min	Absent or no episode of >30 s in 30 min
2. Gross body movements	>3 discrete body/limb movements in 30 min (episodes of active continuous movement considered as single movement)	<2 episodes of body/limb movements in 30 min
3. Fetal tone	>1 episode of active extension with return to flexion of fetal limb(s) or trunk. Opening and closing of hand considered normal tone	Either slow extension with return to partial flexion or movement of limb in full extension or absent fetal movement
4. Reactive fetal heart rate	>2 episodes of acceleration of >15 bpm and of >15 s associated with fetal movement in 10 min	<2 episodes of acceleration of fetal heart rate or acceleration of >15 bpm in 20 min
5. Qualitative amniotic fluid	>1 pocket fluid measuring >1 cm in two perpendicular planes	Either no pockets or a pocket <1 cm in two perpendicular planes

Biophysical Profile Scoring: Interpretation

Score Interpretation	Incidence of Low 5 min Apgar Scores (%)	Incidence of Fetal Distress in Labor (%)	Perinatal Mortality Rate (Per 1000 Live Births)
10 - Normal infant, low risk for chronic asphyxia	2	3	0
8 - Normal infant, low risk for chronic asphyxia	9	9	40
6 - Suspected chronic asphyxia	13	28	0
4 - Suspected chronic asphyxia	27	27	91
2 - Strong suspicion of chronic asphyxia	50	86	125
0 - Strong suspicion of chronic asphyxia	80	100	600

Reference Data

NEUROLOGICAL SIGN	SCORE 0	1	2	3	4	5
POSTURE						
SQUARE WINDOW	90°	60°	45°	30°	0°	
ANKLE DORSIFLEXION	90°	75°	45°	20°	0°	
ARM RECOIL	180°	90-180°	<90°			
LEG RECOIL	180°	90-180°	<90°			
POPLITEAL ANGLE	180°	160°	130°	110°	90°	<90°
HEEL TO EAR						
SCARF SIGN						
HEAD LAG						
VENTRAL SUSPENSION						

Redrawn from Dubowitz L, et al: *J Pediatr* 1970; 77:1.

Techniques of Assessment of Neurologic Criteria (modified from Dubowitz)

POSTURE: Observe infant quiet, supine. Score 0: arms, legs extended; 1: beginning flexion of hips and knees, arms extended; 2: stronger flexion legs, arms extended; 3: arms slightly flexed, legs flexed and abducted; 4: full flexion arms, legs.

SQUARE WINDOW: Flex hand on forearm enough to obtain fullest possible flexion without wrist rotation. Measure angle between the hypothenar eminence and the ventral aspect of the forearm.

ANKLE DORSIFLEXION: Foot is dorsiflexed as much as possible onto anterior aspect of the leg. Measure the angle between the dorsum of the foot and the anterior aspect of the leg.

ARM RECOIL: With infant supine, flex forearms for 5 sec, then fully extend by pulling on hands, then release. Score 2: arms return briskly to full flexion; 1: response is sluggish or incomplete; 0: arms remain extended.

LEG RECOIL: With infant supine, flex hips and knees for 5 sec, then extend by pulling on feet, and release. Score 2: maximal response - full flexion of hips and knees; 1: partial flexion; 0: minimal flexion.

POPLITEAL ANGLE: Hold infant supine with pelvis flat, thigh held in the knee-chest position. Extend leg by gentle pressure and measure popliteal angle.

HEEL TO EAR MANEUVER: With baby supine, draw foot as near to the head without forcing it. Observe distance between foot and head, and degree of extension at the knee. Knee is free and may be down alongside abdomen.

SCARF SIGN: With baby supine, pull infant's hand around the neck around the opposite shoulder. See how far the elbow will go across. Score 0: Elbow reaches opposite axillary line; 1: past midaxillary line; 2: past midline; 3: elbow unable to reach midline.

HEAD LAG: With baby supine, grasp the hands and pull slowly towards the sitting position. Observe the position of head in relation to trunk. In small infant, head may initially be supported by one hand. Score 0: complete lag; 1: partial control; 2: head in line with body; 3: head anterior to body.

VENTRAL SUSPENSION: Suspend infant in prone position. Note back extension, extremity flexion, and head and trunk alignment. Grade according to diagrams.

Assessment of gestational age by physical criteria

External Sign	0	1	2	3	4
Edema	Obvious edema of hands and feet; pitting over tibia	No obvious edema of hands and feet; pitting over tibia	No edema		
Skin texture	Very thin, gelatinous	Thin and smooth	Smooth; medium thickness. Rash or superficial peeling	Slight thickening. Superficial cracking and peeling especially of hands and feet	Thick and parchment-like; superficial or deep cracking
Skin color	Dark red	Uniformly pink	Pale pink; variable over body	Pale; only pink over ears, lips, palms, or soles	
Skin opacity (trunk)	Numerous veins, venules clearly seen, especially over abdomen	Veins and tributaries seen	A few large vessels clearly seen over abdomen	A few large vessels seen indistinctly over abdomen	No blood vessels seen
Lanugo (over back)	No lanugo	Abundant; long and thick over whole back	Hair thinning especially over lower back	Small amount of lanugo and bald area	At least 1/2 of back devoid of lanugo
Plantar creases	No skin creases	Faint red marks over anterior half of sole	Definite red marks over > anterior 1/2; indentations over < anterior 1/3	Indentations over > anterior 1/3	Definite deep indentations over > anterior 1/3
Nipple formation	Nipple barely visible; no areola	Nipple well defined; areola smooth and flat, diameter <0.75 cm	Areola stippled, edge not raised, diameter <0.75 cm	Areola stippled, edge raised, diameter >0.75 cm	
Breast size	No breast tissue palpable	Breast tissue on one or both sides, <0.5 cm diameter	Breast tissue both sides; one or both 0.5-1.0 cm	Breast tissue both sides; one or both >1 cm	

Reference Data   651

Assessment of gestational age by physical criteria (continued).

External Sign	0	1	2	3	4
Ear form	Pinna flat, and shapeless; little or no incurving of edge	Incurving of part of edge of pinna	Partial incurving whole of upper pinna	Well-defined incurving whole or upper pinna	
Ear firmness	Pinna soft, easily folded, no recoil	Pinna soft, easily folded, slow recoil	Cartilage to edge of pinna but soft in places, ready recoil	Pinna firm, cartilage to edge; instant recoil	
Genitals Male	Neither testis in scrotum	At least one testis high in scrotum	At least one testis right down		
Female (with hips 1/2 abducted)	Labia major widely separated, labia minora protruding	Labia majora almost cover labia minora	Labia majora completely cover labia minora		

Dubowitz score and estimation of gestational age

The total Dubowitz score is the sum of the scores based on neurologic and physical criteria. Total score is plotted against gestational age below.

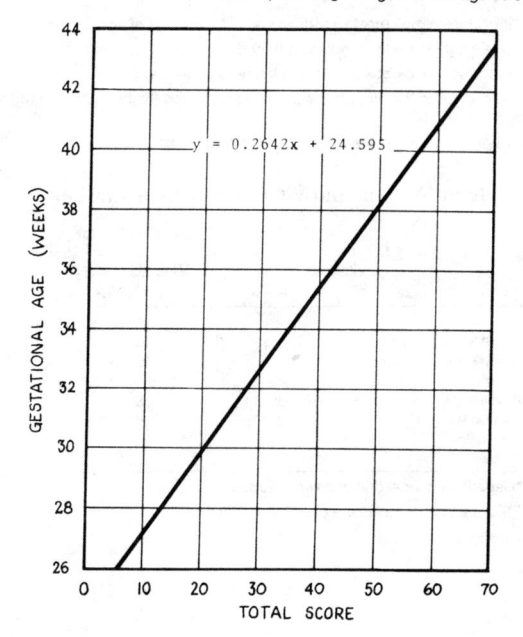

$y = 0.2642x + 24.595$

NOTE: Optimal timing for the Dubowitz exam is within the first 24 hours of life, preferably between 12 and 24 hours of age.

The original population on which Dubowitz scoring was based included only 2 infants with gestational age < 30 wks.

Guide to the Introduction of Supplemental Feedings in Infancy

1. Introduce supplemental foods at about 4-6 months of age.
2. Use single ingredient (not mixed) foods.
3. Introduce foods one at a time at intervals of 3-7 days.
4. Add water to the diet when solids are introduced (higher renal solute load with solids).
5. Begin juices when the infant can drink from a cup.

Guide to Mineral and Vitamin Supplementation

Age	multi	Vitamins D	E	Folate	Minerals Fe	Fluoride*
0-6 months						
(breast fed)		±				±
(formula fed)						±
Preterm						
(breast fed)	+	+	±	±	+	±
(formula fed)	+	+	±	±	+	±
> 6 months		+			±**	±
Children						±

*Depends on local drinking water supply.

**Cereal and formulas are possible sources.

Reference Data

GIRLS
BIRTH TO 36 MONTHS
LENGTH AND WEIGHT

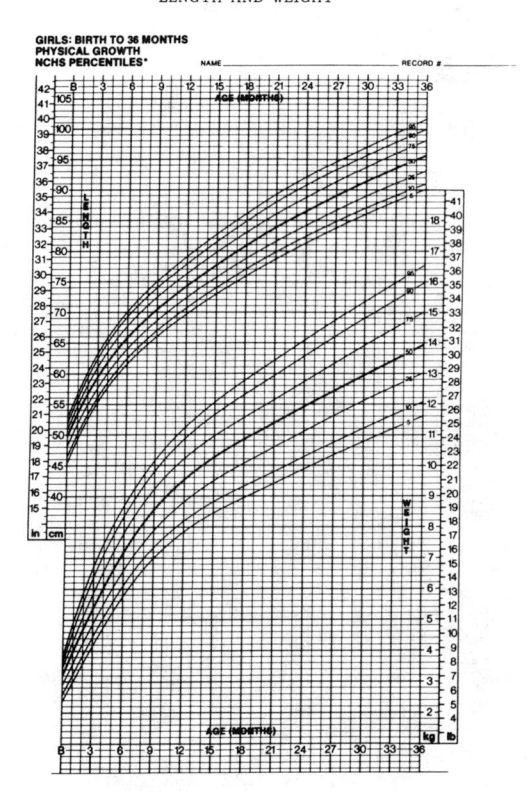

Adapted from National Center for Health Statistics data. Copyright Ross Laboratories, 1976.

GIRLS
2 TO 18 YEARS
STATURE AND WEIGHT

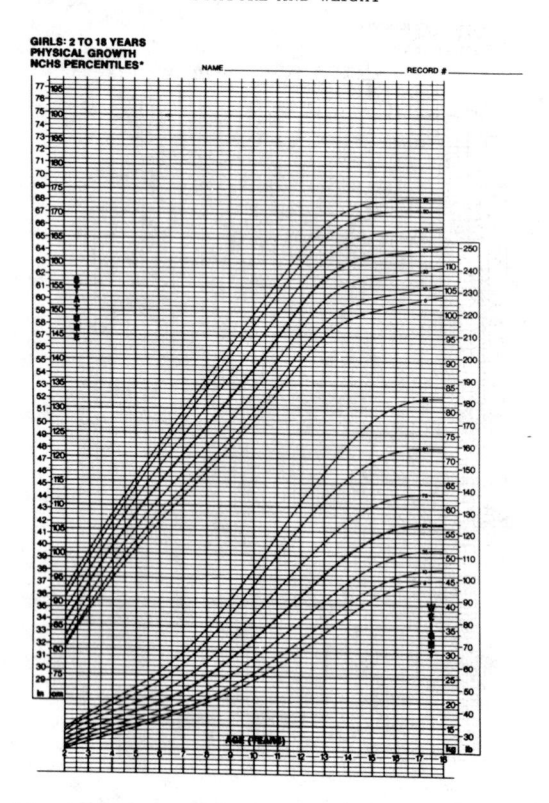

Adapted from National Center for Health Statistics data. Copyright Ross Laboratories, 1976.

Reference Data

BOYS
BIRTH TO 36 MONTHS
LENGTH AND WEIGHT

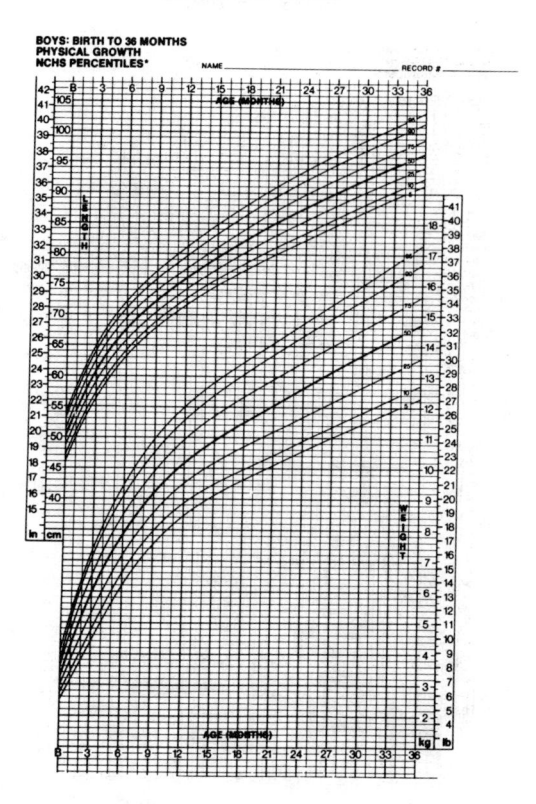

Adapted from National Center for Health Statistics data. Copyright Ross Laboratories, 1976.

BOYS
2 TO 18 YEARS
STATURE AND WEIGHT

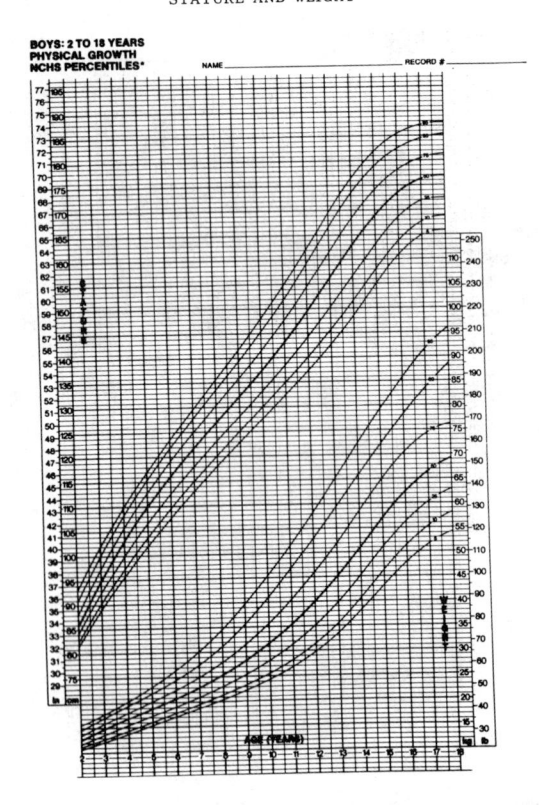

Adapted from National Center for Health Statistics data. Copyright Ross Laboratories, 1976.

Developmental Milestones/Language Skills

Age	Gross Motor	Visual Motor	Language	Social
1 mo	Raises head slightly from prone, makes crawling movements, lifts chin up	Has tight grasp, follows to midline	Alerts to sound (e.g. by blinking, moving, startling)	Regards face
2 mos	Holds head in midline, lifts chest off table	No longer clenches fist tightly, follows object past midline	Smiles after being stroked or talked to	Recognizes parent
3 mos	Supports on forearms in prone, holds head up steadily	Holds hands open at rest, follows in circular fashion	Coos (produces long vowel sounds in musical fashion)	Reaches for familiar people or objects, anticipates feeding
4-5 mos	Rolls front to back, back to front, sits well when propped, supports on wrists and shifts weight	Moves arms in unison to grasp, touches cube placed on table	Orients to voice; 5 mos - orients to bell (localized laterally) says "ah-goo," razzes	Enjoys looking around environment
6 mos	Sits well unsupported, puts feet in mouth in supine position	Reaches with either hand, transfers, uses raking grasp	Babbles; 7 mos - orients to bell (localizes indirectly); 8 mos - "dada/mama" indiscriminately	Recognizes strangers
9 mos	Creeps, crawls, cruises, pulls to stand, pivots when sitting	Uses pincer grasp, probes with forefinger, holds bottle, fingerfeeds	Understands "no", waves bye-bye; 10 mos "dada/mama" discriminately; 11 mos - one word other than	Starts to explore environment, plays pat-a-cake

Developmental Milestones/Language Skills (continued)

Age	Gross Motor	Visual Motor	Language	Social
12 mos	Walks alone	Throws objects, lets go of toys, hand release, uses mature pincer grasp	Follows one-step command with gesture, uses two words other than "dada/mama"; 14 mos - uses three words	Imitates actions, comes when called, cooperates with dressing
15 mos	Creeps upstairs, walks backwards	Builds tower of 2 blocks in imitation of examiner, scribbles in imitation	Follows one-step command without gesture, uses 4-6 words and immature jargoning (runs several unintelligible words together)	
18 mos	Runs, throws toy from standing without falling	Turns 2-3 pages at a time, fills spoon and feeds himself	Knows 7-20 words, knows one body part, uses mature jargoning (includes intelligible words in jargoning)	Copies parent in tasks (e.g. sweeping, dusting), plays in company of other children
21 mos	Squats in play, goes up steps	Builds tower of 5 blocks, drinks well from cup	Points to 3 body parts, uses two-word combinations, has 2-word vocabulary	Asks to have food and to go to toilet

Developmental Milestones/Language Skills (continued)

Age	Gross Motor	Visual Motor	Language	Social
24 mos	Walks up and down steps without help	Turns pages one at a time, removes shoes, pants, etc., imitates stroke	Uses 50 words, two-word sentences, uses pronouns, (I, you, me) Inappropriately, points to 5 body parts, understands 2 step command	Parallel play
30 mos	Jumps with both feet off floor, throws ball overhand	Unbuttons, holds pencil in adult fashion, differentiates horizontal and vertical line	Uses pronouns (I, you, me) appropriately, understands concept of "one", repeats 2 digits forward	Tells first and last names when asked, gets himself drink without help
3 yrs	Pedals tricycle, can alternate feet when going up steps	Dresses and undresses partially, dries hands if reminded, draws a circle	Uses 3 word sentences, uses plurals, past tense. Knows all pronouns. Minimum 250 words, understands concept of "two"	Group play, shares toys, takes turns, plays well with others, knows full name, age, sex
4 yrs	Hops, skips, alternates feet going downstairs	Buttons clothing fully, catches ball	Knows colors, says song or poem from memory, asks questions	Tells "tall tales", plays cooperatively with a group of children

Developmental Milestones/Language Skills (continued)

Age	Gross Motor	Visual Motor	Language	Social
5 yrs	Skips, alternating feet, jumps over low obstacles	Ties shoes, spreads with knife	Prints first name, asks what a word means	Plays competitive games, abides by rules, likes to help in household tasks

SBE Prophylaxis

Indicated for vulvar heart disease, prosthetic valves, congenital heart disease, mitral valve prolapse with regurgitation, IHSS.

	Adult	**Child**
I. <u>Oral</u>:		
A. Dental and Upper Respiratory Procedures:		
1. PCN-V	2 gms 1 hr before and 1 gm 6 hrs later	<60 lbs: 1/2 adult dose
or		
2. Erythromycin	1 gm 2 hrs before and 500 mg 6 hrs later	20 mg/kg 2 hrs before and 10 mg/kg 6 hrs later
B. GI and GU Procedures:		
1. Amoxicillin	3 gms 1 hr before and 1.5 gms 6 hrs later	50mg/kg 1 hr before, 25 mg/kg 6 hrs later

II. <u>Parenteral</u>: recommended for prosthetic valves, previous history or endocarditis.

	Adult	**Child**
1. Ampicillin <u>and</u> Gentamicin	2 gms IM/IV 30 min before 1.5 mg/kg IM/IV 30 min before	50 mg/kg IM/IV 30 min before 2 mg/kg IM/IV 30 min before
or		
2. Vancomycin (gentamicin should be used with vancomycin for GU and GI procedures)	1 gm IV (over 1 hr) starting 1 hr before	20 mg/kg IV (over 1 hr) starting 1 hr before

Modified Coma Scale for Infants

Activity	Best Response	
Eye Opening	Spontaneous	4
	To Speech	3
	To pain	2
	None	1
Verbal	Coos, babbles	5
	Irritable	4
	Cries to pain	3
	Moans to pain	2
	None	1
Motor	Normal spontaneous movements	6
	Withdraws to touch	5
	Withdraws to pain	4
	Abnormal flexion	3
	Abnormal extension	2
	None	1

Index

A

Abdomen
  pain, 408–413
    abdominal exam, 412
    aggravating factors, 410
    associated symptoms, 410–411
    chronology, 409–410
    diagnostic studies, 413
    history, 408–409
    laboratory, 412
    left lower quadrant, 409
    location, 408–409
    medical history, past, 411
    midepigastric, 408
    pelvic exam, 412
    periumbilical, 409
    physical exam, 411–412
    rectal exam, 412
    relieving factors, 410
    right lower quadrant, 409
    right upper quadrant, 408
    treatment, initial, 412–413
    vital signs in, 411
  stab wounds, 21
  trauma, 20–21
    blunt, 21
    penetrating, 20–21
Abortion
  causes, possible, 294
  complete, 294
    treatment, 296
    with vaginal bleeding, 335
  definitions, 294
  incomplete, 294
    treatment, 296
    with vaginal bleeding, 335
  inevitable, 294
    treatment, 296
    with vaginal bleeding, 335
  missed, 294
    treatment, 296
  septic, with vaginal bleeding, 335
  spontaneous, 294–297
    evaluation, 295
    history, 295
    laboratory exam, 295
    physical exam, 295
    treatment, 295–296
  threatened, 294
    treatment, 295–296
    with vaginal bleeding, 335

Index

Abscess
  anorectal (*see* Anorectal abscess)
Abuse
  alcohol (*see* Alcohol abuse)
  drug, clinical manifestations, by class of drug, 560–561
  substance, 559–562
    clinical presentation, 560–561
Accutane: in nodulocystic acne, 524
ACE inhibitors: in hypertension, 77
Acetaminophen
  in otitis in children, 513
  in overdose, 49
  in poisoning, 49
Acetazolamide: in glaucoma, 508
Achalasia, 138
  diagnosis, 138
Acidosis: in kidney failure, 498
Acne, 523–524
  comedonal, 523
    benzoyl peroxide in, 523
    treatment, 523
    vitamin A in, 523
  etiology, 523
  nodulocystic, 524
    corticosteroids in, 524
    isotretinoin in, 524
    treatment, 524
  papulopustular, 523–524
    erythromycin in, 524
    tetracycline in, 524
    treatment, 523–524
Acoustic neuroma, 510–511
Acromioclavicular joint injuries, 242–243
  dislocation, 242–243
  grade I, 242
  grade II, 242
  grade III, 242–243
  sprain, 242
  subluxation, 242
Actinic keratosis, 532
Acyclovir: for herpes simplex genitalis, 486
Adenoma and hyperthyroidism, 198
  treatment, 200
Admit orders: for surgery, 401–402
Adnexal masses (*see* Gynecologic adnexal masses)
Adolescence: vaginal bleeding during, abnormal, 277
Adrenal insufficiency: in hypoglycemia, 182
Adrenalin: and wound repair, 395
Affective disorders, 551–554
  bipolar, 553–554
    antipsychotics in, 554
    evaluation, 553–554
    treatment, 554
Age
  gestational (*see* Gestational age)
  seizure etiology by, 541
Agoraphobia, 557
  characteristics, 557
  treatment, 557
Airway
  CPAP, 98
  in epiglottitis in children, 450
  management, 26–28
    evaluation, 26
    intervention, 26–28
    in resuscitation of infants and children, 12
  obstruction, upper, 35
    treatment, 35
  in overdose, 46
  in poisoning, 46
  pressure, peak, 99

Index **667**

in resuscitation of newborn, 10
after trauma, 15–16
Albumin: in polycythemia in newborn, 435
Alcohol
abuse, 559–560
diagnosis, 559–560
hypoglycemia and, 182
management, 560
during pregnancy, 312
Alcoholic liver disease (*see* Liver disease, alcoholic)
Allergic
conjunctivitis, 502, 506
rhinitis (*see* Rhinitis, allergic)
Allergy: and wounds, 393
Allopurinol: in gout attack prevention, 220
Alpha-fetoprotein, 317–318
elevated, disorders associated with, 317
low, disorders associated with, 317
outcome, projected, 317
risks, 318
Alpha-receptor blocker: in hypertension, 76
Amenorrhea, 276
Aminoglycoside: in endometritis, 390
Aminophylline: dosing, 116
Amitriptyline: in urticaria, chronic, 526
Amniocentesis, 319–320
indications, 319–320
Amnionitis: and premature rupture of membranes, 351
Amniotomy
guidelines for, 365–366
for labor induction, 364
Amoxicillin
in otitis in children, 513
in sinusitis, acute, 518

Ampicillin
in endometritis, 390, 391
in pneumonia in infants and children, 106
Amputation: extremities, 23
Analgesia
in low back pain, 235
in osteoarthritis, 213
Anemia, 165–171
aplastic, 169, 463
clinical manifestations, 169
diagnosis, 169
etiology, 169
treatment, 169
in children, 463–465
definition, 463
etiology, 463
evaluation, 463
management, 465
symptoms, 463
of chronic disease, 166
etiology, 166
laboratory, 166
treatment, 166
Cooley's (*see* β-Thalassemia major)
Fanconi's, 463
hemolytic, 167–168
antibody-induced, 167–168
membrane abnormalities in, 168
hypoplastic, 463
iron deficiency, 165
in children, 463
etiology, 165
exam, 165
laboratory, 165
treatment, 165
of kidney failure, chronic, 169
macrocytic, 169–170
clinical presentation, 169–170
diagnosis, 170
etiology, 169

668 Index

Anemia (*cont.*)
  treatment, 170
  megaloblastic, 463
  microcytic, 165–167
  normochromic-normocytic, 167–169
  sickle cell, 166
    diagnosis, 166
    etiology, 166
  sideroblastic, 165
    etiology, 165
    laboratory, 165
    treatment, 165
  spur cell, 168
Anesthesia
  during labor, 595
  for wound repair, 395–396
    local, 395
    regional, 395
    topical, 395
Angina, 60
  preoperative care and, 403
  prolonged episode, 64–65
    disposition, 65
    management, 64–65
  stable, 63
  unstable, 64
    definition, 64
    management, 64
Angioplasty: PTCA in ischemic heart disease, 62
Angiotensin-converting enzyme: in hypertension, 77
Ankle: in rheumatoid arthritis, 208
Ankylosing (*see* Spondylitis, ankylosing)
Anorectal
  abscess, 157
    diagnosis, 157
    etiology, 157
    treatment, 157
  disease, 156–158
  fissure, 156–157
    classification, 157
    definition, 156–157
    diagnosis, 157
    etiology, 156
    symptoms, 157
    treatment, 157
Anorexia nervosa, 567
  diagnosis, 567
  treatment, 567
Antacids: in duodenal ulcer, 136
Antenatal fetal surveillance, 319–323
Antepartum bleeding (*see* Bleeding, antepartum)
Antibiotics
  after bites in children, 467
  burns and, 425
  in epididymitis, 477
  in epiglottitis in children, 451
  in fever in newborn, 440–441
  in pneumonia, summary, 110–111
  in septic arthritis, 254–255
Antibodies: causing hemolytic anemia, 167–168
Anticholinergic poisoning, 48
Anticoagulant(s)
  in cerebrovascular disease, 546
  lupus, 228
Anticoagulation: in pulmonary embolism, 124–125
Anticonvulsants: in preeclampsia, 332
Antidepressants, 553
  tricyclic
    in anxiety disorders, 555
    in depression, 552
    in overdose, 51–52
    in panic attacks, 556
    in poisoning, 51–52
    in urticaria, chronic, 526
Antihistamines
  in rhinitis, allergic, 520–521

in urticaria
  acute, 525
  chronic, 526
Antihypertensives: in preeclampsia, 332
Anti-inflammatory drugs, nonsteroidal (*see* NSAIDs)
Antimalarials
  in lupus erythematosus, systemic, 229
  in rheumatoid arthritis, 210
Antiplatelet therapy: in cerebrovascular disease, 546
Antipruritics: in poison ivy, oak and sumac, 528
Antipsychotics, 563
  adverse effects, 554
  in bipolar affective disorder, 554
  dose, 554
Anxiety disorders, 555–558
  diagnosis, differential, 555
  generalized, 555–556
    characteristics, 555–556
    treatment, 556
  treatment, 555
Aortic regurgitation, 83
Apgar Score: in asphyxia, intrapartum, 427
Aplastic (*see* Anemia, aplastic)
Apnea in newborn, 428
  causes, 428
  definition, 428
  diagnosis, 428
  treatment, 428
Appendicitis, 414–415
  clinical presentation, 414
  history, 414
  laboratory, 414
  management, 414–415
    atypical presentation, 415
    classical presentation, 414
  physical exam, 414
Arrhythmia
  in myocardial infarction, acute, 69
  preoperative care and, 403–404
  in syncope, 79
Arteries
  coronary, bypass in ischemic heart disease, 62
  of extremities, injury, 23–24
  line (*see* Line, arterial)
Arthritis
  bacterial, 251
  bacterial, nongonococcal, 253–254
    antibiotics in, 255
    causative organisms, 253–254
    prosthetic joint infections, 254
  gonococcal, 252–253
    clinical features, 253
    incidence, 252
    laboratory features, 253
  gouty, chronic, 217
  osteoarthritis (*see* Osteoarthritis)
  rheumatoid (*see* Rheumatoid arthritis)
  septic, 251–256
    antibiotics in, 254–255
    blood cultures in, 252
    clinical appearance, 251–252
    diagnosis, 251–252
    drainage, 255–256
    prognosis, 256
    radiography of, 252
    treatment, 254–256
Arthrocentesis, 628–631
  contraindications, 628
  indications, 628
  steroids and, intra-articular, 629
  technique, 628–629

Index

Arthropathy: neuropathic, in diabetes, 190
Aseptic (*see* Meningitis, aseptic)
Asphyxia, intrapartum, 427
  Apgar Score in, 427
  cause, 427
  treatment, 427
Aspiration
  foreign body (*see* Foreign body aspiration)
  massive, 36
    treatment, 36
  meconium (*see* Meconium aspiration syndrome)
Aspirin
  in cerebrovascular disease, 546
  in rheumatoid arthritis, 210
Asthma, 112–116
  ABGs, 113
  attack severity assessment, 114
  CBC, 113
  diagnosis, differential, 112
  EKG in, 113
  etiology, 112
  evaluation, 112–114
  history, 112
  laboratory for, 113–114
  management, 114–116
    mild attack, 114–115
    moderate attack, 115–116
    severe attack, 115–116
  physical exam, 112–113
  radiography in, 113
  spirometry in, 113
Asystole, 2–3, 4
  in infants and children, 14
Atherosclerosis: and preoperative care, 403
Atony: gastric, in diabetes, 190
Atopy: in eczema, 527
Atrioventricular node: dysfunction causing bradycardia, 8–9
Atrophy: and menopause, 304
Atropine: in resuscitation in infants and children, 13
Autoimmune thyroiditis, 198
  treatment, 200
Autonomic neuropathy: and diabetes, 189–190
AV node: dysfunction causing bradycardia, 8–9
Azotemia, prerenal, 498
  causes, 498
  treatment, 498

B

Bacitracin: in bacterial conjunctivitis, 506
Back (*see* Low back pain)
Bacterial
  arthritis (*see* Arthritis, bacterial)
  conjunctivitis (*see* Conjunctivitis, bacterial)
  cystitis (*see* Cystitis, bacterial)
  meningitis (*see* Meningitis, bacterial)
  prostatitis (*see* Prostatitis, bacterial)
  sepsis (*see* Sepsis, bacterial, in newborn)
  tracheitis, 451–452
Benzodiazepines: in anxiety disorders, 555
Benzoyl peroxide: in comedonal acne, 523
Beta blocker
  in glaucoma, 508
  in heart disease, ischemic, 61
  in hypertension, 76
  in overdose, 50
  in poisoning, 50

Bicarbonate
  in hyperkalemia, 175
  in ketoacidosis, diabetic, 193
  in resuscitation
    in infants and children, 13
    in newborn, 11
Biliary (*see* Colic, biliary)
Biophysical profile scoring
  (*see also* Fetus, biophysical
    profile)
  interpretation, 648
  technique, 647
Biopsy
  breast, fine needle, 624–625
    complications, 625
    contraindications, 624
    indications, 624
    materials, 624
    technique, 624–625
  endometrial, 626–627
    complications, 627
    contraindications, 626
    indications, 626
    materials for, 626
    preparation for, 627
    technique, 627
Bipolar disorder (*see* Affective
    disorder, bipolar)
Bishop score: in labor induction,
    365
Bites, 398–400
  animal, 466
  cat, 398
  in children, 466–469
    (*see also* spider, tick *below*)
    antibiotics for, 467
    etiologic organisms, 466
    evaluation, 466
    history, 466
    management, 466–467
    rabies and, 467
    tetanus status, 466
  dog, 398
  human, 398, 466
  spider, in children, 467–468
    black widow spider, 468
    brown recluse spider, 468
    treatment, 468
  tick, 466
  tick, in children, 467
    prevention, 467
    removal, 467
  wounds, 398–400
Black widow spider bites, 468
Bladder, tap, suprapubic, 608–609
  complications, 609
  contraindications, 608
  indications, 608
  materials, 608
  technique, 608
Bleeding
  antepartum
    early (*see* Vagina,
      bleeding before 20 weeks
      gestation)
    late (*see* Vagina, bleeding
      after 20 weeks gestation)
  classification of, 17
  disorders, 159–164
    clinical presentation, 161
    diagnosis, differential, 159–160
    extrinsic pathway defects, 160
    history, 161
    intrinsic pathway defects, 160
    laboratory studies, 161–162
    management, 162–164
    mixed defects, 160
    physical exam, 161
    vascular defects, 160
  gastrointestinal (*see* Gastrointestinal bleeding)
  postmenopausal, 278
  postpartum, 386–388
    definition, 386

672 Index

Bleeding (*cont.*)
    diagnosis, 386
    etiology, 386
    management, 387–388
    physical exam, 386
    risk factors, 386
    uterine, dysfunctional, 276
    vaginal (*see* Vagina, bleeding)
Block
    digital, 593
    for dilation and curettage, 595
    field, 593
    first-degree, 8
    local and regional, 592–595
        contraindications, 592
        indications, 592
        materials, 592
        technique, 592
    metacarpal, 593
    nerve
        infraorbital, 593–594
        intercostal, 594
        mental, 594
        supraorbital, 593
    paracervical, 594
    pudendal, 595–596
    regional (*see* local and regional *above*)
    second-degree
        type I, 8
        type II, 8
    third-degree, 8
Blocker
    alpha-receptor, in hypertension, 76
    beta (*see* Beta blocker)
    calcium channel (*see* Calcium channel blocker)
    H2, in urticaria, 525
Blood
    cultures in septic arthritis, 252
    in pelvic pain diagnosis, 262
    pressure
        0–12 months, 642
        1–13 years, 643
        13–18 years, 644
    sugar, postprandial, 2-hour, nomogram for interpreting, 186
    vomiting of, 133
Blue bloater: in COPD, 117
Body surface area determination: nomogram for, 641
Bone
    disease, metabolic, 223–225
        clinical features, 223
        laboratory evaluation, 223
        radiography in, 223
    imaging with ^{99m}Tc in stress fracture, 239
    wounds and, 394
Boutonniere deformity: in rheumatoid arthritis, 208
Bowel preparation: for flexible sigmoidoscopy, 637
Bradyarrhythmia
    in infants and children, 14
    in myocardial infarction, acute, 69–70
Bradycardia, 7–9
    atrioventricular node dysfunction causing, 8–9
    sinus, 8
Bradydysrhythmia, 7–9
BRAT diet: in diarrhea in newborn, 444
Breast
    biopsy (*see* Biopsy, breast)
    feeding, 457–458
        failure to thrive in, 458
        nutritional concerns in, 458
    mass
        evaluation, 419–420
        history, 419
        mammography, 419–420
        management, 420
        physical exam, 419
Breathing: after trauma, 16

Breech, 372–374
  complete, 372
  delivery
    buttocks, 372–373
    extremities, 372–373
    head, 373–374
    head, Mauriceau-Smellie-Veit maneuver, 373
    head, Piper forceps extraction, 373
    shoulders, 372–373
  etiology, 372
  frank, 372
  incidence, 372
  incomplete, 372
  types, 372
Bromocriptine: in premenstrual tension syndrome, 303
Bronchitis: chronic, in COPD, 117
Bronchospasm: pharmacotherapy, 115
Brown recluse spider bites, 468
Bulimia nervosa, 567–568
  diagnosis, 567–568
  treatment, 568
Bupivacaine: and wound repair, 396
Burns, 421–426
  antibiotics and, 425
  assessment, 421–423
    initial, 421
  cause of, 422–423
  chemical, 423
    treatment, 424
  contractures after, 424
  depth, 421–422
  electrical, 422
    treatment, 424
  follow up care, 424–425
  nutrition after, 425
  radiation, 423
  severity, 422
  surface area of, 421, 426
  tar, 424
  thermal, 422
  treatment, 423–425
    emergency room, 423–424
Bursa
  greater trochanteric, in bursitis, 240
  olecranon, in bursitis, 240
  subacromial, in bursitis, 240
Bursitis, 240–241
  clinical features, 240
  clinical syndromes, 240–241
  physical exam, 240
  treatment, 241
Buspirone: in anxiety disorders, 555
Bypass: coronary artery, in ischemic heart disease, 62

C

Cafergot: in migraine, 534
Calcitonin: in osteoporosis, 223–224
Calcium
  channel blocker
    in heart disease, ischemic, 61
    in hypertension, 77
  gluconate in hyperkalemia, 175
  during pregnancy, 310
  stones, 492
Calculi (see Stones)
Cancer
  low back pain due to, 232
  skin, 532–533
Candidiasis, 484–485
  lab, 484
  signs and symptoms, 484
  treatment, 485

Cannula: nasal, 97
Captopril: in congestive heart failure, 72
Carbocaine: and wound repair, 396
Carbon monoxide
　in overdose, 50–51
　in poisoning, 50–51
Carcinoma
　skin
　　basal cell, 533
　　squamous cell, 533
　thyroid, 205–206
　　clinical presentation, 205
　　laboratory evaluation, 205
　　treatment, 206
Cardiac (*see* Heart)
Cardiogenic shock, 38
Cardiology, 60–90
Cardioversion, 569–570
　complications, 570
　contraindications, 569
　indications, 569
　materials for, 569
　technique, 570
Care
　after glenohumeral dislocation reduction, 244
　hospital, after prenatal care, 384
　postoperative (*see* Postoperative care)
　postpartum (*see* Postpartum care)
　prenatal (*see* Prenatal care)
　preoperative (*see* Preoperative care)
Cat bites, 398
Catheter
　Foley, in trauma, 17
　intrauterine pressure, 602–603
　　complications, 603
　　contraindications, 602
　　indications, 602
　　interpretations, 603
　　materials, 602
　　technique, 602
Cation-exchange resins: in hyperkalemia, 175
Cefaclor
　in otitis in children, 513
　in sinusitis, acute, 519
Cefazolin: in endometritis, 390
Ceftriaxone
　in chancroid, 485
　in gonorrhea, 485
Cefuroxime: in pneumonia in infants and children, 106
Cell (*see* Anemia, sickle cell)
Central lines (*see* Lines, central)
Central nervous system: in lupus erythematosus, systemic, 227
Cerebrospinal fluid: data on, 646
Cerebrovascular disease, 545–547
　ancillary studies, 546
　definitions, 545
　diagnosis, 545–546
　etiologies, 545
　history, 545–546
　lab, 546
　physical exam, 545–546
　radiography of, 546
　treatment, 546
Cervicitis: ceftriaxone in, 485
Cervix
　in infertility, 285
　palpation in labor evaluation, 355
Cesarean section, 381–382
　indications, 381
　procedure, 381
　risks, 382
Chancroid, 482
　ceftriaxone for, 485
　erythromycin for, 485
　lab, 482

Index

signs and symptoms, 482
Charcoal: activated, after poisoning and overdose, 47–48
Charcot's joint: in diabetes, 190
Chemical burns, 423
  treatment, 424
Chemotherapy: and wounds, 393
Chest trauma, 19–20
Chickenpox, 453
  clinical manifestations, 453
  epidemiology, 453
  treatment, 453
Chilblain, 55
Children, 427–471
  anemia (*see* Anemia in children)
  bites (*see* Bites in children)
  constipation (*see* Constipation in children)
  dyspnea, 450–452
  dysrhythmia, 13–14
  epiglottitis (*see* Epiglottitis in children)
  exanthems, 453–456
  foreign body (*see* Foreign body aspiration in children)
  gynecologic exam, 272
  gynecology, 272–275
  labial adhesions, 273
  life support, advanced, 10–14
  low back pain, 232
  meningitis (*see* Meningitis, in children)
  otitis (*see* Otitis, in children)
  ovarian tumors, 274
  pinworms, 273
  pneumonia (*see under* Pneumonia)
  resuscitation (*see* Resuscitation in infants and children)
  sarcoma botryoides, 274
  seizure (*see* Seizure, febrile, in children)
  stridor, 450–452
  urethral prolapse, 274
  vaginal foreign body, 274
  vulvovaginitis, 272–273
Chlamydia trachomatis
  doxycycline in, 485
  erythromycin in, 485
Chlorpromazine
  in migraine, 535
  in narcotic withdrawal in newborn, 435
Cholecystitis, acute, 417–418
  treatment 418
Cholecystography: in cholelithiasis, asymptomatic, 416
Cholelithiasis, asymptomatic, 416–417
  gallbladder evaluation in, 416
  imaging in, 416
  management, 416–417
Cholestyramine: in hypercholesterolemia, 88
Cholinergic poisoning, 48
Chondrocalcinosis, 215–216
  clinical features, 215–216
  laboratory, 215–216
  radiography of, 216
  treatment, 216
Chymopapain: in low back pain, 235
Circulation
  in overdose, 46
  in poisoning, 46
  in resuscitation in infants and children, 12–13
  in syncope, 78–79
  after trauma, 16, 168
Circumcision, 589–591
  Gomco clamp technique, 589–591
    complications, 591
    contraindications, 589
    follow-up, 591

676 Index

Circumcision (*cont.*)
    indications, 589
    materials, 589
    technique, 589–591
Clavulanic acid: in otitis in children, 513
Clicks: of heart, 81
Clindamycin: in endometritis, 390
Clinoril: in gout, 219
Clomiphene citrate: in infertility, 286
Clotrimazole: in vaginal infection, 485
Coagulation
    disseminated intravascular, management, 164
    disseminated intravascular, in newborn, 436
        diagnosis, 436
        heparin in, 436
        initiating factors, 436
        treatment, 436
    factor deficiencies, 162–164
Cocaine: and wound repair, 395
Colchicine
    in chondrocalcinosis, 216
    in gout
        acute attack, 218
        prevention, 219
Cold
    common, 102
        management, 102
    injury
        peripheral, 55–57
        systemic, 57–58
    -related illnesses, 55–58
Colic, biliary, 417
    laboratory evaluation, 417
    physical exam, 417
    treatment, 417
Colorectal tumors, 154–155
    clinical manifestations, 154–155
    diagnosis, 155
    epidemiology, 154
    predisposing factors, 154
    prognosis by Duke's classification, 155
    screening measures, 155
    types of polyps, 154
Coma, 41–45
    coma scale, modified, for infant, 664
    disposition, 44–45
    etiology, 41
    evaluation, 41–44
    Glasgow Coma Scale, 44
    management, 41–44
    myxedema, 202–203
    after overdose, 46
    after poisoning, 46
    resuscitation, in, 42
    survey
        primary, 41–42
        secondary, 43–44
Compulsive (*see* Obsessive compulsive disorder)
Condyloma acuminata, 483
    lab, 483
    signs and symptoms, 483
    treatment, 483
Conjunctivitis, 505–506
    allergic, 502, 506
    bacterial, 502, 505–506
        acute, 505
        chronic, 505
        diagnosis, 505–506
        local measures, 506
        treatment, 506
    definition, 505
    diagnosis, differential, 505
    Neisseria in, 506
    toxic, 506
    TRIC, 506
    viral, 502, 506
Connective tissue disorders: hereditary, 160

Constipation, 152–153
  in children, 461–462
    diagnosis, 461
    etiology, 461–462
    management, 462
    management, long standing, 462
    management, simple constipation, 462
  complications, 152
  definition, 152
  etiology, 152
  treatment, 152
Continuous positive airway pressure, 98
Contraception, 258–261
  action mechanism, 258–259
  contraindications, 258–261
  failure rate, optimal/typical, 258–259
  during lupus erythematosus, systemic, 229
  method, 258–259
  oral
    contraindications, 260–261
    contraindications, absolute, 260
    contraindications, relative, 260
    in dysmenorrhea, 280
    side effects, possible, 260–261
Contraction stress testing (*see* Fetus, contraction stress testing)
Contractures: after burns, 424
Cooley's anemia (*see* β-Thalassemia major)
COPD (*see* Lung, COPD)
Cornea
  abrasion, 503
  injury and infection, 502
  lesions, 503

Coronary artery bypass: in ischemic heart disease, 62
Corticosteroids
  in acne, nodulocystic, 524
  in gout, 219
  in lupus erythematosus, systemic, 229
  osteopenia due to, 225
  in poison ivy, oak and sumac, 538
  in rheumatoid arthritis, 210
Cortisone: in tendonitis, 237
Counseling
  format, 548–549
  primary care, goals of, 548
  principles of, 548–550
  techniques, 549–550
Cramps: heat, 53–54
Creatinine: evaluation in hypertension, 75
Cricothyrotomy, 33–34
  advantages, 33
  complications, 34
  contraindications, 33
  disadvantages, 33
  technique, 34
Crotamiton: for scabies, 484
Croup, 451
  atypical, 451–452
  clinical presentation, 451
  diagnosis, differential, 450
  etiology, 451
  lab, 451
  treatment, 451
Cryotherapy, 615–617
  complications, 616
  contraindications, 615
  follow-up, 616
  indications, 615
  materials, 615–616
  technique, 616
Culdocentesis, 579–581
  complications, 580

678 Index

Culdocentesis (*cont.*)
  contraindications, 579
  in ectopic pregnancy, 299
  indications, 579
  left handers' approach, 580
  materials for, 579
  in pelvic pain, 262
  procedure, 579–580
  results, 581
  technique, 579–580
Curettage: anesthesia for, 595
Cushing's syndrome, 160

Cyanosis: and resuscitation of newborn, 11
Cyproheptadine: in chronic urticaria, 526
Cyst: ovarian, 267
Cystitis
  bacterial, in males, 474
    lab, 474
    signs and symptoms, 474
    treatment, 474
  interstitial, in female, 472–473

D

Danazol
  in endometriosis, 289
  in premenstrual tension syndrome, 302
Decubitus (*see* Ulcer, decubitus)
Defibrillation, 569–570
  attempt
    pulse after, 3
    rhythm after, 3
  complications, 570
  contraindications, 569
  indications, 569
  materials for, 569
  technique, 569–570
Delivery
  breech (*see* Breech)
  compound presentation, 377
    definition, 377
    management, 378
  forceps, 368–369
    definition, 369
    indications, 368–369, 370
    low, 369
    midforceps, 369
    outlet, 369
    Piper, in breech, 373
    requirements, 369
    technique, 369–370
  malpresentation, 377–378
    brow, 377

  face, 377
  face, diagnosis, 377
  face, incidence, 377
  face, management, 377
  postpartum care (*see* Postpartum care)
  shoulder dystocia (*see* Dystocia, shoulder)
  transverse lie/shoulder presentation, 377
  vacuum extraction, 370
    advantages, 370
    disadvantages, 370
    technique, 370–371
  vaginal, 367–371
    of body, 368
    cardinal movements, 367
    of head, 367–368
    normal spontaneous, 367–368
    of shoulders, 368
  vertex, management, 367
Dementia, 537–538
  diagnosis, differential, mnemonic for, 537
  etiologies, 537
    nontreatable, 537
    treatable, 537
  evaluation, 537, 538
  treatment, 538

Depression, 551–553
  diagnosis, 551
  electroconvulsive therapy, 552
  evaluation, 551–552
  examination in, 551–552
  history, 551
  hospitalization for, 552
  psychotherapy of, 552
  treatment, 552
Dermatitis
  contact, 528–529
    causes, 528–529
  diaper, 273
Dermatology, 523–533
Dermatomes: spinal, 640
Developmental milestones: language skills, 659–662
Dexamethasone
  in croup, 451
  in poison ivy, oak and sumac, 528
Diabetes mellitus, 184–194
  arthropathy in, neuropathic, 190
  classification, 184
  complications, 189–190
  diagnosis, 185–186
  diet in, 186–187
  drug interactions in, 188
  drugs in, 187
  early, 182
  feet in, 190
  gastroparesis in, 190
  gestational (*see* with pregnancy *below*)
  hypoglycemic agents in, oral, 188
  insulin in, 187–188
  insulin-dependent, 184
  ketoacidosis of (*see* Ketoacidosis, diabetic)
  myopathy in, 190
  neuropathy of, 189–190
  with pregnancy, 184, 326–329
    definition, 326
    diet in, 327
    evaluation, 326–327
    glucose challenge test in, 326
    glucose tolerance test in, 326–327
    management, 327–328
    morbidity, potential, 327
    obstetric surveillance, 327–328
    risk, factors, 326
  presentation, 184
  retinopathy of, 190
  treatment, 186–188
  White's classification, 328–329
  wounds and, 393
Dialysis in kidney failure, 498
  chronic, 499
Diaper dermatitis, 273
Diarrhea
  acute, 147–149
    definition, 147
    diagnosis, 147–148
    invasive, 147
    noninvasive, 147
    supportive measures, 148–149
    treatment, 148–149
  chronic, 150–151
    definition, 150
    diagnosis, 150–151
    etiology, 150
    evaluation, 150
    treatment, 151
  in newborn, 444
    BRAT diet in, 444
    evaluation, 444
    exam, 444
    history, 444
    lab, 444
    treatment, 444
  with vomiting in newborn, 442–443

Diarrhea (*cont.*)
 disposition, 442–443
 evaluation, 442
 exam, 442
 lab, 442
DIC (*see* Coagulation, disseminated intravascular)
Diet
 BRAT, in diarrhea in newborn, 444
 in diabetes, 186–187
  with pregnancy, 327
 after gastrectomy, 183
 in ketoacidosis, diabetic, 194
 postoperative care and, 405
 in premenstrual tension syndrome, 302
 preoperative, 401
 in renal failure, chronic, 499
 in vomiting in newborn, 443
Digital block, 593
Digitalis: in heart failure, congestive, 72–73
Digoxin
 in overdose, 51
 in poisoning, 51
Dihydroergotamine: in migraine, 534–535
Dilation and curettage: anesthesia for, 595
Diphenhydramine: in acute urticaria, 525
Disc injury, 231
Discharge: after normal vaginal delivery, 384–385
Dislocation
 acromioclavicular joint, 242–243
 elbow, 244–245
  clinical features, 244
  reduction, 244–245
  reduction, care after, 245
 extremities, 23
 glenohumeral, 243–244

care after reduction, 244
clinical features, 243
reduction, 243–244
 interphalangeal joint, 246–247
  proximal, 246–247
  proximal, reduction, 246
  proximal, reduction, care after, 247
 metacarpophalangeal joint, 246
  clinical features, 246
  reduction, 246
 patella, 247–248
  clinical features, 247
  reduction, 247–248
  reduction, care after, 248
Diuretics
 in heart failure, congestive, 71–72
 in hypertension, 76
 hypokalemia and, 172–173
 in premenstrual tension syndrome, 302
 thiazide (*see* Thiazide diuretics)
Diverticulum: Zenker's, 138
Dizziness (*see* Vertigo)
Dobutamine: in congestive heart failure, 73
Dog bites, 398
Dopamine: in myocardial infarction with hypotension, 68
Doxycycline: for *Chlamydia trachomatis*, 485
Dressings, 397
Drug(s)
 abuse, clinical manifestations by class of drug, 560–561
 in diabetes, 187
 interactions, 188
 lupus erythematosus due to, systemic, 228
 in postoperative care, 405–406

during pregnancy, 312
purpura due to, vascular, 160
Dubowitz modification: in neurologic criteria technique assessment, 650
Dubowitz score: in gestational age assessment, 653
Duke's classification: of colorectal tumors, 155
Duodenal (see Ulcer, duodenal)
Dysentery, 147
Dyslipidemia, 85–89
  classification, 85–87
  evaluation, 87–88
  treatment
    initial, 87–88
    pharmacologic, 88–89
Dysmenorrhea, 279–282
  diagnosis, 279
  evaluation, 280
  history, 279
  importance of, 279
  primary, 279–281
    clinical features, 279–280
    definition, 279
    etiology, 279
    treatment, 280–281
  secondary, 281–282
    clinical features, 281
    definition, 281
    etiology, 281
    evaluation, 281
    treatment, 282
  types, 279
Dyspareunia, 268–271
  deep, 269
  diagnosis, differential, 268–269
  evaluation, 269–270
  history, 269
  laboratory exam, 270
  physical exam, 270
  psychologic, 269
  superficial, 268
  treatment, 270–271
  types, 268
Dyspepsia, 136–137
Dysphagia, 138
  causes, 38
  evaluation, 138
Dyspnea: in children, 450–452
Dysrhythmia
  in children, 13–14
  in infant, 13–14
  life-threatening, 4–7
Dystocia, shoulder, 379–380
  diagnosis, 379
  incidence, 379
  management, 379

E

Ear, 501–522
  foreign body removal (see Foreign body removal, ear)
Eating
  disorders, 567–568
Echocardiography: in syncope, 80
Eclampsia, 330
Ectopic pregnancy (see Pregnancy, ectopic)
Eczema, 527
  atopic, 527
  definition, 527
  dyshidrotic, 527
  endogenous, 527
  nummular, 527
  seborrheic, 527
  treatment, basic principles, 527
  types, 527
Edema
  heat, 53
  pulmonary, 36

Edema (*cont.*)
   in myocardial infarction, acute, 68–69
   treatment, 36
Education: prenatal patient, 310–313
Elbow
   dislocation (*see* Dislocation, elbow)
   joint access, 630
   nursemaid's, 245
   in rheumatoid arthritis, 208
Electrical burns, 422
   treatment, 424
Electrocardiography
   in asthma, 113
   in myocardial infarction, 66
Electroconvulsive therapy: for depression, 552
Electrode (*see* Fetus, scalp electrode)
Electrodesiccation, 618–619
   complications, 618
   contraindications, 618
   indications, 618
   materials for, 618
   technique, 618
Electroencephalography: in syncope, 80
Electrolyte(s)
   disorders, 159–206
   in hyperglycemic-hyperosmolar nonketotic syndrome, 196
Electromechanical dissociation, 2, 4
   in infants and children, 14
Embolism (*see* Pulmonary embolism)
Emergency
   care of burns, 423–424
   medicine, 1–59
   procedures, 569–584
Emesis
   in overdose, 47
   in poisoning, 47
Emphysema: in COPD, 117
Endocarditis: lupus erythematosus and, systemic, 227
Endometriosis, 288–290
   definition, 288
   diagnostic aids, 288
   evaluation, 288
   history, 288
   hospital admission criteria, 292
   management, 289–290
   pathogenesis, 288
   physical exam, 288
Endometritis, 390–391
   etiology, 390
   risk factors, 390
   treatment, 390–391
Endometrium (*see* Biopsy, endometrial)
Enterobius vermicularis (*see* Pinworms)
Environmental illnesses, 53–59
Enzyme(s)
   angiotensin-converting, in hypertension, 77
   heart, 65
   pancreatic enzyme supplements in chronic diarrhea, 151
Epididymitis, 476–477
   diagnosis, differential, 477
   etiology, 476–477
   lab, 477
   with scrotal pain, acute, 493
   signs and symptoms, 477
   treatment, 477
Epiglottitis, in children, 450–451
   antibiotics in, 451
   clinical presentation, 450
   diagnosis, differential, 450
   etiology, 450

Index **683**

lab, 450
treatment, 450–451
Epileptic seizure: classification, 542
Epinephrine
  in glaucoma, 508
  racemic, in croup, 451
  in resuscitation
    in infant and children, 13
    in newborn, 11
Epiphyseal plate: fracture, 249–250
Episiotomy, 375–376
  advantages, 375
  mediolateral, 375
  midline, 375
    repair, 375–376
  types, 375
Equipment
  for fetal contraction stress testing, 321
  for fetal non-stress testing, 320
Ergotamine: in migraine, 534
Erythema infectiosum, 455
  clinical manifestations, 455
  epidemiology, 455
Erythromycin
  in acne, papulopustular, 524
  in chancroid, 485
  for *Chlamydia trachomatis*, 485
  in otitis
    in children, 513
    media, acute, 514
  in pneumonia in children 5–14, 108
  in sinusitis, acute, 519
Esophagitis, 139
  complications, 139
  diagnosis, 139
  predisposing factors, 139
  treatment, 139
Esophagus
  disease, 138–140
  gastroesophageal (*see* Gastroesophageal)
  spasm, 139
    diagnosis, 139
    treatment, 139
Estrogen replacement
  in osteoporosis, 224–225
  therapy (*see* Menopause, hormone replacement therapy)
Exanthems: in children, 453–456
Exchange transfusion (*see* Transfusion, exchange)
Exercise during pregnancy, 310–311
  contraindications, 311
Extremities
  amputation, 23
  arterial injury, 23–24
  dislocations, 23
  fractures, 23
    open, 23
  trauma, 22–24
Eye, 501–522
  foreign body removal (*see* Foreign body removal, eye)
  red, 501–504
    evaluation, 501–503
    exam, 501
    history, 501
    lab, 503
    management, 503

F

Face (*see* Delivery, malpresentation, face)
Factor
  deficiencies, 162–164
  VIII concentrate, 163
  XI deficiency, 160

Factor (*cont.*)
　IX deficiency, management, 163
　replacement therapy, 163
　XIII deficiency, management, 163
Failure to thrive, 459–460
　in breast feeding, 458
　diagnosis, differential, 459
　evaluation, 460
　general groups, 459
　observation period, 460
Fallopian tube
　in gynecologic adnexal masses, 265
　in infertility, 285
Fanconi's anemia, 463
Febrile (*see* Seizure, febrile)
Feeding
　breast (*see* Breast feeding)
　supplemental, for infant, 654
Feet
　in diabetes, 190
　in rheumatoid arthritis, 208
Felty's syndrome, 209
Ferrous sulfate: in iron deficiency anemia, 165
Fetoprotein (*see* Alpha-fetoprotein)
Fetus
　antenatal surveillance, 319–323
　biophysical profile, 322
　　indications for, 320
　　interpretation, 322
　　management protocol in, 322–323
　cesarean section and, 381
　　risks, 382
　contraction stress testing, 321–322
　　contraindications, possible, 321
　　equipment, 321
　　indications for, 320, 321
　　interpretations, 321–322
　　management, 321–322
　distress, management, 359–360
　heart rate, 358–360
　　accelerations, 359
　　baseline, 358
　　decelerations, 359
　　monitoring, 358
　　monitoring, indications, 358
　　patterns, 360
　　patterns, abnormal, management, 359–360
　　patterns, common periodic, 359
　　tracing interpretation, 358–359
　　variability, 358
　non-stress testing, 320–321
　　equipment, 320
　　indications, 320
　　interpretations, 320–321
　scalp electrode, 585–586
　　complications, 586
　　contraindications, 585
　　indications, 585
　　materials, 585
　　technique, 585–586
　scalp pH, 361
　scalp pH sampling, 587–588
　　complications, 588
　　contraindications, 587
　　indications, 587
　　materials, 587
　　results, 587–588
　　technique, 587
　ultrasound of, 319
　　indications, 319
　　timing, 319
Fever
　in newborn (*see* Newborn, fever)
　postoperative, 406

puerperal (*see* Puerperal fever)
scarlet (*see* Scarlet fever)
Fibrillation (*see* Ventricle, fibrillation)
Field bloc, 593
Fifth disease (*see* Erythema infectiosum)
Finger, mallet, 247
  treatment, 247
Fissure (*see* Anorectal fissure)
Fluid: in renal failure, chronic, 499
Fluoride
  breast feeding and, 458
  in osteoporosis, 224
Folate deficiency, 170
  treatment, 170
Foley catheter: in trauma, 17
Folic acid: during pregnancy, 310
Forceps (*see* Delivery, forceps)
Foreign body
  aspiration in children, 452
    clinical presentation, 452
    course, 452
    Heimlich maneuver for, 452
    treatment, 452
  removal, ear, 610
    complications, 610
    contraindications, 610
    indications, 610
    materials, 610
    technique, 610
  removal, eye, 611–612
    complications, 611–612
    contraindications, 611
    indications, 611
    materials, 611
    technique, 611
  vaginal, in infants and children, 274
  wounds and, 394
Fracture, 249–250
  epiphyseal plate, 249–250
  extremities, 23
    open, 23
  pelvis, 21–22
  Salter I, 249
  Salter II, 249–250
  Salter III, 250
  Salter IV, 250
  Salter V, 250
  stress, 238–240
    clinical features, 238
    CT of, 239
    physical exam, 238
    prevention, 240
    radiography, 238–239
    treatment, 239–240
  terminology for, 249
Frostbite, 56
Furosemide: in congestive heart failure, 72

G

Gallbladder
  disease, 416–418
  evaluation in cholelithiasis, asymptomatic, 416
Gallstones, 417
Gastrectomy: diet after, 183
Gastric (*see* Stomach)
Gastroenterology, 133–158
Gastroesophageal reflux, 139
  complications, 139
  diagnosis, 139
  predisposing factors, 139
  treatment, 139
Gastrointestinal bleeding, 133–134
  diagnosis, 134
  etiology, 133
  lower, 135
  radiography in abdominal pain, 413

686 Index

Gastrointestinal bleeding (*cont.*)
  treatment, 134
  types, 133
  upper, 134
Gastroparesis diabeticorum, 190
Gemfibrozil: in hypercholesterolemia, 89
Genital herpes (*see* Herpes simplex genitalis)
Genitourinary
  disorders, 472–500
  trauma, 21–22
Genotypes: in lipoprotein disorder classification, 86
German measles (*see* Rubella)
Gestational age
  assessment
    by neurologic criteria, 649
    physical criteria, 651–652
  Dubowitz score estimation, 653
Gestational diabetes (*see* Diabetes mellitus with pregnancy)
Glasgow Coma Scale, 44
Glaucoma, 507–508
  acetozolamide in, 508
  acute, 502, 503
  beta blockers in, 508
  clinical presentation, 507–508
  definition, 507
  epinephrine in, 508
  laser trabeculoplasty in, 508
  management, 508
    angle closure, acute, 508
    open angle, 508
  ophthalmoscopy in, 507
  pathophysiology, 507
  pilocarpine in, 508
  prevalence, 507
  screening methods, 507
  tonometry in, 507
  visual fields in, 507
Glenohumeral (*see* Dislocation, glenohumeral)

Glucocorticoids: causing osteopenia, 225
Glucose
  challenge test in diabetes with pregnancy, 326
  in coma resuscitation, 42
  tolerance test in diabetes with pregnancy, 326–327
Goiter, 204
  multinodular, 204–205
    clinical presentation, 204
  toxic, 198
  toxic, treatment, 200
  treatment, 204–205
Gold: in rheumatoid arthritis, 210–211
Gomco clamp (*see* Circumcision, Gomco clamp technique)
Gonadotropin: human menopausal, in infertility, 286
Gonococcal
  arthritis (*see* Arthritis, gonococcal)
  urethritis (*see* Urethritis, gonococcal)
Gonorrhea, 482
  ceftriaxone in, 485
  lab, 482
  in newborn, 432
    ophthalmia and, 432
    presentation, 432
    prevention, 432
    treatment, 432
  signs and symptoms, 482
Gout, 217–220
  acute attack, 217
    prevention, 219–220
    treatment, 218–219
  chronic, tophaceous, 217
  clinical features, 217–218
  course, 217
  diagnostic features, 217–218
  radiography in, 218

Granuloma inguinale, 483
  lab, 483
  signs and symptoms, 483
  tetracycline for, 486
Grave's disease, 198
  iodine in, 199
  ophthalmopathy of, 200
  propranolol in, 199–200
  treatment, 199–200

Growth (*see* Intrauterine growth retardation)
Gynecologic adnexal masses, 265–267
  diagnosis, differential, by organ system, 265–266
  evaluation, 266
Gynecology, 258–306
  pediatric, 272–275

H

Haloperidol: in bipolar affective disorder, 554
Hands
  in osteoarthritis, 212
  in rheumatoid arthritis, 207–208
HBSAg positive mothers: infants of, 316
Head trauma, 18
Headache, 534–536
  clinical features, 536
  cluster, 536
  etiologies, 534
  muscle contraction, 534
  tension, clinical features, 536
  treatment, 534–535
Healing: of wound, 395
Heart
  block (*see under* Block)
  disease and diabetes, 189
  disease, ischemic, 60–67
    beta blockers in, 61
    calcium channel blocker in, 61
    diagnosis, 60–61
    etiology, 60
    history, 60
    inpatient, 64–67
    laboratory, 60–61
    nitrates in, 61–62
    nitroglycerin in, 62
    revascularization in, 62
    stable, 60

  treatment, 61–62
  types, 60
  unstable, 60
  variant, 60
enzymes, 65
factors in preoperative care, 403
failure, congestive, 71–73
  diuretics in, 71–72
  evaluation, 71
  history, 71
  laboratory exam, 71
  physical exam, 71
  preoperative care and, 404
  treatment, 71–73
  treatment, chronic condition, 73
life support, advanced, 1–9
in lupus erythematosus, systemic, 227
monitor after trauma, 17
rate
  fetal (*see* Fetus, heart rate)
  in resuscitation of newborn, 10–11
in rheumatoid arthritis, 209
sounds (*see* Sounds)
in syncope, 78–79
Heat
  cramps, 53–54
  edema, 53
  exhaustion, 54
  -related illnesses, 53–55

Index

Heat (cont.)
  stroke, 54–55
  syncope, 53
Heel: bursitis, 241
Heimlich maneuver: in foreign body aspiration in children, 452
Hematemesis, 133
Hematochezia, 133
Hematologic disorders, 159–206
  in newborn, 434–438
  preoperative care and, 402
Hematology: normal values, 645
Hematuria, 489–490
  etiology, 489
  evaluation, 489
  history, 489
  infectious, 489
  laboratory, 489
  physical exam, 489
  treatment, 489–490
Hemoglobinuria, paroxysmal nocturnal, 168
  congenital, 168
Hemolytic anemia (see Anemia, hemolytic)
Hemophilia
  A, 160
  B, 160
  management, 163
Hemoptysis, 129–131
  evaluation, 129–130
  history, 129
  laboratory exam, 129–130
  management, 130–131
    massive hemoptysis, 130
    minimal hemoptysis, 130–131
    moderate hemoptysis, 130
  physical exam, 129
Hemorrhage (see Bleeding)
Hemorrhoids, 156
  classification, 156
  complications, 156
  definition, 156
  etiology, 156
  symptoms, 156
  treatment, 156
Heparin: in disseminated intravascular coagulation in newborn, 436
Hepatitis, 144–145
  A in newborn, 431
  B in newborn, 431
  clinical features, 144
  comparisons of A, B and non-A, non-B, 144–145
  complications, 145
  diagnosis, 144
  etiology, 144
  laboratory features, 144
  management, 145
  screening during pregnancy, 316
Hernia: in acute scrotal pain, 493
Herpes simplex
  genitalis, 483
    acyclovir for, 486
    lab, 483
    signs and symptoms, 483
  keratitis, 503
Hip
  in osteoarthritis, 213
  in rheumatoid arthritis, 208
Hormone (see Menopause, hormone replacement therapy)
Hospital care: after normal delivery, 384
Hospital procedures, 585–609
H2 blocker: in acute urticaria, 525
Huhner test: in infertility, 285
Hyaline membrane disease, 428–429
  diagnosis, 428
  treatment, 428–429

Hydrocele, 495
Hydrothorax (*see* Pleural effusion)
Hydroxyzine hydrochloride: in acute urticaria, 525
Hypercholesterolemia, 88–89
Hyperemesis gravidarum, 324–325
  definition, 324
  etiology, 324
  management, 324–325
    hospital, 324–325
    outpatient, 324
Hyperglycemic-hyperosmolar nonketotic syndrome, 195–196
  clinical presentation, 195
  electrolytes in, 196
  evaluation, 195
  insulin in, 196
  laboratory, 195
  resuscitation, initial, 195
  treatment, 195–196
    continuing, 195–196
Hyperkalemia, 174–175
  bicarbonate in, 175
  calcium gluconate in, 175
  cation-exchange resins in, 175
  etiology, 174
  insulin and, 175
  presentation, 174–175
  treatment, 175
Hypernatremia, 177–178
  etiology, 177
  signs and symptoms, 177
  treatment, 177–178
Hyperosmolar (*see* Hyperglycemic-hyperosmolar nonketotic syndrome)
Hyperplastic anemia, 463
Hypertension, 74–77
  causes, 74
  education of patient, 75
  essential, 74
  evaluation, 74–75
  follow-up, 77
  life-style intervention, 75
  medications for, 75–77
  menopause with hormone replacement therapy and, 305
  physical exam, 74–75
  in pregnancy, 330–334
  pregnancy-induced, 330
    antihypertensives in, 332
    chronic, 333–334
    chronic, management, 333–334
    chronic, risks, 333
    evaluation, 331
    laboratory studies, 331
    management, 331–333
    management, ambulatory, 331
    management, hospital, 331–332
    physical exam, 331
    risk factors for, 330
  preoperative care and, 403
  secondary, 74
  treatment, 75–77
Hyperthyroidism, 197–200
  etiology, 198–199
  exam in, 197
  laboratory evaluation, 197–198
  signs and symptoms, 197
  treatment, 199–200
Hypertriglyceridemia, 89
Hypertrophy (*see* Prostate, hypertrophy)
Hypocalcemia in newborn, 434–435
  diagnosis, 435
  treatment, 435
Hypoglycemia, 180–183
  causes, 180–181
  diagnosis, 180–181

Hypoglycemia (*cont.*)
  fasting, 181–182
  idiopathic, 181
  in newborn, 434
    cause, 434
    definition, 434
    diagnosis, 434
    treatment, 434
  postprandial, 181
  symptoms, 180
  treatment, 182–183
Hypoglycemic agents: oral, in diabetes, 188
Hypokalemia, 172–174
  diuretics and, 172–173
  etiology, 172–173
  K^+ supplement in, 173–174
  presentation, 173
  treatment, 173–174

Hyponatremia, 178–179
  etiology, 178
  signs and symptoms, 178–179
  treatment, 179
Hypotension
  in myocardial infarction, 68
  orthostatic, 78
  in shock, 38
Hypothermia, 57–58
  disposition, 58
  mild, 57
  moderate, 57
  severe, 57
  treatment, 57–58
Hypothyroidism, 201–202, 463
  etiology, 201
  laboratory findings, 202
  levothyroxine in, 202
  signs and symptoms, 202
  treatment, 202

I

Ibuprofen: in gout, 219
Imaging
  bone, with ^{99m}Tc, in stress fracture, 239
  in cholelithiasis, asymptomatic, 416
  MRI in low back pain, 123
Imipramine: in anxiety disorders, 555
Immersion injury, 55–56
Immunosuppression: in lupus erythematosus, systemic, 229–230
Immunotherapy: in allergic rhinitis, 521
Imodium: in diarrhea, acute, 148–149
Indocin: in gout, 219
Infant
  coma scale for, modified, 664
  feedings, for, supplemental, 654
  gynecologic exam, 272

  of HBSAg positive mothers, 316
  labial adhesions, 273
  ovarian tumors, 274
  pinworms, 273
  pneumonia (*see* Pneumonia in infants)
  resuscitation (*see* Resuscitation, of infant)
  roseola (*see* Roseola infantum)
  sarcoma botryoides, 274
  urethral prolapse, 274
  vaginal foreign body, 274
  vulvovaginitis, 272–273
Infarction (*see* Myocardial infarction)
Infertility, 283–287
  cervical factor, 285
  evaluation, overview of, 283
  luteal phase defect in, 286–287

male, causes, 284
male factor in, 284–285
male, treatment, 284–285
ovulation factor, 286–287
tubal factor, 285
Influenza, 102–103
  clinical presentation, 102–103
  management, 103
Ingrown toenail, 632–633
  complications, 633
  contraindications, 632
  indications, 632
  materials for, 632
  technique, 632–633
Innervation: sensory, of skin, 640
Insulin
  in diabetes, 187–188
    ketoacidosis of, 192–193
  in hyperglycemic-hyperosmolar nonketotic syndrome, 196
  hyperkalemia and, 175
  hypoglycemia and, 182
Insulinoma, 182
Integument disorders: and preoperative care, 402–403
Interphalangeal joint (*see* Dislocation, interphalangeal joint)
Intestine (*see* Gastrointestinal)
Intraosseous infusion, 576–578
  complications, 578
  contraindications, 576
  indications, 576
  materials for, 576
  technique, 576–578
Intrapartum
  asphyxia (*see* Asphyxia, intrapartum)
  management, 358–361
  monitoring, 358–361
Intrauterine growth retardation, 341
  definition, 341
  diagnosis, 341
  management, 341
  risk factors, 341
Intrauterine pressure catheter (*see* Catheter, intrauterine pressure)
Intubation
  nasotracheal, 29–30
    advantages, 29
    complications, 30
    contraindications, 29–30
    disadvantages, 29
    technique, 30
  orotracheal, 28–29
    advantages, 28
    complications, 28
    contraindications, 28
    disadvantages, 28
  orotracheal, tactile, 30–32
    advantages, 30–31
    complications, 31
    contraindications, 31
    disadvantages, 31
    technique, 31
  orotracheal, technique, 28–29
Iodine: in Grave's disease, 199
Iritis, 502, 503
Iron
  deficiency anemia (*see* Anemia, iron deficiency)
  during pregnancy, 310
  stores and breast feeding, 458
Ischemic
  heart disease (*see* Heart disease, ischemic)
  transient ischemic attacks, 545
    preoperative care and, 402
  tubular necrosis, 497
Isoimmunization: and Rh, 314–315
Isotretinoin: in nodulocystic acne, 524

692 Index

J

Jaundice in newborn
  complications, 437
  non-physiologic, 437
  pathologic, evaluation of, 437
  transfusion in, exchange, 437
  treatment, 437
Joint(s)
  acromioclavicular (see Acromioclavicular joint)
  Charcot's, in diabetes, 190
  elbow, access, 630
  interphalangeal (see Dislocation, interphalangeal joint)
  knee, access, 631
  in low back pain, 231
  in lupus erythematosus, systemic, 226
  metacarpophalangeal (see Dislocation, metacarpophalangeal joint)
  in osteoarthritis, 212–213
  prosthetic joint infections, 254
  in rheumatoid arthritis, 207
  shoulder, access, 629
  wrist, access, 630
Jugular vein access, 600

K

Kayexalate: in hyperkalemia, 175
Keratitis: herpes simplex, 503
Keratosis: actinic, 532
Ketoacidosis, diabetic, 192–194
  bicarbonate in, 193
  diagnosis, 192
  diet in, 194
  evaluation, 192
  insulin in, 192–193
  phosphate in, 193
  potassium in, 193
  treatment, 192–194
    continuing, 193–194
Kidney
  failure, 497–500
  failure, acute, 497–498
    diagnosis, 497
    etiology, 497
    treatment, 498
  failure, chronic, 498–499
    anemia of, 169
    clinical manifestations, 499
    diet in, 499
    etiology, 499
    syndrome, 498
    transplant in, 499
    treatment, 499
  insufficiency, 499
  in lupus erythematosus, systemic, 227
  transplant, 499
  tubular necrosis, 497–498
    causes, 497
    evaluation, 497–498
    ischemic, 497
    toxic, 497
Knee
  bursitis, 240–241
  joint access, 631
  in osteoarthritis, 212–213
  in rheumatoid arthritis, 208
K^+ supplement: in hypokalemia, 173–174

L

Labial adhesions: in infants and children, 273
Labor
  abnormal patterns, management, 355, 357
  anesthesia during, 595

arrest disorder, 357
defining, 354
evaluation, 354–357
history, 354
induction, 364–366
  Bishop Score in, 365
  contraindications, 364
  indications, 364
  methods, 365–366
  risks, 364–365
normal pattern, 355, 356
physical examination, 354–355
preterm, 345–349
  cause, 345
  definition, 345
  magnesium in, 348
  management, 346–348
  protocol for, 347–348
  risk determination, system for, 345–346
  risk factors, 345–346
  ritodrine in, 348
  terbutaline in, 348
  tocolysis score, 346–347
  ultrasound in, 346
protraction disorder, 357
stages of, 356
uterine activity in (*see* Uterus, activity during labor)
VBAC and, 343
Labyrinthitis, viral, 510
treatment, 510
Language skills: developmental milestones, 659–662
Laryngotracheobronchitis (*see* Croup)
Laser trabeculoplasty: in glaucoma, 508
Lavage (*see* Peritoneal lavage)
Length, birth to 36 months in boys, 657
in girls, 655
Levothyroxine: in hypothyroidism, 202

Lice (*see* Pediculosis)
Lidocaine
for arrhythmia in acute myocardial infarction, 69
wound repair and, 395
Life support, advanced
cardiac, 1–9
pediatric, 10–14
Lindane
in pediculosis pubis, 484
for scabies, 484
Line(s)
arterial, 597–599
  complications, 598
  contraindications, 597
  indications, 597
  materials, 597
  technique, 597–598
central, 599–601
  complications, 600–601
  contraindications, 599
  indications, 599
  materials, 599
  technique, 599–600
Lipid metabolism, 85
Lipoprotein disorders: classification by phenotypes and genotypes, 86
Liver
disease, 144–146
  alcoholic (*see below*)
  hypoglycemia in, 182
  management, 164
disease, alcoholic, 145–146
  clinical features, 145–146
  diagnosis, 146
  etiology, 145
  treatment, 146
Local block (*see* Block, local)
Lomotil: in diarrhea, acute, 148
Lovastatin: in hypercholesterolemia, 89
Low back pain, 231–236
analgesia for, 235

Low back pain (*cont.*)
  in children, 232
  chronic, 236
  etiology, 231–232
  laboratory evaluation, 234
  physical exam, 232–234
  physical therapy, 235
  steroids in, 235
  treatment, 234–236
Lumbar puncture
  adult, 606–607
    complications, 607
    contraindications, 606
    indications, 606
    materials, 606
    technique, 606–607
  in cerebrovascular disease, 546
  in febrile seizure in children, 445
Lung
  capacities, 91–92
    definitions, 92
    values, average, 92
  COPD, 117–121
    blue bloater in, 117
    centrilobular, 117
    clinical manifestations, comparison of, 117–119
    evaluation, 119–120
    history, 119
    hospitalization indications, 121
    infection in, 120–121
    laboratory in, 119–120
    management, 120–121
    outpatient management, 121
    panlobular, 117
    physical exam, 119
    pink puffer, 117
    respiratory failure in, 120
  disease
    obstructive, 37
    obstructive, chronic (*see* COPD *above*)
    obstructive, severity assessment, 94
    restrictive, severity assessment, 94
  function tests, 91–95
    interpretation, 92–94
  history and preoperative care, 404
  in lupus erythematosus, systemic, 227
  mechanics, 92
  in rheumatoid arthritis, 209
  volumes, 91–92
    definitions, 92
    values, average, 92
Lupus anticoagulant, 228
Lupus erythematosus, systemic, 226–230
  ANA negative, 228
  clinical features, 226–227
  CNS in, 227
  diagnosis, 228
  discoid, 226
  drug induced, 228
  gastrointestinal manifestations, 227
  heart in, 227
  joints in, 226
  kidney in, 227
  laboratory tests, 228
  lung in, 227
  prevention, 229
  skin in, 226
  subacute, 226
  treatment, 229
Luteal phase defect: in infertility, 286–287
Lymphogranuloma venereum, 482–483
  doxycycline in, 485
  erythromycin in, 485
  lab, 482
  signs and symptoms, 482

Index **695**

M

Magnesium
 in preeclampsia, 332–333
 in preterm labor, 348
Magnetic resonance imaging: in low back pain, 234
Mallet finger, 247
 treatment, 247
Malpresentation (*see* Delivery, malpresentation)
Mammography: of breast mass, 419–420
Mania, 553
Marcaine: and wound repair, 396
Marrow failure, 159
Masks
 reservoir, 97
 Venturi, 97
Mauriceau-Smellie-Veit maneuver: for breech delivery of head, 373
Measles, 453–454
 clinical manifestations, 454
 epidemiology, 453
 German (*see* Rubella)
 treatment, 454
Mebendazole: for pinworms, 470
Meconium aspiration syndrome, 427–428
 diagnosis, 427
 treatment, 427–428
Medications (*see* Drugs)
Medicine
 emergency, 1–59
 pulmonary, 91–132
Megaloblastic anemia, 463
Melanoma: malignant, 532
Melena, 133
Meniere's disease, 510
 treatment, 510
Meningitis, 539–540
 aseptic, 448–449, 540

 clinical presentation, 540
 etiology, 540
 evaluation, 540
 treatment, 540
 bacterial, acute, 539–540
 clinical presentation, 539
 etiology, 539
 evaluation, 539
 treatment, 539–540
 bacterial, in children, 447, 448
 in children, 447–449
 bacterial, 447
 bacterial, management, 448
 complications, 447–448
 etiology, 447–448
 evaluation, 448
 lab, 448
 management, 448–449
 presentation, 447
 prophylaxis, 449
 stabilization, 448
 viral, management, 448–449
 viral (*see* aseptic *above*)
Menopause, 304–306
 clinical features, 304
 hormone replacement therapy, 305–306
 initial assessment for, 305–306
 risks, 305
 standard therapy, 306
 management, 305
 osteoporosis and, 304
 postmenopausal bleeding, 278
 symptoms
 atrophic, 304
 psychologic, 304
 vasomotor, 304
Menorrhagia, 276

696 Index

Mental status: alteration in shock, 38
Meperidine: in migraine, 535
Mepivacaine: and wound repair, 396
Metabolic bone disease (*see* Bone disease, metabolic)
Metabolic disorders, 159–206
  in newborn, 434–438
Metacarpal block, 593
Metacarpophalangeal joint (*see* Dislocation, metacarpophalangeal joint)
Methotrexate: in rheumatoid arthritis, 211
Methylprednisolone: in asthma, 115
Methysergide: for migraine prophylaxis, 535
Metronidazole
  in endometritis, 390
  in vaginal infection, 485
Metrorrhagia, 276
Midrin: in migraine, 535
Migraine, 534–535
  acute, 534
  classic, clinical features, 536
  common, clinical features, 536
  prophylaxis, 535
  status, 535
Minoxidil: in congestive heart failure, 72
Molar pregnancy: with vaginal bleeding, 336
Molluscum contagiosum, 484
  lab, 484
  signs and symptoms, 484
  treatment, 484
Monitor: of heart after trauma, 17
Monitoring
  fetal heart rate, 358
  intrapartum, 358–361

Morbidity
  in postdate pregnancy, 352
  potential, in diabetes with pregnancy, 327
  puerperal febrile, differential diagnosis, 389–390
Morphine: in myocardial infarction, 66
Mortality: from trauma, 15
Motor neuropathy: and diabetes, 189
Murmurs, 82–84
  diastolic flow, 83–84
  diastolic regurgitant, 83
  grading of, 82
  maneuvers to differentiate, 84
  systolic ejection, 82–*83*
  systolic regurgitant, 83
Muscle: contraction headache, 534
Myocardial infarction, 65–70
  acute
    arrhythmia in, 69
    bradyarrhythmia in, 69–70
    complications, 68–70
    hypotension in, 68
    pulmonary edema in, 68–69
    shock in, 68
    ventricular fibrillation in, 69
    ventricular tachycardia in, 69
  definition, 65–66
  history of, and preoperative care, 403
  location of infarct by EKG, 66
  lupus erythematosus and, systemic, 227
  management, 66–67
  morphine in, 66
  nifedipine in, 66
  nitroglycerin in, 66
  thrombolytic therapy in, 66, 67

Index **697**

Myocarditis: lupus erythematosus and, systemic, 227

Naloxone for resuscitation
 in coma, 42
 in newborn, 11
Naproxen: in premenstrual tension syndrome, 302
Narcan (*see* Naloxone)
Narcotic withdrawal in newborn, 435
 diagnosis, 435
 treatment, 435
Nasogastric tube: in trauma, 17
Nasopharyngoscopy, flexible, 622–623
 complications, 623
 indications, 622
 materials, 622
 technique, 622
Nasotracheal intubation (*see* Intubation, nasotracheal)
Nebulizer, 97
Neck
 in rheumatoid arthritis, 208
 swan neck deformity in rheumatoid arthritis, 207
 trauma, 19
  blunt, 19
  penetrating, 19
Necrosis: tubular (*see* Kidney, tubular necrosis)
Neisseria: in conjunctivitis, 506
Neonate (*see* Newborn)
Nerve
 block (*see* Block, nerve)
 skin innervation, sensory, 640
Nervous system: central, in SLE, 227
Neurologic criteria: assessment techniques, Dubowitz modification, 650
Neurologic exam: and wounds, 394

Myopathy: diabetic, 190
Myxedema: coma of, 202–203

N

Neurologic history: and preoperative care, 402
Neurology, 534–547
Neuroma: acoustic, 510–511
Neuromuscular paralysis: and sedation, 99
Neuropathy, diabetic, 189–190
 autonomic, 189–190
 motor, 189
Nevi
 common, 532
 congenital, 532
Newborn
 apnea (*see* Apnea in newborn)
 diarrhea (*see* Diarrhea in newborn)
 DIC (*see* Coagulation, disseminated intravascular, in newborn)
 fever, 439–441
  antibiotics for, 440–441
  definition, 439
  evaluation, 439–440
  exam, 440
  history, 439–440
  infection, bacterial, 439
  keys, 439
  lab, 440
  treatment, 440–441
 gonorrhea (*see* Gonorrhea, in newborn)
 gynecologic exam, 272
 hematologic disorders, 434–438
 hypocalcemia (*see* Hypocalcemia in newborn)
 hypoglycemia (*see* Hypoglycemia in newborn)
 infection, 430–433
  bacterial, with fever, 439

Newborn (*cont.*)
    congenital, 430–433
    jaundice (*see* Jaundice in newborn)
    metabolic disorders, 434–438
    narcotic withdrawal (*see* Narcotic withdrawal in newborn)
    pneumonia (*see* Pneumonia in newborn)
    polycythemia (*see* Polycythemia in newborn)
    in postdate pregnancy, 352
    respiratory problems, 427–429
    resuscitation (*see* Resuscitation, of newborn)
    sepsis (*see* Sepsis, bacterial, in newborn)
    tachypnea (*see* Tachypnea, transient, of newborn)
    thrombocytopenia (*see* Thrombocytopenia in newborn)
    vaginal bleeding, 274
    vomiting (*see* Vomiting in newborn)
Niacin: in hypercholesterolemia, 88–89
Nifedipine
    in heart failure, congestive, 72
    in myocardial infarction, 66
Nitrates
    in heart disease, ischemic, 61–62
    in heart failure, congestive, 72
Nitroglycerin
    in heart disease, ischemic, 62
    in myocardial infarction, 66
Nomogram: for body surface area determination, 641
Nonsteroidal anti-inflammatory drugs (*see* NSAIDs)
Nose, 501–522
    cannula, 97
NSAID's
    in gout, 219
    in lupus erythematosus, systemic, 229
    in rheumatoid arthritis, 210
Nursemaid's elbow, 245
Nursing
    postoperative care and, 405
    preoperative surgical care and, 401
Nutrition
    breast feeding and, 458
    after burns, 425
    during pregnancy, 310
    status in preoperative care, 403

O

Oak (*see* Poison ivy, oak)
Obesity: and preoperative care, 403
Obsessive compulsive disorder, 557
    characteristics, 557
    treatment, 557
Obstetric(s), 307–391
    risk factor analysis, 308–309
Office procedures, 610–638
Oligomenorrhea, 276
Ophthalmia: with gonorrhea in newborn, 432
Ophthalmologic manifestations: of rheumatoid arthritis, 209
Ophthalmopathy: of Grave's disease, 200
Ophthalmoscopy: in glaucoma, 507
Opiate poisoning, 48
Orotracheal intubation (*see* Intubation, orotracheal)
Orthopedic(s), 207–257
    injuries, 242–248

Orthostatic hypotension, 78
Osteitis fibrosa: causing osteopenia, 225
Osteoarthritis, 212–214
  clinical features, 212–213
  diagnostic tests, 213
  laboratory, 213
  radiography in, 213
  signs and symptoms, 212
  treatment, 213–214
Osteomalacia: causing osteopenia, 225
Osteopenia, 223–225
Osteoporosis, 223–225
  menopause and, 304
  prevention, 224–225
  treatment, 223–224
Otitis, 512–515
  in children, 512–514
    course, clinical, 512
    diagnosis, 512–513
    drugs for, 513
    follow-up, 513–514
    treatment, 513
  media, 512–515
  media, acute, 514
    diagnosis, 514
    erythromycin in, 514
    penicillin V in, 514
    treatment, 514
  serious, 514
    diagnosis, 514
    treatment, 514
Ovaries
  cysts, 267
  in gynecologic adnexal masses, 265
  masses, treatment, 266–267
  tumors in infants and children, 274
Overdose, 46–52
  acetaminophen in, 49
  airway in, 46
  antidepressants, tricyclic, 51–52
  beta blocker in, 50
  carbon monoxide in, 50–51
  charcoal in, activated, 47–48
  circulation in, 46
  decontamination, 47–48
  diagnosis, 47
  digoxin in, 51
  emesis in, 47
  lavage in, gastric, 47
  management, initial, 46
  neurologic status after, 46
  resuscitation in, 46
  salicylates in, 50
  stimulants in, 49
  treatment, 49–52
Overuse syndromes, 237–241
Ovulation: and infertility, 286–287
Oxygen
  delivery systems, 97
  therapy, 96
Oxytocin for labor induction, 364–365
  guidelines for, 366

P

Pain
  abdominal (*see* Abdomen, pain)
  back (*see* Low back pain)
  pelvic (*see* Pelvis, pain)
  scrotal (*see* Scrotum, pain)
Pancreas: enzyme supplements in chronic diarrhea, 151

Pancreatitis
  acute, 141–142
    clinical features, 141
    complications, 142
    diagnosis, 141
    etiology, 141
    management, 142

700 Index

Pancreatitis (*cont.*)
    prognosis based on Ranson's criteria, 141
  chronic, 143
    clinical features, 143
    complications, 143
    diagnosis, 143
    etiology, 143
    management, 143
Panic attacks, 556
  characteristics of, 556
  treatment, 556
Paracentesis, 582–584
  complications, 583
  contraindications, 582
  indications, 582
  materials for, 582–583
  results, 583–584
  technique, 583
Paracervical block, 594
Paralysis: neuromuscular, and sedation, 99
Parasites, 470–471
Patella (*see* Dislocation, patella)
Pediatrics (*see* Children)
Pediculosis, 470–471
  evaluation, 470
  pubis, 484
    lab, 484
    signs and symptoms, 484
    treatment, 484
  treatment, 471
PEEP, 99
Pelvimetry, 362–363
  hazards, potential, 362–363
  pelvic inlet, 362
  pelvic midplane, 362
  pelvic outlet, 362
  radiographic, 362–363
    advantages, 362
    chart, 363
    indications, 362
    parameters, 363
Pelvis
  exam
    in abdominal pain, 412
    in labor evaluation, 354–355
    prenatal, 307–308
  fracture, 21–22
  inflammatory disease, 291–293
    complications, 292–293
    diagnosis, 291–292
    diagnosis, differential, 291
    pathogenesis, 291
    predisposing factors, 291
    treatment, 292
    treatment, inpatient, 292
    treatment, outpatient, 292
  pain, 262–264
    diagnosis, differential, 263
    diagnostic aids, 262–263
    diagnostic approach, 262–263
    history, 262
    management, 263
    physical exam, 262
  trauma, 21–22
Penicillamine: in rheumatoid arthritis, 211
Penicillin
  G
    benzathine for syphilis, 485
    in endometritis, 390
    in gonorrhea in newborn, 432
    in septic arthritis, 254
  V in otitis media, acute, 514
Peptic ulcer, 136–137
Perfusion
  studies, 94–95
  /ventilation tests, 94–95
    interpretation, 95
Pericarditis;
  lupus erythematosus and, systemic, 227
Peritoneal lavage, 582–584

Index

complications, 583
contraindications, 582
fluid, evaluation criteria, 583–584
indications, 582
materials for, 582–583
results, 583–584
technique, 583
Permethrin: for pediculosis, 471
pH (*see* Fetus, scalp pH)
Pharyngitis, 516–517
complications, 517
etiology, 516
evaluation, 516–517
Phenergan: for vomiting in newborn, 444
Phenobarbital: in narcotic withdrawal in newborn, 435
Phenotypes: in lipoprotein disorder classification, 86
Phobia
simple, 557
characteristics, 557
treatment, 557
social, 557
characteristics, 557
treatment, 557
Phosphate
in diabetic ketoacidosis, 193
stones, triple, 492
Physical therapy
low back pain, 235
in osteoarthritis, 213–214
in tendonitis, 237–238
Pigmented lesions, 532
Pilocarpine: in glaucoma, 503, 508
Pink puffer, in COPD, 117
Pinworms, 470
examination for, 470
in infants and children, 273
symptoms, 470
treatment, 470
Pituitary insufficiency: causing hypoglycemia, 182

Placenta
abruption, 338–339
classification, 338
diagnosis, 339
incidence, 338
management, 340
previa, 338
classification, 338
diagnosis, 338
incidence, 338
management, 339–340
Platelet
disorders
qualitative, 159
quantitative, 159
transfusion in thrombocytopenia in newborn, 439
Pleural effusion, 126–128
differentiation of transudate from exudate, 127
evaluation, 126–127
history, 126
laboratory, 126–127
management, 127–128
physical exam, 126
pleurocentesis in, 126
Pleurocentesis, in pleural effusion, 126
Pneumonia, 104–111
antibiotics in, summary, 110–111
causative agents by types of patient, 105
in children 5–14, 107–108
evaluation, 107–108
management, 108
presentation, 107
15 and over, 108–111
evaluation, 109
management, 109
presentation, 108
in infants and children, 104–107
evaluation, 106

Pneumonia (*cont.*)
  presentation, 104–106
  management, 106–107
  in newborn, 104
    evaluation, 104
    management, 104
    presentation, 104
Pneumothorax, 35–36
  treatment, 36
Podophyllin: in condyloma acuminata, 483
Poison ivy, oak and sumac, 528
  antipruritics in, 528
  steroids in, 528
  treatment, 528
Poisoning, 46–52
  acetaminophen in, 49
  airway in, 46
  anticholinergic, 48
  antidepressants in, tricyclic, 51–52
  beta blocker in, 50
  carbon monoxide in, 50–51
  charcoal in, activated, 47–48
  cholinergic, 48
  circulation in, 46
  decontamination, 47–48
  diagnosis, 47
  digoxin in, 51
  emesis in, 47
  lavage in, gastric, 47
  management, initial, 46
  neurologic status after, 46
  opiate, 48
  resuscitation in, 46
  salicylates in, 50
  stimulants in, 49
  treatment, 49–52
Polycythemia in newborn, 435–436
  diagnosis, 435
  treatment, 435–436
Polymenorrhea, 276
Polyps: in colorectal tumors, 154

Positive end-expiratory pressure, 99
Postdate pregnancy (*see* Pregnancy, postdate)
Postoperative care
  diet, 405
  drugs, 405–406
  laboratory, 406
  nursing, 405
  orders, 405
Postoperative fever, 406
Postpartum bleeding (*see* Bleeding, postpartum)
Postpartum care, 383–385
  discharge, 384–385
  hospital care, 384
  orders after routine vaginal delivery, examples of, 383
Post-traumatic stress disorder, 558
Potassium, 172–176
  in ketoacidosis, diabetic, 193
Prazosin: in congestive heart failure, 72
Precancer: of skin, 532–533
Prednisone: in asthma, 115
Preeclampsia, 330
  anticonvulsants in, 332
  evaluation, 331
  magnesium in, 332–333
  laboratory studies, 331
  management, 331–333
    ambulatory, 331
    hospital, 331–332
  physical exam, 331
Pregnancy
  activity during, 311–312
  calcium during, 310
  with diabetes (*see* Diabetes mellitus with pregnancy)
  ectopic, 298–300
    culdocentesis in, 299
    etiology, 298

evaluation overview, 298–299
history, 298
incidence, 298
laboratory exam, 299
physical exam, 298
treatment, 300
ultrasound in, 299
with vaginal bleeding, 335–336
work-up of stable patient, 299–300
work-up of unstable patient, 299
exercise during, 310–312
contraindications, 311
folic acid during, 310
habits and, 312
hepatitis screening during, 316
hypertension in (*see* Hypertension in pregnancy)
infections during, 312
iron during, 310
molar, with vaginal bleeding, 336
nutrition during, 310
postdate, 352–353
definitions, 352
etiology, 352
management, 352–353
morbidity, potential, 352
postmature, 352
problems, potential, 312
prolonged, 352
test in pelvic pain, 262
vaginal infection during, 485
Premature rupture of membranes, 350–351
amnionitis and, 351
definitions, 350
diagnosis, 350
management, 350–351
preterm, 350–351
term, 350

Premenstrual tension syndrome, 301–303
diagnosis, 301–302
diet in, 302
epidemiology, 301
etiology, 301
symptoms, physical and emotional, 302
treatment, 302–303
Prenatal
care, 307–309
history at initial evaluation, 307
laboratory evaluation, 308
laboratory evaluation during pregnancy, 308
pelvic exam, 307–308
physical examination, 307–308
risk factor analysis, 308–309
weight gain, expected, 308
course, review of, 354
fetal surveillance, 319–323
patient education, 310–313
Preoperative care, 401–404
laboratory, 402
medical history of major importance, 402–404
Preoperative evaluation, 401–404
Preterm labor (*see* Labor, preterm)
Probenecid: in gout attack prevention, 219–220
Progesterone
luteal phase in infertility and, 287
in premenstrual tension syndrome, 302
Promethazine;
in migraine, 535
for vomiting in newborn, 444
Propranolol: in Grave's disease, 199–200

Propylthiouracil: in thyroid storm, 201
Prostaglandin inhibitors
  in dysmenorrhea, 280
  in premenstrual tension syndrome, 302
Prostate, hypertrophy, benign, 487–488
  clinical presentation, 487
  etiology, 487
  lab, 487
  radiography of, 487
  treatment, 487–488
Prostatitis, bacterial, 474–476
  acute, 474–475
    lab, 474
    management, 475
    signs and symptoms, 474
    treatment, 474–475
  chronic, 475–476
    lab, 476
    signs and symptoms, 475
    treatment, 476
Prostatitis, nonbacterial, 476
  etiology, 476
  lab, 476
  signs and symptoms, 476
  treatment, 476
Prostatodynia, 475, 476
  lab, 476
  signs and symptoms, 476
  treatment, 476
Prosthetic joint infections, 254
Prothrombin complex concentration, 163
Pseudogout, 215
Pseudohyponatremia, 178
"Pseudo-menopause:" in endometriosis, 289
Pseudo-osteoarthritis, 215
"Pseudo-pregnancy:" in endometriosis
Pseudorheumatoid arthritis, 215
Psychiatry, 548–568

Psychologic
  dyspareunia, 269
  symptoms of menopause, 304
Psychosis
  acute, 563–564
    diagnosis, differential, 563
    treatment, 563
  brief reactive, 566
    diagnosis, differential, 566
    treatment, 566
Psychotherapy
  in anxiety disorders, generalized, 556
  of depression, 552
PTCA: in ischemic heart disease, 62
Pudendal block, 595–596
Puerperal febrile morbidity: differential diagnosis, 389–390
Puerperal fever, 389–391
  definition, 389
  diagnosis, differential, 389–390
Pulmonary
  edema (see Edema, pulmonary)
  embolism, 122–125
    anticoagulation in, 124–125
    diagnosis, differential, 122
    evaluation, 122–123
    history, 122
    laboratory, 123
    management, 123–125
    physical exam, 122
    predisposing factors, 122
    re-embolization in, 125
    thrombolytic therapy of, 124
  medicine, 91–132
  regurgitation, 83
Pulse: after defibrillation attempt, 3
Purpura

ITP, management, 162
senile, 160
simplex, 160
TTP, management, 162
vascular, drug induced, 160
Pyelonephritis
  acute, 479–480
    clinical presentation, 479
    definition, 479
    etiology, 479
    lab, 479
    treatment, 479–480
  chronic, 480
Pyrantel pamoate: for pinworms, 470
Pyrethrins: for pediculosis, 471

R

Rabies
  bites in children and, 467
  treatment, 398–400
Radial head: subluxation, 245
Radiation burns, 423
Radiography
  acromioclavicular joint dislocation, 242
  in asthma, 113
  in bone disease, metabolic, 223
  of cerebrovascular disease, 546
  in cholelithiasis, asymptomatic, 416
  in chondrocalcinosis, 216
  in fracture, stress, 238–239
  gastrointestinal, in abdominal pain, 413
  glenohumeral dislocation, 243
  in gout, 218
  in osteoarthritis, 213
  in pelvic pain, 263
  in pelvimetry (*see* Pelvimetry, radiographic)
  in pleural effusion, 126
  of prostatic hypertrophy, benign, 487
  in septic arthritis, 252
  in spondylitis, ankylosing, 221–222
  after trauma, 24
  ulcer, duodenal, 136
Rash
  in chickenpox, 453
  in measles, 454
  in rubella, 454
  in scarlet fever, 456
Rebreathing: partial, 97
Rectum
  anorectal (*see* Anorectal)
  colorectal (*see* Colorectal)
  exam in abdominal pain, 412
Red eye (*see* Eye, red)
Reference data, 639–664
Reflux (*see* Gastroesophageal reflux)
Regional (*see* Block, local and regional)
Regurgitation
  aortic, 83
  pulmonary, 83
Reiter's syndrome, 478
Renal (*see* Kidney)
Respiratory
  arrest after trauma, 15–16
  distress, 35–37
    evaluation, initial, 35
    intervention, 35
    syndrome (*see* Hyaline membrane disease)
  failure in COPD, 120
  postoperative fever, 406
  problems of newborn, 427–429
  tract infection, upper viral, 102–103
Resuscitation
  in coma, 42

Resuscitation (cont.)
  in hyperglycemic-hyperosmolar nonketotic syndrome, 195
  in infants and children, 12–14
    airway management, 12
    assessment, 12
    atropine, 13
    circulation 12–13
    epinephrine, 13
    sodium bicarbonate, 13
  of newborn, 10–11
    assessment, 10–11
    epinephrine, 11
    heart rate, 10–11
    naloxone, 11
    sodium bicarbonate, 11
    volume expanders, indications for, 11
  in overdose, 46
  in poisoning, 46
  after trauma, 16–17
Retin-A: in comedonal acne, 523
Retinopathy: diabetic, 190
Revascularization: in heart disease, ischemic, 62
Rh screening: protocol for, 314
Rheumatoid arthritis, 207–211
  articular involvement, 207–208
  clinical features, 207–210
  course, 207
  extra-articular, 208–209
  initial presentation, 207
  laboratory, 209–210
  treatment, 210–211
Rheumatology, 207–257
Rhinitis, 520–522
  allergic, 520–521
    antihistamines in, 520–521
    diagnosis, 520
    exam, 520
    history, 520
    immunotherapy in, 521
    steroids in, 520
    treatment, 520–521
  medicamentosa, chronic
    diagnosis, 521
    treatment, 521
  vasomotor, 521
Rho-GAM, 314
Rhythm
  after defibrillation attempt, 3
  pulseless, 1–4
Ritodrine: in preterm labor, 348
Roseola infantum, 455
  clinical manifestations, 455
  epidemiology, 455
Rubella, 431, 454
  clinical manifestations, 454
  epidemiology, 454
  treatment, 454
Rubeola (*see* Measles)
Rupture
  of membranes (*see* Premature rupture of membranes)
  uterine, 339

S

Salicylates
  in overdose, 50
  in poisoning, 50
Salter fracture (*see* Fracture, Salter)
Saphenous vein: cutdown, 574
Sarcoma botryoides: in infants and children, 274
SBE prophylaxis, 663
Scabies, 484
  lab, 484
  signs and symptoms, 484
  treatment, 484
Scalp (*see* Fetus, scalp)
Scanning (*see* Imaging)
Scarlet fever
  clinical manifestations, 455–456

epidemiology, 455
treatment, 456
Schizophrenia, 565–566
  diagnosis, differential, 565
  subtypes, 565
  treatment, 566
Schizophreniform disorder, 566
  characteristics, 566
Scleroderma, 139
  diagnosis, 139
  treatment, 139
Scrotum
  masses, painless, 495–496
  pain, acute, 494–495
    causes, 493–495
    epididymitis in, 493
    etiology, 493
    evaluation, 493
    hernia in, 493
    testicular torsion in, 493–495
    trauma in, 493
    urolithiasis in, 493
Scurvy, 160
Seatbelts: during pregnancy, 312
Seborrheic eczema, 527
Sedation: and neuromuscular paralysis, 99
Seizure, 541–544
  absence, 543
  diagnosis, 541
  epileptic, classification, 542
  etiology, 541
    by age, 541
  febrile, in children, 445–446
    chemistries, 445
    evaluation, 445
    exam, 445
    history, 445
    lab, 445
    lumbar puncture in, 445
    treatment, 446
    treatment, chronic, 446
    treatment, emergent, 446
  grand mal, 543
  after overdose, 46
  partial, 543
  petit mal, 543
  after poisoning, 46
  primary generalized, 543
  secondarily generalized, 543
  tonic-clonic, 543
  treatment, 541–543
Semen analysis: in infertility, 284
Sepsis, bacterial, in newborn, 432–433
  etiology, 432
  presentation, 432
  treatment, 433
  work-up, 432–433
Septic
  abortion (*see* Abortion, septic)
  arthritis (*see* Arthritis, septic)
Sexually transmitted diseases, 481–486
Shock, 38–40
  cardiogenic, 38
  cause, determination of, 39–40
  diagnosis, 38
  distributive, 38
  etiology, 38
  hypoperfusion with, 38
  hypovolemic, 38
  management, 39–40
    immediate, 39
  mental status alteration in, 38
  mild, 39
  moderate, 39
  in myocardial infarction, acute, 68
  orthostatic changes, 38
  severe, 39
  severity, clinical, 39
  trauma and, 40
  treatment, 39–40
Shoulder

Index

Shoulder (*cont.*)
dystocia (*see* Dystocia, shoulder)
joint access, 629
in rheumatoid arthritis, 208
Sickle cell (*see* Anemia, sickle cell)
Sideroblastic (*see* Anemia, sideroblastic)
Sigmoidoscopy, flexible, 636–638
bowel preparation for, 637
complications, 638
contraindications, 636
documentation, 637–638
indications, 636
interpretation, 637
materials, 636–637
technique, 637
Sinus bradycardia, 8
Sinusitis, 518–519
acute, 518
complications, 519
decongestants in, topical, 519
diagnosis, 518
drugs for, 518–519
management, 519
treatment, 518–519
chronic, 519
diagnosis, 519
treatment, 519
Skin
cancer, 532–533
carcinoma (*see* Carcinoma, skin)
innervation, sensory, 640
lesion excision, 613–614
complications, 614
contraindications, 613
indications, 613
materials, 613
technique, 613–614
in lupus erythematosus, systemic, 226
precancer, 532–533
in rheumatoid arthritis, 209
Smoking: during pregnancy, 312
Social phobia (*see* Phobia, social)
Sodium, 177–179
bicarbonate (*see* Bicarbonate)
deficiency, 179
excess, 179
in renal failure, chronic, 499
Sounds, 81
clicks, 81
ejection, 81
S_1, 81
S_2, 81
S_3, 81
S_4, 81
systolic, 81
Spasm; (*see* Esophagus, spasm)
Sperm penetration assay: in infertility, 284
Spermatocele, 495
Spider (*see* Bites, spider)
Spinal
canal stenosis, 231
dermatomes, 640
Spirometry, 92, 93
in asthma, 113
Spironolactone;
in heart failure, congestive, 72
in premenstrual syndrome, 302
Spondylitis, ankylosing, 221–222
clinical features, 221–222
history, 221
laboratory tests, 222
physical exam, 221
radiography in, 221–222
treatment, 222
Spondylolisthesis: in low back pain, 231
Spondylosis: in low back pain, 231

Sprain: of acromioclavicular joint, 242
Stab wounds: of abdomen, 21
Stature, 2 to 18 years
  in boys, 658
  in girls, 656
Status epilepticus, 543–544
  treatment protocol, 543–544
Stenosis: spinal canal, 231
Steroids
  intra-articular, and arthrocentesis, 629
  in low back pain, 235
  in poison ivy, oak and sumac, 528
  in rhinitis, allergic, 520
Stimson reduction: modified, of glenohumeral dislocation, 243
Stimulants
  in overdose, 49
  in poisoning, 49
Stomach
  (see also Gastrointestinal)
  atony in diabetes, 190
  lavage in poisoning and overdose, 47
  ulcer (see Ulcer, gastric)
Stones
  calcium, 492
  gallstones, 417
  phosphate, triple, 492
  uric acid, 492
Streptokinase: in pulmonary embolism, 124
Stress
  contraction stress testing (see Fetus, contraction stress testing)
  fracture (see Fracture, stress)
  post-traumatic stress disorder, 558
Stridor: in children, 450–452
Stroke, 545
  heat, 54–55
Subclavian vein access, 600
Substance abuse, 559–562
  clinical presentation, 560–561
Sucralfate: in duodenal ulcer, 137
Sugar: postprandial blood, 2-hour, nomogram for interpreting, 186
Sulfacetamide: in bacterial conjunctivitis, 506
Sulfamethoxazole (see Trimethoprim-sulfamethoxazole)
Sulfisoxazole: in otitis in children, 513
Sumac (see Poison ivy, oak and sumac)
Sun exposure: lesions related to, 532–533
Suprapubic (see Bladder tap, suprapubic)
Supraventricular tachycardia, 5–7
  paroxysmal, 6–7
Surgery
  general, 392–426
  medical history of major importance, 402–404
Suture(s), 399
  removal, 398
Suturing, 397
Swan neck deformity: in rheumatoid arthritis, 207
Sympatholytics: in hypertension, 76
Sympathomimetics: in preterm labor, 348
Syncope, 78–80
  arrhythmia in, 79
  causes, 78–79
    cardiac, 78–79
    circulatory, 78–79
    metabolic, 79
    neurological, 79

Syncope (*cont.*)
  definition, 78
  evaluation, 79–80
  heat, 53
  history, 79–80
  laboratory studies, 80
  near, 78
  physical exam, 80
  treatment, 80
  vasodepressor, 78
  vasovagal, 78

Syphilis, 481
  in newborn, 431
  penicillin G benzathine for, 485
  primary, 481
    lab, 481
    signs and symptoms, 481
    treatment, 481
  secondary, 481
    lab, 481
    signs and symptoms, 481

T

Tachycardia
  with shock, 38
  supraventricular, 5–7
    paroxysmal, 6–7
  ventricular
    in infants and children, 14
    in myocardial infarction, acute, 69
    pulseless, emergency care, 1–2
    sustained, 4–5, 6
    sustained, in infants and children, 13–14
  wide-complex, 5
Tachypnea, transient, of newborn, 429
  diagnosis, 429
  treatment, 429
Tar burns, 424
Technetium-99m: for bone scan in stress fracture, 239
Tendon(s): and wounds, 394
  Tendonitis, 237–238
    clinical features, 237
    physical therapy, 237–238
    prevention, 238
    treatment, 237–238
Tension
  headache, clinical features, 536
  premenstrual (*see* Premenstrual tension)
Terbutaline: in preterm labor, 348
Testes
  torsion in acute scrotal pain, 493–495
  tumor, 496
Tetanus
  after bites in children, 466
  status, 393
Tetany, 53–54
Tetracaine: and wound repair, 395
Tetracycline
  in acne, papulopustular, 524
  in conjunctivitis, bacterial, 506
  for granuloma inguinale, 486
Thalassemia, 166–167, 463
  α-Thalassemia, 166
  β-Thalassemia
    major, 167
      clinical presentation, 167
      diagnosis, 167
      treatment, 167
    minor, 166–167
      clinical presentation, 166
      diagnosis, 167
      treatment, 167
Theophylline: in asthma, 116

Index

Thiamine: in coma resuscitation, 42
Thiazide diuretics
  in heart failure, congestive, 71–72
  in hypertension, 76
Thoracentesis, 604–605
  complications, 605
  contraindications, 604
  indications, 604
  materials, 604
  technique, 604–605
Thoracostomy, tube, 571–572
  complications, 572
  contraindications, 571
  indications, 571
  materials, 571
  technique, 571–572
Throat, 501–522
Thrombocytopenia, 162
  in newborn, 436
    diagnosis, 436
    treatment, 436
Thrombocytosis, 159
Thrombolytic therapy
  in myocardial infarction, 66, 67
  in pulmonary embolism, 124
Thrombophlebitis: postoperative, 406
Thyroid, 197–203
  carcinoma (*see* Carcinoma, thyroid)
  enlargement, 204–206
  nodule, solitary, 205
  storm, 201
    etiology, 201
    propylthiouracil in, 201
    signs and symptoms, 201
    treatment, 201
Thyroiditis
  autoimmune, 198
    treatment, 200
  subacute, 198–199, 205

treatment, 200
TIAs, 545
  preoperative care and, 402
Tick bites (*see* Bites, tick)
Ticolysis score: in preterm labor, 346–347
Tobacco: during pregnancy, 312
Toenail (*see* Ingrown toenail)
Tomography, computed
  in cerebrovascular disease, 546
  in fracture, stress, 239
  in low back pain, 234
Tonometry: in glaucoma, 507
Tonsillitis: recurrent, 517
TORCHS, congenital, 430–431
  diagnosis, maternal, 430
  evaluation, 430
  laboratory, 430–431
  presentation in newborn, 430
  prevention, 431
  treatment, 431
Torsade de pointes, 5
Toxic
  conjunctivitis, 506
  tubular necrosis, 497
Toxidromes, 48–49
Toxoplasmosis: in newborn, 431
Trabeculoplasty: laser, in glaucoma, 508
Trachea
  nasotracheal (*see* Intubation, nasotracheal)
  orotracheal (*see* Intubation, orotracheal)
  transtracheal (*see* Ventilation, transtracheal)
Tracheitis: bacterial, 451–452
Transfusion
  exchange
    in disseminated intravascular coagulation in newborn, 436
    in jaundice in newborn, 437

Transfusion (*cont.*)
  platelet, in thrombocytopenia in newborn, 436
Transplantation: kidney, in kidney failure, 499
Trauma, 15–25
  abdomen (*see* Abdomen, trauma)
  assessment, 15
  breathing after, 16
  cardiac monitor after, 17
  chest, 19–20
  in circulation, 168
  circulation after, 16
  decompression after, 17
  diagnostic procedures, 24
  disability after, 16
  extremities, 22–24
  genitourinary, 21–22
  head, 18
  laboratory procedures, 24
  mortality, 15
  neck (*see* Neck trauma)
  paracentesis and, 582
  pelvis, 21–22
  peritoneal lavage and, 582
  post-traumatic stress disorder, 558
  radiography after, 24
  resuscitation after, 16–17
  in scrotal pain, acute, 493
  shock and, 40
  survey
    primary, 15–16
    secondary, 18
Triamcinolone: in nodulocystic acne, 524
TRIC conjunctivitis, 506
Trichomoniasis, 485
  clotrimazole for, 485
  lab, 485
  metronidazole for, 485
  signs and symptoms, 485
Tricyclics (*see* Antidepressants, tricyclic)
Trimethoprim-sulfamethoxazole
  in otitis in children, 513
  in sinusitis, acute, 519
Tubal (*see* Fallopian tube)
Tube
  nasogastric, in trauma, 17
  thoracostomy (*see* Thoracostomy, tube)
Tubule (*see* Kidney, tubular necrosis)
Tumors
  colorectal (*see* Colorectal tumors)
  ovarian, in infants and children, 274
  testes, 496
Tympanometry, 620–621
  contraindications, 620
  indications, 620
  interpretation, 620–621
  materials for, 620
  technique, 620

U

Ulcer
  decubitus, 530–531
    clinical presentation, 530
    predisposing factors, 530
    prevention, 530
    stages in development, 530
    treatment, 530–531
  duodenal, 136–137
    clinical presentation, 136
    history, 136
    laboratory, 136
    physical exam, 136
    radiography of, 136
    treatment, 136–137
  gastric, 137
    clinical presentation, 137

evaluation, 137
peptic, 136
Ultrasound
  in abdominal pain, 413
  in cholelithiasis, asymptomatic, 416
  in ectopic pregnancy, 299
  fetal (*see* Fetus, ultrasound of)
  in pelvic pain, 263
  in preterm labor, 346
Urethra: prolapse in infants and children, 274
Urethral syndrome: in female, 472
Urethritis
  ceftriaxone in, 485
  gonococcal, in males, 477–478
    lab, 477
    signs and symptoms, 477
    treatment, 477
  in males, 475
  nongonococcal, in males, 478
    etiology, 478
    lab, 478
    signs and symptoms, 478
    treatment, 478
  postgonococcal, 478
Uric acid stones, 492
Urinalysis
  in hypertension, 75
  in pelvic pain, 262
Urinary
  (*see also* Genitourinary)
  disorders, 472–500
  tract infection, lower, in female, 472–473
    etiology, 472
    lab findings, 472
    signs and symptoms, 472

    single-dose regimens, 473
    standard oral regimens, 473
    three-day regimens, 473
    treatment, 473
  tract infection, lower, in males, 474–478
    etiology, 474
    localization, 474
  tract infection, postoperative, 406
Urine collection, 608
  technique, 608
Urokinase: in pulmonary embolism, 124
Urolithiasis, 491–492
  clinical presentation, 491
  continuing care, 492
  history, 491
  laboratory, 491
  physical exam, 491
  in scrotal pain, acute, 493
  treatment, initial, 491–492
Urticaria, 525–526
  acute, 525
    antihistamines in, 525
    causes, 525
    treatment, 525
  chronic, 525
    amitriptyline in, 526
    etiology, 525
    evaluation, 525
    treatment, 526
Uterus
  activity in labor, 360–361
    configuration, 361
    contractility, 360
    resting tone, 360
    rhythmicity, 361
  adnexal masses, 265
  bleeding, dysfunctional, 276
  rupture, 339

V

Vacuum extraction (*see* Delivery, vacuum extraction)

Index

Vagina
  bleeding, abnormal, 276–278
    during adolescence, 277
    etiology, 276–277
    evaluation, 277
    history, 277
    laboratory evaluation, 277
    physical exam, 277
    postmenopausal, 278
    terminology, 276
    treatment, 277–278
  bleeding after 20 weeks gestation, 338–340
    diagnosis, differential, 338–339
    laboratory evaluation, 339
  bleeding before 20 weeks gestation, 335–337
    diagnosis, differential, 335–336
    management, 336–337
  bleeding in newborn, 274
  delivery by (*see* Delivery, vaginal)
  foreign body in infants and children, 274
  infection
    clotrimazole for, 485
    metronidazole for, 485
    during pregnancy, 485
Varicella (*see* Chickenpox)
Varicocele, 495
Vasectomy, 634–635
  complications, 635
  contraindications, 634
  indications, 634
  materials for, 634
  postoperative instructions, 635
  technique, 6734–635
Vasodepressor syncope, 78
Vasodilators: in hypertension, 76–77
Vasomotor rhinitis, 523
Vasovagal syncope, 78

VBAC, 342–344
  advantages, 342
  contraindications, 342
  decision to attempt, 342
  definition, 342
  disadvantages, 342
  management, 343
  risks, 343
  success probability, 342
Vein
  cutdown, 573–575
    complications, 574–575
    contraindications, 573
    indications, 573
    materials for, 573
    technique, 573–574
  jugular, access, 600
  saphenous, cutdown, 574
  subclavian, access, 600
Ventilation
  controlled, 96
  in COPD, 121
  mandatory, intermittent, 98
  mechanical
    modes, 96–98
    withdrawal, 99–100
    withdrawal of, guidelines for, 100
  minute, 98
  /perfusion tests, 94–95
    interpretation, 95
  in resuscitation in infants and children, 12
  studies, 94
  transtracheal, percutaneous, 32–33
    advantages, 32
    complications, 32
    contraindications, 32
    disadvantages, 32
    technique, 32–33
Ventilators, 96–101
  assist-control, 96–98
  indications for, 96

management, 98–99
weaning from, 100
Ventricle
fibrillation, 3
emergency care, 1–2
in myocardial infarction, acute, 69
tachycardia (*see* Tachycardia, ventricular)
Venturi Mask, 97
Vertigo, 509–511
benign paroxysmal positional, 510
treatment, 510
central, 509
diagnosis, differential, 509
evaluation, 509–510
peripheral, 509
Vessels
cerebral (*see* Cerebrovascular)
defects, 160
disease and diabetes, 189
Virus(es)
conjunctivitis due to, 502, 506
herpes (*see under* Herpes)

labyrinthitis due to, 510
treatment, 510
meningitis (*see* Meningitis, aseptic)
respiratory tract infection due to, upper, 102–103
Visual fields: in glaucoma, 507
Vital signs: in abdominal pain, 411
Vitamin
A in acne, comedonal, 523
B12 deficiency, 170
signs and symptoms, 170
treatment, 170
D and breast feeding, 458
K, 163–164
Vomiting
of blood, 133
with diarrhea (*see* Diarrhea, with vomiting)
in newborn, 443–444
diet in, 443
evaluation, 443
treatment, 443
von Willebrand's disease, 159
management, 163

W

Water
deficiency, 179
excess, 179
Weaning: from ventilator, 100
Weight
birth to 16 months, in boys 657
birth to 36 months, in girls, 655
gain, expected during pregnancy, 308
2 to 18 years
in boys, 658
in girls, 656
White's classification: of diabetes, 328–329

narcotic (*see* Narcotic withdrawal)
ventilation, mechanical, 96–98
guidelines for, 100
Wound
allergy and, 393
chemotherapy and, 393
closure, 396–397
tape, 396
diabetes and, 393
dressings, 397
follow up care, 397–398
healing, 395
infections, postoperative, 406
injury
mechanism, 392

Index

Wound (*cont.*)
 time of, 392
 management, 392–398
  history, significant, 392–393
 open, care of, 396–397
 physical exam, 393–394
 prep, 396
 repair, 395–397
  anesthesia for, 395–396
 social factors in, 393
 suture removal, 398
 suturing, 397
 tetanus status and, 393
Wrist
 joint access, 630
 in rheumatoid arthritis, 208

X

X-ray exam (*see* Radiography)

Z

Zenker's diverticulum, 138